Progress in Human Nutrition

Volume 2

Progress in Human Nutrition
Editorial Board

Progress in Human Nutrition

Volume 2

Editors: SHELDON MARGEN, M.D.

Professor of Human Nutrition
Department of Nutritional Sciences
University of California, Berkeley

and

RICHARD A. OGAR, M.A.

Bibliographer
Department of Biomedical and Environmental Health Sciences
University of California, Berkeley

Symposium on the Biological and Cultural
Sources of Variability in Human Nutrition

Sponsored by the Malnutrition Panel of the United States–Japan Cooperative
Medical Sciences Program, the National Institutes of Health, and the University
of California, Berkeley

THE AVI PUBLISHING COMPANY, INC.
WESTPORT, CONNECTICUT

Library of Congress Cataloging in Publication Data

Symposium on the Biological and Cultural Sources of Vari-
    ability in Human Nutrition, University of California, Berke-
    ley, 1975.
    Symposium on the Biological and Cultural Sources of
Variability in Human Nutrition.
    (Progress in human nutrition; v. 2)

    Updated papers of the symposium held Dec. 3-5, 1975.
    Includes bibliographical references and index.
    1. Malnutrition—Congresses. 2. Nutrition—Congresses.
3. Human evolution—Congresses. 4. Food habits—Congresses. I. Margen, Sheldon. II. Ogar, Richard A. III. United
States-Japan Cooperative Medical Science Program. Malnutrition Panel. IV. United States. National Institutes of
Health. V. California. University.

RC623.S95   1975   362.5   78-948
ISBN 0-87055-255-4

Contributors to this Volume

TSUNEO ARAKAWA, M.D., Chairman and Professor of Pediatrics, Department of Pediatrics, Tohoku University School of Medicine, Sendai, Japan.

JOSEF BROŽEK, Ph.D., Professor of Psychology, Department of Psychology, Lehigh University, Bethlehem, Pennsylvania.

ROBERT H. CAGAN, M.D., Veterans Administration Hospital, Philadelphia, and Monell Chemical Senses Center, University of Pennsylvania, Philadelphia, Pennsylvania.

DORIS CALLOWAY, Ph.D., Professor of Nutrition, Department of Nutritional Sciences, University of California, Berkeley, California.

SOL CHAFKIN, Division of National Affairs, Social Development, The Ford Foundation, New York, New York.

C. WEST CHURCHMAN, Ph.D., Professor of Business Administration, Department of Business Administration, University of California, Berkeley, California.

HERNÁN DELGADO, M.D., M.P.H., Division of Human Development, Institute of Nutrition of Central America and Panama (INCAP), Guatemala City, Guatemala.

TIMOTHY FARRELL, Division of Human Development, Institute of Nutrition of Central America and Panama (INCAP), Guatemala City, Guatemala.

C. GOPALAN, M.D., D.Sc., F.R.C.P.E., Director, Indian Council of Medical Research, New Delhi, India.

BRIAN HAYDEN, Ph.D., Professor of Archaeology, Department of Archaeology, Simon Fraser University, Burnaby, British Columbia, Canada.

ROBERT F. HEIZER, Ph.D., Professor and Coordinator, Archaeological Research Facility, Department of Archaeology, University of California, Berkeley, California.

S. HORI, Department of Physiology, Hyogo College of Medicine, Hyogo-Prefecture, Japan.

DERRICK B. JELLIFFE, M.D., Division of Population, Professor of Family and International Health, School of Public Health, University of California, Los Angeles, California.

E.F.P. JELLIFFE, M.P.H., Division of Population, Family and International Health, School of Public Health, University of California, Los Angeles, California.

J. LEONARD JOY, Ph.D., Institute of Developmental Studies, University of Sussex, Sussex, England.

MORLEY R. KARE, M.D., Veterans Administration Hospital, Philadelphia, and Monell Chemical Senses Center, University of Pennsylvania, Philadelphia, Pennsylvania.

ROBERT E. KLEIN, Ph.D., Division of Human Development, Institute of Nutrition of Central America and Panama (INCAP), Guatemala City, Guatemala.

NORMAN KRETCHMER, M.D., Director, National Institute of Child Health and Human Development, National Institutes of Health, Bethesda, Maryland.

AARÓN LECHTIG, M.D., M.P.H., Division of Human Development, Institute of Nutrition of Central America and Panama (INCAP), Guatemala City, Guatemala.

MARGARET MACKENZIE, Ph.D., R.N., Professor of Anthropology, Department of Anthropology, University of California, Berkeley, California.

SHELDON MARGEN, M.D., Professor of Nutrition, Department of Nutritional Sciences, University of California, Berkeley, California.

REYNALDO MARTORELL, Ph.D., Division of Human Development, Institute of Nutrition of Central America and Panama (INCAP), Guatemala City, Guatemala.

LEONARDO J. MATA, Ph.D., Director, Institute of Research in Health (INISA), University of Costa Rica, Cuidad Universitaria "Rodrigo Facio," Costa Rica.

PANATA MIGASENA, M.D., Faculty of Tropical Medicine, Mahidol University, Bangkok, Thailand.

ASOK MITRA, Ph.D., Professor and Director for ICSSR and FPF Projects, Center for Regional Development, Jawaharlal Nehru University, New Delhi, India.

EDGAR MOHS, Hospital Nacional de Niños, Costa Rica.

EDWARD MONTGOMERY, Ph.D., Assistant Professor, Department of Anthropology, Washington University, St. Louis, Missouri.

v

TOSHIO OISO, M.D., Consultant, International Medical Foundation of Japan, National Institute of Nutrition, Tokyo, Japan.

GILBERT OMENN, M.D., Ph.D., Associate Professor of Medicine, Division of Medical Genetics, Department of Medicine, University of Washington, Seattle, Washington.

S. ONAKA, Department of Nutrition, Tokushima University School of Medicine, Tokushima, Japan.

RICHARD ORRACA-TETTEH, Ph.D., Professor and Head, Department of Nutrition and Food Science, University of Ghana, Legon, Ghana.

ROBERTA PALMOUR, Ph.D., Assistant Professor of Genetics, Department of Genetics, University of California, Berkeley, California.

JOHN PLATT, Ph.D., Mental Health Research Institute, University of Michigan, Ann Arbor, Michigan.

N. SAITO, Department of Nutrition, Kyoto University School of Medicine, Kyoto, Japan.

NEVIN S. SCRIMSHAW, M.D., Ph.D., Professor and Head, Department of Nutrition and Food Science, Massachusetts Institute of Technology, Cambridge, Massachusetts.

K. SHIRAKI, Department of Nutrition, Tokushima University School of Medicine, Tokushima, Japan.

OSAMU SINODA, Director, Japan Society for Historical Research of Manners and Customs, Kyoto, Japan.

PHILIP E.L. SMITH, Ph.D., Professor of Anthropology, Department of Anthropology, University of Montreal, Quebec, Canada.

CHARLES YARBROUGH, Ph.D., Division of Human Development, Institute of Nutrition of Central America and Panama (INCAP), Guatemala City, Guatemala.

VERNON R. YOUNG, Ph.D., Professor of Nutrition and Biochemistry, Department of Nutrition and Food Science, Massachusetts Institute of Technology, Cambridge, Massachusetts.

HISATO YOSHIMURA, M.D., Department of Physiology, Hyogo College of Medicine, Hyogo-Prefecture, Japan.

PREFACE

The U.S.-Japan Cooperative Medical Sciences Program was developed more than ten years ago as an expression of the joint concern by those two governments for a variety of health problems of particular significance to Asians.

Over the years, it has become increasingly apparent that many of these problems—and particularly those of malnutrition—are not merely Asian concerns, but have worldwide significance. As a result, the Panel's activities have become increasingly more global in the effort to conduct research in its primary areas of concern. Among these primary areas of concern are the effects of nutrition on infection, the relationship of nutrition and anemia, the impact of nutrition on physical and mental growth and performance, and the various effects of a host of environmental factors on human nutritional requirements.

During the past ten years, the U.S.-Japan Malnutrition Panel has supported a number of very productive research projects in these areas, and has generated a great deal of significant information in each. *Progress in Human Nutrition* Volume 1, published in 1971, summarized our earlier meetings. For the convenience and interest of readers, we have included the Contents of Volume 1 following the Contents of this volume.

The present volume is based upon a symposium entitled "The Biological and Cultural Sources of Variability in Human Nutrition," held at the University of California, Berkeley, December 3-5, 1975. All of these papers have been reviewed and brought up to date by their authors.

The meeting was sponsored by the U.S.-Japan Malnutrition Panel of the U.S.-Japan Cooperative Medical Sciences Program, and its title emphasizes what many of us believe to be the next important step for the field of nutrition, namely the enlargement of its scope from the strict confines of nutritional science into the ramifications that nutrition has for human health and welfare, a process which would involve the interaction of nutritionists with individuals from other disciplines in a mutual effort to clarify their interrelationships.

In a sense, this book is devoted to an examination of the history and evolution of man and his food. First, we view man and food in terms of history and ethnography. Second, we turn our attention to present-day man and his genetic and cultural relationships to food, as well as to his ability (or inability) to adapt. Finally, we direct our attention to trying to determine why malnutrition (whether undernutrition in the developing world, or overnutrition in the developed nations) has become such a serious problem, and what areas might prove most fruitful in our search for solutions. We feel certain that the symposium raised more questions than it answered; in large part, this was the intent of its framers. But we are equally certain that the reader will find great value in this book, and that it will become a landmark for those seeking new directions in their search for solutions to the problems of malnutrition.

The organizers of the Berkeley program would like to thank all the members of the U.S.-Japan Malnutrition Panel for their superb cooperation in the effort to carry this project through. In addition, we wish to express special thanks to our assistant, Mrs. Dale Ogar, who was really the principal organizer of the symposium.

Lastly, as noted elsewhere in this volume, we wish to dedicate the symposium to the memory of Dr. Richard L. Lyman, Professor of Nutrition at the University of California, who died virtually on the eve of its inception. Dr. Lyman was a quiet, intense, internationally known nutritionist and biochemist who, like so many of us, was groping toward some understanding of the relationship between food and biological process. Although principally a laboratory scientist, in recent years Dr. Lyman had become increasingly interested in the problems to which this symposium was addressed. It was therefore a great loss that he could not be present with us. In view of his commitment to the field of human nutrition and of our love for the man himself, we dedicate this volume to him.

Sheldon Margen, M.D.
Richard Ogar, M.A.

November 1977   *Editors*

Dedicated to the memory of
Professor Richard L. Lyman

Contents of Volume 2

Contents of Volume 1

SECTION I

MAN'S HISTORICAL AND SOCIOCULTURAL EVOLUTION AND THE EFFECT OF NUTRITION

Sheldon Margen

Prologue: Notes on a Strange Journey

Survival is a question which has concerned mankind almost from the time the species began its uncertain march through history. And many of us who are mindful of ecology and concerned with the various threats to man's existence feel that *homo sapiens* may in fact be the most endangered species of them all. Endangered by what? Allow me to withdraw from the immediate subject and fantasize a bit. As children, we felt perfectly comfortable doing this. We were able to share our deepest thoughts and fears with our parents and with our friends. But as adults, we tend to keep our fantasies to ourselves for fear of being carried off to some grim institution. Despite the obvious risks, I shall take the plunge.

Within my fantasy world, I am a superbeing (undoubtedly from Outer Space, the birthplace of all superbeings), able to defy the laws of physics and to move at will through the space/time continuum. As Super Sheldon, I also have the power to alter the magnification of any object at will.

In my wanderings through the void, I suddenly spy a small, rotating globe which seems rather different from others I have passed. It has a bluish tinge to it, but its surface is obscured by white swirls of some substance I cannot identify. Popping through the top layer, I notice a peculiar odor which I recognize as that of ozone. But farther down, I discover an atmosphere composed principally of oxygen and nitrogen (although I also note small amounts of carbon dioxide and other gases).

As I get closer to the surface, I can see (by slightly increasing the magnification) that this globe (or "planet," as I later learn it is called) is largely populated by a curious form of biped. In some places the concentration of these bipeds is very dense, while in others they seem to be relatively scattered. As I approach one of the more crowded communities, I find an almost equal concentration of primitive four-wheeled vehicles which seem to be in constant motion. I also notice that the atmosphere has changed drastically—the blue I had noticed before is now largely brown, and the freshness has been supplanted by a foul profusion of odors. Once I actually set foot on the surface, my eyes begin to water, my throat turns raw and my nose starts to run.

Oddly enough, this foul air seems to have no effect at all on either the bipeds or their vehicles. My curiosity piqued by this fact, as well as their rather outlandish apparel, I approach one of the bipeds. Immediately it begins to utter a series of incomprehensible sounds. At first I am uncertain whether

3

these sounds are a cry of alarm or an attempt to communicate with me. When I fail to respond, the biped begins to draw a number of odd characters on thin sheets of hide or tissue, using a sharp stick which seems to have been manufactured for this purpose. Using my highly developed translational abilities, I quickly learn the rudiments of this unusual form of communication.

Trying my hand at the language, I ask who or what this creature is. She tells me her name, and explains that a name is what distinguishes her from the other bipeds in her group. She also tells me that this larger group has been called *homo sapiens* by a biped subgroup known as scientists. When I ask her how she got to this place, she explains that she has always been there, that her species evolved over millions of years and now dominates the planet.

Unsure of what "evolution" meant (but taking a clue from the phrase "millions of years"), I rush back through the eons until I reach a point where the sky nearly vanishes. At this time, there is little oxygen in the atmosphere, and the surface seems unstable. Volcanoes erupt at various places, and occasionally there are tremors under my feet. Since there are no signs of biped life (or, indeed, of any other), I feel that I have reached a good starting point.

Moving slowly forward in time, I notice deep ponds of water begin to form. Later, a greenish substance begins to appear in the water. All of this is taking place very slowly, so I make a fast forward leap through the time belt and arrive at a time when this green material has begun to proliferate. At the same time, I notice that the atmosphere contains much more oxygen and far less carbon dioxide. This material gradually rises to the surface, filling the atmosphere with even more oxygen.

Intrigued by this substance, I magnify it to the point where I can see the cells within which this green material resides, and I realize that these cells are actually removing energy from the cosmos and storing it in chemical bonds.

Farther down the time line, other cells appear which incorporate the ability to break down the chemical bonds created by the green cells. The electrons which are released by this process are used to generate energy for the cell's various functions, including one called "life." This breakdown also releases carbon dioxide and water, which are reused by the green cells.

As I move further along this "evolutionary" line, I discover something truly remarkable—a new substance appears which contains within itself all sorts of knowledge and directions. This new substance is able to combine with some of the spherules of green material or the small spherules carrying out the products of oxidation to carbon dioxide, water and other elements swimming about in the environment, often by a twisting, spiral motion.

These various elements are encapsulated by a complex series of layers which allow some materials from the environment to enter the newly formed spherule and keep other elements out. Clearly this is a new form of creation, one which is integrated and somewhat independent. From this point on in my time travels, I find this same sort of basic structure wherever I look.

Over time, I learn that this "thing" tends to conglomerate itself into masses of various shapes and sizes, and seems able to survive in all parts of the globe. (Later, the "she" will explain to me that these spherules are called cells, and that she herself is composed of billions of them, each different from the other but sharing a common link.)

Events seem to be occuring more quickly, and I slow my pace through the continuum. Wherever I set down on the planet, I notice that the living creatures there survive in an environment which changes slowly, despite their presence and without their active intervention. On closer examination, however, I realize that the living masses and the environment are an integrated system. One, in fact, could not be separated from the other.

Suddenly I notice the appearance of the bipeds which "she" had called *homo sapiens*. Initially their numbers are small and their impact upon the environment slight. But they increase their population at a dizzying rate, changing the surface of the globe wherever they spread. Old waterways disappear; new ones are created. The vast green surface becomes pitted with areas of yellow and brown where the bipeds have congregated. Their masses become so great that I no longer have to search them out by magnification.

Not only do they change the surface of the globe, they dig beneath it to remove the rubble of earlier times and earlier lives, which they convert into energy, thereby greatly intensifying their ability to alter their environment.

More disturbing than this rupturing and pitting of the global surface is the emergence of a phenomenon stranger than any I have encountered on my journey through time—I begin to see groups of bipeds attack and kill each other for reasons I cannot understand. Unlike other life masses I have seen, they do not eat their prey, although occasionally they do carry off the possessions of their victims.

While there are a seemingly infinite number of life masses on this planet, only *homo sapiens* seems to behave in this strange fashion. Unable to come up with an explanation on my own (the question defies even superbeings like myself), I return to what the bipeds call "the present" and ask my "she" for an answer.

"You call yourself a superbeing?" she says disdainfully. "The answer is simple. We of the species *homo sapiens* have invented language. We can speak with one another. We can also remember the past and record it in books. And while no one can see into the future (although some claim that they can), we know that there will be one. This allows us to plan.

"We have learned to control the physical environment, and we have even created an environment of our own which we call 'culture.' That's what makes us different from all other living things, and that is why we are the dominant force on this globe we call the planet Earth."

At first I had to agree that it was all very simple, and I could have kicked myself for not having discovered the answer myself. But as I traveled around this globe, poking into this great city and that remote village, I discovered that the problem was actually more complex. For one thing, these bipeds had not one language in which to converse, but many. And rarely was a biped from one region able to understand a biped from another. And in fact, even among those bipeds speaking the same language, there were often differences of opinion over the meaning of words. So great were these differences in some cases that the bipeds involved tried to destroy each other.

Nor is their control of the environment all that "she" made it out to be. While in some areas the environment was so well controlled that everyone seemed to have food and shelter, other areas were marked by starvation and deprivation. And even in those areas of control, the environment seemed disrupted to the point of utter disequilibrium.

The disharmony was so great (and it scarcely took a superbeing like myself to perceive it) that several large groups of bipeds had dug mammoth holes in the ground, lined them with a substance called concrete, and placed death-dealing weapons called "missiles" into these "siloes." (Oddly enough, I also encountered "siloes" on places called "farms," where the substances which nourish the bipeds are produced.) After a quick count, I decided that there were enough of these missiles to destroy every living thing on the planet.

I was further struck by the fact that very few of these bipeds seemed to be at all concerned about these matters. Stranger yet was the fact that I cared even if they didn't. But try as I might, I couldn't find any way to help them out of their predicament.

Then off somewhere in the distance I saw a small, seemingly tranquil area. Moving closer, I observed a group of bipeds—part of that subgroup known as scientists—entering a great hall. I joined them impulsively, and awoke to find that I was in fact attending a symposium in which those scientists were about to examine the very questions that had arisen during my dream voyage.

I hope that we shall discover some answers so that I do not have to revert to my fantasy world. But whether I remain here as Dr. Margen or resume my life as Super Sheldon, I realize that I cannot exist simply as *I*. As Martin Buber so eloquently phrased it, I can only exist as *I-Thou*. And only through the *I-Thou* can I hope that *homo sapiens* may see the threat it poses to itself.

CHAPTER 1

Man as a Biological and Cultural Species

Josef Brožek

Nutrition is an aspect of the mode of life, with complex sources and with implications for fitness and health, including the development of noninfectious degenerative diseases. Its study includes a number of disciplines. The models need to be multivariate, with special attention given to the phenomena of interaction.

Considered on a worldwide scale, man's problems of food and nutrition must be viewed in relation to the other great problems facing contemporary society and the society of the future. These include the energy crisis and, perhaps most critically, the population crisis.

The intricacy of the issues may be illustrated by the acute and long-range problems of the Sahel. In his introduction to a 1975 report of the National Academy of Sciences Advisory Panel on Arid Lands of Sub-Saharan Africa, John McKelvey refers to rehabilitation of the Sahel as a "very large, complex and intractable set of social, economic and political, as well as technical, problems."

The first consideration is, of course, food—"food security," in the language of the report. But this is one link in a long chain. Increased food production involves, clearly, both dry-land and irrigated agriculture, planned for a better utilization and management of soils and water resources. However, an adequate infrastructure calls for much more than schemes to make water available. The report points out the need to improve the transport and communication system in the Sahel region to facilitate the movement of goods and services and, in the case of emergency, the movement of relief supplies. One cannot forget the role of health services in dealing with endemic infectious diseases, controlling the hazards associated with the new bodies of water, and improving the work potential. From concern with health it is a short step to concern with the acquisition of required information and skills, and modification of attitudes—the large and critical area of education, in the broad sense. To quote the report, "the delivery of educational opportunity is the crucial element in successful organization of all parts of the system."

In short, we have to think of the climate, the land, the man, ending with "a modification of the economic-marketing systems within countries and integration of the economic system in the whole West African region." The complexity of the "Sahel problem" is inescapable. Clearly a systems approach is essential for arriving at an integrated strategy for the long-term development of the region.

At the same time, the offers of assistance must be sensitive to the cultural context within which the proposed measures are to be applied and the implications of these measures. The Senegalese government and the Western relief agencies believe that it is a good idea to transform a part of the Sahelian bush and marginal grasslands into an area raising beef calves for Senegalese urban markets. However, as Jacques May warned, "Any transformation of the geographical environment may be pregnant with unsuspected consequences that can and will affect nutrition." The proposed development would affect many aspects of traditional life, including the techniques people use to grow food, to harvest it, to store it, to market it, and to prepare it for consumption (cf. May 1974).

J. M. Teitelbaum (1975) indicates that the seminomadic Fulani cattlekeepers of the Sahel of Senegal are not as enthusiastic about a transformation of their subsistence culture into a "cash crop" system as we might expect. Rapid implementation of the plan may have undesirable nutritional consequences for the poor, small-scale stock-raising people of the Sahel whose living standards and health are meant to be improved by it. Most important, there is the danger that milk, a critical human foodstuff in this region, would be diverted to the feeding of calves. With the herds assigned to specified range areas from which they would not return to the villages overnight, the cattle dung used to fertilize soil for grain cultivation would no longer be available in the areas where it is needed. The project calls for ending the traditional use of brushfires to provide ash and clear the land for cultivation. Teitelbaum stresses that the use of fertilizers and the practices of intensive agriculture are alien to the Fulani way of life, which is threatened in various other ways by the proposed range-livestock project, including disruption of the social organization of the villages, closely tied to the present occupational activities: "Children take care of the calves near the village; women milk the cows morning and evening and prepare the milk products for consumption; old men braid ropes and do ancillary, often mystical tasks to protect the herds; adult and adolescent males drive the animals to pasture, take them to water, shelter them at night, and control the herd during transhumance" (the seasonal moving of the livestock to areas containing underground or river water, during the dry season).

Our concern here is not with the validity of Teitelbaum's critique of the project but rather with the general point that it is essential to consider the human factors, cultural and nutritional, that are important for the population at risk. Economics and efficiency are not enough; the whole system must be considered.

REFERENCES

MAY, J. M. 1974. The geography of nutrition. *In* The Geography of Health and Diseases. J. M. Hunter (Editor). Univ. North Carolina Press, Chapel Hill, N.C.

NATIONAL ACADEMY OF SCIENCES. 1975. Arid Lands of Sub-Saharan Africa. Staff Final Report on an Advisory Panel of the Board on Science and Technology for International Development, Commission on International Relations, NAS-NCR, Washington D.C.

TEITELBAUM, J. M. 1976. Human versus animal nutrition: A development project among Fulani cattlekeepers of the Sahel of Senegal. *In* Nutrition and Anthropology in Action. T. Fitzgerald (Editor). Royal Van Gorcum, Assen, Netherlands. (In press).

CHAPTER 2

Robert F. Heizer

Man, The Hunter-Gatherer: Food

Availability vs Biological Factors

There is one flat statement that can be made about the technologically and economically simpler human societies which have characterized over 99% of man's history—that these societies solved the basic survival problem of finding enough to eat, and that their diets were sufficient in quantity and quality to maintain the group's reproductive viability. In short, it can be argued that, for the near totality of human history on earth, man as a genus and species has been a biological success. Until recently, the threats to the species' continuance have not been a matter of practical concern. When the Babylonian civilization declined, or when Assyria and Persia imposed their domination over Egypt, or when the Macedonian Greeks conquered the known world, only to be succeeded and exceeded by the Romans, a lot of textbook history may have been registered.

But it should be remembered that these were essentially local political events within the literate Old World *Oikumene*; that is, events which had nothing to do with the continuance of the human species which, by 12,000 years ago, had occupied the habitable portions of the earth, and was distributed into a series of linguistically, politically, territorially and economically-ecologically adjusted units classed as "bands," "tribes," "nations" or "states." In the larger terms of man's history, it did not really matter when one of these nations succeeded in eliminating its neighbor (or even several neighbors), since the continuum of culture was not affected.

When Columbus discovered the New World in October 1492, a series of events was set in motion which, within four and a half centuries, would lead to the near total extinction of the tribal cultures that had been developing for at least 2,000,000 years. The extinguishers, in the form of the Atlantic European powers, were well-equipped with sailing vessels, guns and an unbounded ambition to impose their domination (by "right of discovery") over the "uncivilized" peoples of the earth. The discovery of the New World was only the opening gun for the "discovery" by European nations of a world outside the limited known earth at the time of the Renaissance—a world whose very existence came as a surprise. In my opinion, the cultural significance—or perhaps better, the consequence—of Columbus' discovery is the destruction of a world of other cultures which possessed an invaluable store of knowledge which was recorded, if at all, in only the most superficial and descriptive manner. Thus, at the present time we can understand these thousands of extinct societies only through the imperfect accounts of explorers and ethnographers, and from the investigations of archeologists.

The label "hunter-gatherer" accurately characterizes the main food procurement techniques of pre-Neolithic societies, as well as the partial or secondary activities of many of the simpler agricultural tribal societies. If people hunt or fish for meat and gather wild plant foods, they do this with tools and devices which are part of their technological repertoire. The artifact—something which is conceived in the mind, made with the hands and put to use for survival purposes—is therefore a critical factor in the pre-food-producing history of man. While there are some examples of tool use among lower animals—the Galapagos finch, for example, which uses a cactus thorn held in its beak to spear grubs and extract them from their holes; or the African vulture, which uses a stone, again held in the beak, to hammer open ostrich eggs; or the sea otter, which uses pebbles to break apart mollusk shells—none of these animals actually forms or fashions implements from wood or stone to serve a specific purpose. Only man does this. It is perhaps significant, however, that most (and possibly all) of these anticipatory tool-using examples among birds and lower mammals are directly concerned with food-getting.

It has been calculated that the earliest pebble tools, dating from about 2,000,000 years ago, provided 5 cm of cutting edge per pound of flint. In the Lower Paleolithic (500,000 to 1,000,000 years ago), the implement cutting edge per pound of raw material rises to 20 cm; in the Middle Paleolithic, the figure is 100 cm; and in the Upper Palolithic, it reached 300 to 1200 cm. But since we can only guess at the obviously varied uses of specific stone tool forms, the best we can say is that, over time, they were more efficiently produced, and that some proportion of this stone tool use must have been directed toward food catching or collecting, and toward food preparation. In other words, improved efficiency in food-getting over time probably meant a more assured (as well as more varied) diet.

The oldest known artifacts or tools are pebbles which have been purposefully struck with another stone to remove flakes and produce a cutting edge or piercing point. The most ancient forms known at present (from the Omo area in Ethiopia) were made about 2,500,000 years ago. While their specific uses are not known, it seems likely that they served either as weapons to capture food or tools for food preparation (cutting up animals, smashing nuts, cutting through tough fruit rinds, etc.). After all, with his limited dentition, man cannot tear a animal apart with his teeth—he needs a knife, however simple, to cut through the tough hide and reduce the animal to manageable bits. As time goes on, the tool inventory expands both in number and function, which probably reflects the increasing sophistication in food-getting methods.

The progressive development of tools presumably mirrors both the enlargement of catching and collecting methods, as well as an improved chance (or even assurance) of success. For the 2,000,000 years and more of pre-Neolithic human history, we are talking about small social groups which traditionally exploit a territory with which they are familiar in terms of terrain, plants and animals. At heart, territoriality rests on the staking out and defense of a specific area from which the group obtains its food supply. Among primitive societies the world over, the basic cause of warfare is trespassing, usually for the purpose of poaching food (cf. James and Graziani 1975).

Coon (1959) uses the analogy of "modern Stone Age" hunter-gatherers and concludes that the size of such groups probably did not exceed 80 to 100 family units. In California, the tribelet averaged about 250 persons (Kroeber 1962). Deevey (1960) proposes that population density in the Paleolithic probably did not exceed .04 persons per square km, and that Early Pleistocene numbers may not have exceeded 500,000 persons. By the end of the Pleistocene, the human population may have been in excess of 3,000,000; and by the early Neolithic there were probably 100,000,000 people alive. Of course these are estimates. But while they are not to be taken as actual figures, their orders of magnitude indicate a great expansion in population in post-Pleistocene times. What such a steady increase in numbers means, quite simply, is that more people are living than are dying. That is a crude measure of life success.

Information on prehistoric diet can be obtained from a variety of sources:

(1) Painted or engraved representations of plants and animals on rock surfaces or interior cave walls which presumably indicate the artist's special interest in such forms; one would assume that this interest includes nutritional use.

(2) Palpable residues of food, such as animal bones, carbonized plant remains, or negative impressions ("casts") of seeds in clay (Helbaek 1961) found in archaeological sites.

(3) Analysis of stomach or intestinal contents of deliberately mummified individuals, or of naturally mummified corpses preserved under conditions of extreme dryness, immersion in cold and acid peat bogs or perpetual freezing.

(4) Prehistoric fecal pellets, usually called coprolites, and most commonly preserved in dry cave occupation deposits.

(5) Inferences on what prehistoric social groups were doing about food-getting based on the practices of recently surviving peoples in the Old and New Worlds.

(6) "Chemical archaeology," a potentially useful method for determining the former presence of plant materials in archaeological soils by detecting high levels of certain trace elements known to be concentrated in specific plants.

If we turn to the archaeological record of ancient nutrition, we find a great mass of evidence (cf. Heizer 1960), but its utility is beset with limitations. On any time level, whether we are dealing with contemporary societies or cultural stages such as Lower or Middle or Upper Paleolithic, there is a wide variation in tool types, size of settlement, habitat and food remains (which are almost exclusively limited to preserved bones of food animals). And despite the totality of the evidence, the amount of information on discrete time levels is always minimal, as so clearly pointed out by F. Clark Howell (Lee 1968). Therefore, it is hazardous to try to generalize on the basis of limited data. Added to the difficulties in tracing the history of human nutrition is the fact that the vegetable element in the diet is perishable. Palpable residues are preserved only under special conditions, such as immersion in water, carbonization, or deposition in completely dry caves or shelters. In open sites subject to alternating wet and dry conditions, bacterial decay soon causes the total decomposition of plant materials.

The oldest plant materials found in prehistoric sites which may be considered to be food remains are hackberry seeds from Chou-kou-tien in China about 500,000 years old (Chaney 1935); seeds from the site of Terra Amata on the French Riviera, about 300,000 years old; and a half dozen varieties of seeds and nuts from the Kalambo Falls site in Africa, about 100,000 years old. This is pretty slim evidence of vegetal dietary elements from man's very ancient past. In contrast, hunting may be disproportionately evident in the archaelogical record because stone tools were used for killing and butchering, and the bones of the killed animals were preserved. For the most part, gathering or food collecting is done with the hands, or with the aid of wooden tools which leave no traces; and, as mentioned earlier, any residues of vegetal foods in open sites will disappear completely. Pollen analysis of archaeological site soils can tell us much about the vegetation cover in the vicinity during the time the site was occupied, but it does not tell us whether any of the available nutritional opportunities were actually being exploited.

Brothwell and Brothwell (1969) have published a well-documented survey of the evidence regarding foods used in prehistoric times, but this is no more than a sampling of the very large amount of such information contained in archaelogical reports. Ethnologists, working with primitive societies all over the world, have recorded a great mass of information on food-getting (Mountford 1960; Sullivan 1942; Riviera 1949; Sweeney 1947; Roth 1901; Krogh 1951; Hawley et al. 1943; Stefansson 1937) which has thus far been examined and synthesized in only the most superficial way (Simoons 1960; Lowie 1938; Heizer 1960).

Presumably man has always been an omnivore, although his teeth and long gut mark him as primarily a vegetarian. Lower primates catch and eat small animals and birds with apparent relish, so they are not averse to meat. Gorillas in captivity adapt readily to meat eating, even though they are primarily vegetarians (or more precisely, herbivores) in nature. Meat eating is documented at Olduvai Gorge in Bed I, dated at roughly 1,800,000 years ago. Some Olduvai localities emphasize the bones (assumed to be food refuse) of one animal, while others may feature different animals. It would seem, then, that even at this early time, there was some kind of selective effort (or "cropping") in securing what was eaten. While no clear evidence of the collecting and eating of plant foods is discernible on this time level, it is difficult to assume that there was not a significant amount of plants (such as nuts, berries, roots and leaves) being used as food.

Even though we have no certain evidence concerning the importance of plant foods to early man, we *do* have opinions and argument. Leopold and Ardrey (1972A, B) hold that toxic or poisonous substances are so common in plants that not until man was able to use fire to remove them through cooking could the phytic element in human nutrition become significant, and that anthropologists have overestimated the importance of plant foods to early human groups. In my opinion, Dornstreich (1973) has argued effectively against this view, pointing out that there are plenty of vegetal foods that can be eaten raw (as judged from the nutritional regimes of many primitive societies), and that there are other methods (e.g., drying, soaking, leaching and pressing) to remove the toxic principles from plants (cf. Gifford 1936).

Jolly (1970) argues that we still lack a "convincing causal model of homonid origins," and believes that there is currently an "obsession with hunting and carnivorousness" which inhibits correct interpretation of the fossil evidence and primate behavior studies. Using abundant supportive data on ecology and dental features, he further argues that "the diet of basal homoids was probably centered upon cereal grains as that of the chimpanzee is upon fruit and that of the gorilla is on herbage."

As Washburn and Avis (1958) have pointed out, the bipedal gait was presumably a precondition to the emergence of man as a new form. But here, too, the opinions are varied. Whether the earliest men adopted an upright posture because they were using tools which required free use of the hands, or whether bipedalism freed the hands for useful activity is not as yet known (Jolly 1970; McHenry 1975). Whichever the case, bipedalism and the free use of the hands for tool use and tool making brought with it an increase in intelligence, although the physiological–mental–cultural–psychological syncretism or synergism involved in this evolutionary process is not understood. What we see in the fossil record is the evidence of great and rapid change, but thus far, I believe, we simply have no idea of what caused it.

Bipedalism, tool making and hunting were important in expanding the subsistence potential of early man—they added protein to his diet and gave him the opportunity to exploit more northerly latitudes and climates. In tropical and subtropical zones, a relatively weak and hairless animal such as man can live comfortably outdoors. But beyond those zones, some additional equipment was needed for survival—items like clothing, shelter, fire, and some knowledge of storing surplus foods to be used in the lean seasons when provender could not be collected. Almost certainly, food storage was one of the preconditions to the effective organization of human groups into societies and to man's worldwide migration. In some environments, food in sufficient quantity to support the population is available all year. But in temperate and colder zones, where seasonal contrasts strongly affect the plant and animal life, it is necessary to accumulate and store a sufficient nutritional surplus to tide the group over until fresh food is again available in quantity.

We do not know whether the earliest men of a couple of million years ago regularly stored food; probably they did not. But as the geographical range of homonids expanded, some knowledge of the need to accumulate and hoard food surpluses toward the lean winter months would seem to have been needed. North of 45°–50° N. Latitude it is cold enough in the winter to preserve meat by freezing. We do not know when the geographical expansion of man from Africa began, but he was living in China and Java 500,000 years ago, and he was in possession of fire (Breuil 1932-33; Oakley 1956A, B). This is the earliest known evidence of fire in man's hands. Fire is useful and efficient as a way to cook meat directly (i.e., to broil it). But it is not essential, as we know from the example of the Eskimos, who eat their meat raw.

The amount of meat (whether cooked or raw) that people can eat is impressive. Holmberg (1950) reports that among the Siriono of Brazil he observed 4 men eat a 60-lb peccary in a single sitting. Since 70% of this animal is usable meat (White 1953), each man consumed about 10 lb of food. In other instances, Holmberg says that a man can eat up to 30 lb of meat in 24 hours; he once observed 2 men eat 6 spider monkeys, each weighing 10–15 lb, in a single day. Stefansson (1937) noted that Pt. Barrow Eskimo ate 9.25 lb of raw seal meat per day.

Aside from roasting meat, the application of fire makes some otherwise inedible foods ingestible. But since cooking can also lead to a loss of nutrients, the advantages of fire are not altogether positive (Barnicot 1969). Small, hard seeds cannot be digested unless they have been cooked in some manner; roasting or boiling begins the conversion of starch which promotes the digestibility of such seeds (which must also be ground, as a means of breaking through the tough outer hull). Boiling is accomplished either by setting a stone or pottery vessel directly over a fire, or by dropping heated stones into a basket or skin "pot." Roasting can be done either by baking the seeds on a heated stone, or by tossing them onto a tray full of glowing coals (which causes the seed kernel to expand, bursting the hull at the same time the heat begins to convert the starchy interior).

Poisonous or unpleasantly bitter constituents—such as the tannic acid in acorns (*Quercus* sp.), saponin in the soaproot plant bulb (*Chlorogalum* sp.) or prussic acid in buckeye nuts (*Aesculus californica*)—can be removed by roasting in an underground oven, which volatilizes the objectionable substances while cooking the nuts or bulbs. We have no way of judging the antiquity of these (and scores of other) special methods of food preparation, but some of them must be very old indeed, judging from their worldwide distribution. The oldest flat milling stones used to grind seeds into flour were recovered from Mousterian sites in Spain and date back some 50,000 years.

We might presume that cooking food introduced new patterns of mastication, nutrition and digestion. Moreover, it might have instituted new social features once the family hearth existed, to which one had to bring firewood. Fire provided a focus for social and economic activities (Movius 1966). Breaking down plant and animal fibers through cooking helped to liberate protein and carbohydrate elements. The increased softness and digestibility of cooked foods must have been a significant benefit to the very old and the very young who might have had problems chewing or digesting raw and coarse foods (Brothwell and Brothwell 1969).

With fire, clothing and shelter, man was able to become the most wide-ranging of all animal species because he was able to fashion his own environment wherever he went. The cooking fire not only allowed him to make more efficient use of whatever the natural environment offered, but could also be used as a defense against predatory animals which greatly surpassed him in strength and ferocity. Somewhere in the history of man, various cultural controls were developed to aid in the continuation of the food supply. Among these were conservation measures (Heizer 1955), and the management of plant and animal food resource acquisition through ritualists (Swezey 1975).

Food-sharing may have been equally important in making the hearth the focus of home and family activity for our earliest ancestors (Heizer 1963). Food-sharing as a social rule on a regular basis is unique to man. The chimpanzee and the red spider monkey have been seen to share food in a free-ranging (i.e., noncaptive) state, but so far as we can tell they are the only lower primates that do so even occasionally (Dare 1974). Probably *Sinanthropus* practiced food-sharing, judging from the evidence of communal living and debris-scatter in the cave at Chou-kou-tien; likewise, the so-called "living floors" of *Homo habilis* can be seen as group living spots to which the food acquired by hunting was brought and consumed (Isaac 1971, 1973; Clark 1972). *Australopithecus*, not yet man, may have done the same, based on the abundance of food bone in his cave sites. Food-sharing is highly significant in the formation of family bonds, since children can be cared for and trained in a settled locus, even if it is frequently changed (Howell 1965). Given verbal communication under these conditions, members of the group could make their food preferences known; thus, the hunters or collectors who ranged out from the base camp could choose selectively from the available foods. Of course, this is all speculation. But even on the time level of a couple of million years ago, the scanty evidence can be interpreted in this manner with some confidence.

Ardrey (1961) and others have argued that the assumed predatory activities of early man are the cause of human violence; and further, that while man is now civilized, he continues to act out a torn flesh and flowing blood routine because of an ingrained evolutionary response which allowed him to survive throughout the immense span of the Paleolithic. While the idea is appealing, it may have no real basis in fact. Although admittedly scant, the evidence we have from Pleistocene archaeology (covering the past 2,000,000 years) does not offer strong support for this position when it is interpreted through analogy with recent hunting and gathering societies around the world. As pointed out long ago (by Kropotkin, I think) in answer to Darwin and Spencer, man may have found that survival owed as much to cooperation as to competition. Take, for example, the sexual division of labor among hunter-gatherers around the world: the men hunt and perform those tasks which are dangerous and require a high outlay of energy; women collect vegetal food and maintain the home (Murdock 1937; Willoughby 1963). This is a distinctively human socioeconomic pattern, and it is cooperative in the full sense of the word. It may also date back to the very beginnings of man (Jolly 1970), although there is no way to demonstrate this at present.

Cannibalism and human sacrifice are occasionally referred to as evidence of man's ingrained tendency toward violence. This may indeed be the case, but more likely it is not. Most human sacrifice is ritualistic, and, as Kroeber pointed out long ago, can be more readily interpreted as a mark of civilization than one of savagery. The first concrete evidence of cannibalism seems to date back to *Sinanthropus,* some 500,000 years ago (Brothwell and Brothwell 1969). Those humans who were eaten may have been poachers who were caught, killed and brought home as part of the day's haul of edibles, rather than fellow Sinanthropines who dropped off to sleep and were killed to make a meal.

Among the Aztecs of Mexico, first seen and described by the Spanish conquistadores of the first quarter of the 16th century, more than 500,000 humans were sacrificed each year (Cook 1946). The reason may have been the desire (perhaps unconscious) to mitigate the effects of overpopulation. But it is equally possible, given the fact that the immolated victims were eaten by the audience, that human sacrifice was a ritualized means of increasing to a significant degree the amount of animal protein available to people who had practically extinguished wild game. I cannot forbear adding one other comment concerning cannibalism—one taken from the pen of Oscar Ameringer, a journalist who ran the *American Guardian* in Oklahoma: "Cannibalism gave way to Capitalism," he wrote, "when man discovered it was more profitable to exploit his neighbor than to eat him."

If we knew anything definite about the organization of social groups in

Paleolithic times, we might be able to make better informed guesses about such things as territoriality, individual vs communal ownership, the exploitation of food resources and the like. Contemporary primitive peoples vary from loosely bound bands to strong lineal descent or clan groups, and from free community access to any and all resources to systems of private ownership (either individual or familial) of certain economic items. The Bushmen of the Kalahari Desert of southwest Africa (Lee 1970) and the Uto-Aztecan (or Shoshonean) Paiute and Shoshone tribes of the Great Basin area of the western United States (Steward 1938) have served as "models" of the Paleolithic hunter–gatherer—as, for example, in the "site catchment" reconstruction of the Upper Paleolithic Mt. Carmel (Palestine) area by Vita-Finzi and Higgs (1970). In this scenario, a radius of six miles from an occupied site is taken as the free-ranging site-catchment or economic exploitation zone.

However, not all hunters and collectors are like the Bushmen. I can cite one example from the Yurok tribe of northwestern California, where private ownership of economic resources was practiced. We have a specific record of one man who owned the exclusive rights to one offshore sea stack where sea lions were hunted, two long stretches of ocean beach, fifteen acorn-bearing oak groves, four salmon-fishing pools, and two deer-snaring spots (Waterman 1920). While this degree of individually controlled food potential seems unusually great, it is clear that even lesser levels of personal control over the tribal food supply would impose restrictions on open hunting and free gathering within the group.

But since we know nothing about how Paleolithic groups were organized, and cannot tell if they controlled the exploitation or management of their resources in any way, it is impossible to even begin to understand how the food supply system operated. All we really know (and this we conclude from the fact that Paleolithic sites were occupied for long periods) is that the systems which were in operation worked effectively in terms of the group's continued existence.

Health conditions related to nutrition among primitive societies and prehistoric populations can be crudely estimated through skeletal remains (Hoffman and Brunker 1976; Crain 1971; Armelagos et al. 1971). Hunting and gathering groups have an intimate knowledge of the food resources within their own territories. Modern primitives seem to emphasize those nutritional resources which are most assured, and for which they have developed taste preferences (Yudkin 1969). Such taste preferences may also be directly locked into the technological apparatus devised to collect, prepare and cook specific items. Is it not true, one might ask, that the simpler and less specialized the technology associated with food getting and preparation, the wider the range of tastes will be? Viewed in their totality, recently living primitive peoples exhibit a very wide range of food tastes, and it seems likely that the very early men of the Pleistocene were little concerned with food preferences—at least not to the point of going hungry simply because they did not particularly care for some nutritional food resource. When food is scarce, humans eat whatever is available, and have presumably done so for a long while (Howe 1939).

Brothwell and Brothwell (1969) note that the extraction of bone marrow dates back to the very beginnings of man, and the fact is attested to in the archaeological record of all groups engaged in hunting. What reasons can we find for this practice? Splitting open long bones to extract the marrow may have been done simply because people considered the substance a delicacy. Or the marrow might have represented a secondary (and final) utilization of the killed animal, once all of the available flesh had been consumed. Bone marrow might have been a very important (perhaps even critical) dietary item for young children being weaned, or for the old who had lost too many teeth to eat much of anything else. Hrdlicka (1908) observed that fat and marrow were much relished by the Southwestern Indians, where meat was in short supply. But nothing is clear, however interesting it might be to know what really lies behind the human penchant for eating bone marrow.

Human fecal pellets, usually referred to as coprolites, can be preserved in dessicated form in dry deposits such as caves, or even open occupation sites in such places as the rainless coast of Peru and Chile. Unfortunately, it is only within the past 15 years that archaeologists have begun to appreciate how much detailed information these humble objects can provide about diet, endoparasites and the like among prehistoric peoples. A considerable body of published coprolite analyses has now accumulated, covering Israel, Peru, Chile, the western United States (Texas, Arizona, Nevada, Utah and California), Mexico, Kentucky and Arkansas. This geographical coverage is spotty, and—given the total number of coprolites presumably voided by local populations over centuries of occupation in certain sites—the number recovered is relatively small.

Nonetheless, the opportunity to determine in great detail the nutritional habits of some hunter-gatherers in the centuries (or even millenia) prior to the advent of Europeans to the New World provides us with a unique datum in the history of human nutrition. At Berkeley, there is a collection of some 6000 prehistoric human coprolites from one dry cave site in Nevada. The literature on the dietary aspects of prehistoric coprolites is referred to in the bibliographies of several papers (Heizer 1969; Heizer and Napton 1969; Bryant 1974); parasitological examinations are listed in the bibliography of Wilke and Hall (1975). Kliks (1975) has studied the parasite-free coprolites of Lovelock Cave, Nevada, and suggested that the absence of intestinal worms may be attributed to the dietary intake of high levels of anthelmintic substances contained in chenopod seeds; he also examined (1976) the fiber content of these coprolites, finding up to 30% by dry weight of fibrous residues.

Another, albeit rarer, source of such information derives from the stomach or intestinal contents of mummified, frozen or "pickled" corpses found in acid peatbogs (Ruffer 1921; Wakefield and Dellinger 1936; Mostny 1957; Helbaek 1950, 1951).

In regard to the way in which technology can lock human groups into a particular food resource, we need only think of farmers who have forgotten, through simple inattention, how to hunt or to identify edible wild plant products. A case in point concerns the aboriginal California Indians who placed their primary subsistence attention on the acorns yielded by a dozen or so species of *Quercus*. The acorn nutrition complex involved a specialized set of technological apparatus which included carrying baskets, grinding mortars, baskets in which the ground acorn meal was boiled by means of heated stones and basketwork storage granaries that held up to 50 bushels.

The chief drawback to the highly nutritious acorn is its tannic acid content, which was removed by percolating warm water through the ground meal. This leaching process is time-consuming, and one can guess that the women, whose lot it was to prepare the food, found the hulling, grinding and water-percolating rather onerous. The acorn bears heavily in the fall, and was gathered in great quantity during that season and stored for winter use. Through contacts with other native peoples living on and east of the Colorado River, the California Indians almost certainly were exposed to maize agriculture, and had the opportunity to accept this as a surrogate for—or at least an adumbration to—collecting, grinding, leaching and stone-boiling acorns. Yet this was not done in aboriginal times, probably because the adjustment in their routine activities (basketmaking, grinding, leeching, etc.) would have been too great.

The "proof" of the latter proposition is afforded by an historical event—Franciscan missionization of the coastal California tribes from 1769 to 1834, with secularization of the missions constituting one of the anticlerical acts involved in Mexico's independence from Spain in 1821. Many of the Indians released in 1834 withdrew to the interior, taking with them maize seeds and a knowledge of planting and cultivation. This demonstates that maize farming was environmentally feasible, and implies that it took something as drastic as the mission experience to break through the acorn complex so that it could be replaced with Spanish-introduced maize farming (cf. Heizer 1958). S.F. Cook (1941) carried this history of nutritional adaptation one step farther by tracing the shift among California Indians from the acorn economy to the modern American diet in the years since the Gold Rush of the 1850s.

Another approach to ancient nutrition is through skeletal remains. Bones may (but do not always) display directly visible effects of diet, or they may bear mute witness to food-getting activities. Thus, the prehistoric Patagonians suffered from extensive arthritis of the shoulders and elbows, a condition attributed to the use of the bola as a hunting weapon (Wells 1964). Prehistoric skeletons from west and south African archaeological sites commonly show heavy lipping of the small bones in the wrist and at the base of the right thumb, probably as a result of the continous jarring of these joints through the use of the hoe and mattock required to break up the heavy, sun-baked soil for planting. Skeletal remains of pastoral groups that lived in the same area do not show these lesions (Wells 1964).

A study by J. Roney (1959) of a prehistoric Pacific Coast cemetery population from Bodega Bay, California, showed an unusually high frequency of limb and bone fractures, as well as lumbosacral and sacraliliac arthritis. The suggested cause was from falls suffered while collecting mussels (*Mytilis*), a staple food, from the slippery, seaweed-covered rocks which were exposed at low tide.

The teeth can also serve as a register of the dietary regime. The Australopithecines of southern Africa commonly have dental caries, which is generally taken to indicate either an unbalanced or an inadequate diet. The dental problems of ancient men of the Pleistocene were similar (Brothwell 1959). Cereal eaters tend toward greater tooth loss, more dental caries and less tooth wear than do preagricultural hunting and gathering peoples (Wells 1964; Brothwell and Brothwell 1969). An illustration of this can be found in the prehistoric populations of the Clarksville and Tollifero sites in Virginia— the Tollifero people being preagricultural hunters and collectors, while the Clarksville groups were maize farmers (Table 2.1).

Yudkins (1969) argues that widespread nutritional diseases—such as protein deficiency, beriberi, pellagra, riboflavin deficiency and rickets— appear only with the Neolithic revolution. A good deal has been written about defects in tooth enamel (enamel hypoplasia) thought to result from childhood malnutrition (Wells 1964, 1967; Allison *et al.* 1974; Park 1964). A second presumed skeletal effect of food deprivation or malnutrition during childhood is the formation of Harris lines, i.e., thin bands of increased bone density

TABLE 2.1

DENTAL CONDITIONS OF THE PREHISTORIC HUNTER-
COLLECTOR TOLLIFERO POPULATION AND THE LATER
MAIZE-FARMING CLARKSVILLE POPULATION, VIRGINIA

Series	Degree of Wear				
	0 (Absent)	1	2	3	4 (Greatest)
Tollifero series (18)	–	1	6	9	2
Dentitions with caries	–	0	1	3	2
Dentitions with lost teeth	–	0	1	3	2
Clarksville series (38)	7	17	12	2	–
Dentitions with caries	7	15	12	2	–
Dentitions with lost teeth	2	12	12	2	–

From Hoyme and Bass (1962)

formed during stress periods at the epiphyseal ends of immature bones; these can be seen radiographically. Since malnutrition is alleged to be the single cause of both pathologies, one would expect to find both enamel hypoplasia and Harris lines in the same skeletons; but according to Wells (1967), this is usually not the case (Brothwell and Brothwell 1969).

A study by McHenry and Schulz (1975) of Harris lines and enamel hypoplasia in a large series of prehistoric central California skeletons dating from 2000 B.C. to 1500 A.D. shows a 50% decrease in Harris lines from earliest to latest times, along with a significantly greater increase in dental caries. They correlate this with a decrease in dependence on hunting and an increasing dependence on the acorn (whose carbohydrate element took its toll on teeth) as a staple food. This study fails to show a significant correlation in individuals exhibiting both Harris lines and dental hypoplasia. *If* malnutrition is indeed responsible for both conditions, it would appear that factors related to age, sex or genetics must be intimately involved in the skeletal registration of this experience.

Mortality rates for infants and children in primitive societies are high. Polunin (1967) presents data from 16 contemporary primitive groups in Asia, North America and Africa. In 4 of these societies, infant mortality averages 28%; in 2, death before the age of 5 runs to 50%; and in 4 groups, 34% die before reaching the age of 18. Brothwell and Brothwell (1969) think that the critical survival period lies between 1.5 and 2.5 years of age, when the child is making the transition from breast-feeding to solid food. If the latter is inadequate, either in quantity or composition (especially in terms of protein), the child may not gain enough weight and thus be subject to disease. It is impossible to verify such assumptions using prehistoric skeletal materials, but Kunitz and Euler (1972) have suggested that the drought in the American Southwest during the 13th century A.D. may have seriously reduced the production of beans (*Phaseolus vulgaris*), a food source with a protein content of 21%, which would account (at least in part) for the observed infant mortality rate of 50% during that time. Cora DuBois' (1941) observations of childhood experiences among the agricultural Atimelang people of Alor in Indonesia provide one example of the extraordinarily complex interplay of psychological and physiological tensions surrounding hunger and food. Whether such complicated social situations could have prevailed in the Paleolithic seems doubtful. But it might be suggested that survival on the Paleolithic/Stone Age level required a continual maximum effort which offered few amenities for children.

Among non-food-producing hunters and collectors, population numbers are maximized in terms of the least amount of food in a generation. When there is too little food, some will not survive; thus, at some level, the critical limiting factor of minimal nutritional needs for individual survival is always present. Presumably this condition operated throughout the Pleistocene and accounts in no small degree for the relatively low population density for all hunters and gatherers—and especially among those in higher latitudes, where strong seasonal changes in climate exist (Deevey 1958).

With the appearance, some 8000–9000 years ago, of Neolithic food-producers, the food supply may have been more assured, populations may have increased, and infant mortality might have been reduced. The invention of pottery may have caused a revolution in diet, since food was probably cleaner, food mixtures could be tested, and the first cookbooks could have been compiled. But town living also introduced hitherto unknown health hazards, such as poor sanitation, overemphasis on one staple crop which may have been nutritionally deficient (thereby opening the door to disease), famine resulting from unexpected changes in weather, or insect and rodent disease vectors. In short, Neolithic man began to create many of the same problems in health and nutrition that plague us today.

Through the long tunnel of time, a considerable body of knowledge concerning preagricultural diets has been given to us. Ignoring meat, hundreds of nutritious high protein plant foods are known (Bell and Castetter 1937; O. F. Cook 1919; Earle and Jones 1962; Smith *et al.* 1958; Wolf 1945). Many of these grasses, shrubs and trees can be easily cultivated on land which is otherwise useless for agriculture, especially on poor upland soils and in desert areas (cf. Hackenberg 1962; Gardener 1965), and would produce enough food to alleviate a good deal of world hunger.

Solutions to current problems may have already been achieved by past societies, and we might learn much from them. For as Goethe said, "Everything has been thought of before—the difficulty is to think of it again."

REFERENCES

ALLISON, M. J., MENDOZA, D., and PEZZIA, A. 1974. A radiographic approach to child-hood illness in pre-Columbian inhabitants of Southern Peru. Am. J. Phys. Anthrop. *40*, 409–416.
ARDREY, R. 1961. African Genesis. Literat S. A., London.
ARMELAGOS, G. J., MIELKE, J. H., and WINTER, J. 1971. Bibliography of human paleo-pathology. Res. Rep. *8*, Dep. Anthrop., Univ. Mass., Amherst, Mass.
BARNICOT, N. A. 1969. Human nutrition: Evolutionary perspectives. *In* The Domestication of Plants and Animals. P. J. Ucko and G. Dimbleby (Editors). Aldine Publishing, Chicago.
BELL, W. H., and CASTETTER, E. F. 1937. The utilization of mesquite and screwbean by the aborigines in the American Southwest. Bull. *314*, Univ. New Mexico, Albuquerque, N. M.
BREUIL, H. 1932–33. The Sinanthropus deposit at Chou-Kou-Tien (China) and its remains of fire and tools. Anthropos *27*, 1–8. (French)
BROTHWELL, D. R. 1959. Teeth in earlier human populations. Proc. Nutr. Soc. *18*, 59–65.
BROTHWELL, D. R. 1967. The bio-cultural background to disease. *In* Diseases in Antiquity. D. Brothwell and A. T. Sandison (Editors). C. C. Thomas, Springfield, Ill.
BROTHWELL, D., and BROTHWELL, P. 1969. Food in Antiquity: A survey of the diet of early peoples. Thames and Hudson, London.
BRYANT, V. M. 1974. The role of coprolite analysis in archaeology. Texas Archaeol. Soc. Bull. *45*, 1–28.
CHANEY, R. W. 1935. The food of Peking Man. Carnegie Inst. Wash. Bull. *3*, 199–202.

CLARK, J. D. 1972. Paleolithic butchery practices. *In* Man, Settlement and Urbanism. P. J. Ucko, R. Tringham and G. W. Dimbleby (Editors). G. Duckworth, London.

COOK, O. F. 1919. Olneya beans: A native food product of the Arizona desert worthy of domestication. J. Hered. *10*, 321–331.

COOK, S. F. 1941. The mechanism and extent of dietary adaptation among certain groups of California and Nevada Indians. Ibero-Americana *18*.

COOK, S. F. 1946. Human sacrifice and warfare as factors in the demography of pre-colonial Mexico. Hum. Biol. *18*, 81–102.

COON, C. S. 1959. Race and ecology in man. Cold Spring Harbor Symp. on Quant. Biol. *24*, 153–159.

CRAIN, J. B. 1971. Human paleopathology: A bibliographic list. Sacramento Anthrop. Soc. Paper *12*, Sacramento, Calif.

DARE, R. 1974. The ecology and evolution of food sharing. Calif. Anthrop. *2*, 13–25.

DEEVEY, E. S. 1958. The equilibrium population. *In* The Population Ahead. R. G. Francis (Editor). Univ. Minn. Press, Minneapolis, Minn.

DEEVEY, E. S. 1960. The human population. Sci. Am. *203*, 194–204.

DORNSTREICH, M. D. 1973. Food habits of early man: Balance between hunting and gathering. Science *179*, 306–307.

DU BOIS, C. 1941. Attitudes toward food and hunger in Alor. *In* Language, Culture and Personality: Essays in Memory of Edward Sapir. L. Spier, A. I. Hallowell and S. S. Newman (Editors). Sapir Memorial. Publ. Fund, Menasha, Wisc.

EARLE, F. R., and JONES, Q. 1962. Analyses of seed samples from 113 plant families. Econ. Bot *16*, 221–250.

GARDNER, J. L. 1965. Native plants and animals as resources in arid lands of the Southwestern United States. Comm. on Desert and Arid Zones Res., Southwestern and Rocky Mt. Div., AAAS, Contribution *8*. Ariz. State Coll., Flagstaff, Ariz.

GIFFORD, E. W. 1936. California balanophagy. *In* Essays in Anthropology. Robert H. Lowie (Editor). Univ. Calif. Press, Berkeley, Calif.

HACKENBERG, R. A. 1962. Economic alternatives in arid lands: A case study of the Pima and Papago Indians. Ethnology *1*, 186–196.

HAWLEY, F. M., PIJOAN, M., and ELKIN, C. A. 1943. An inquiry into the food economy in Zia Pueblo. Am. Anthrop. *45*, 547–556.

HEIZER, R. F. 1955. Primitive man as an ecological factor. Kroeber Anthrop. Soc. Papers *13*, 1–31.

HEIZER, R. F. 1958. Prehistoric Central California: A problem in historical-developmental classification. Univ. Calif. Archaeol. Surv. Rep. *63*, 1–9.

HEIZER, R. F. 1960. Physical analysis of habitation residues. *In* The Application of Quantitative Methods in Archaeology. R. F. Heizer and S. F. Cook (Editors). Viking Fund Publ. in Anthrop. *28*, Quadrangle Books, Chicago.

HEIZER, R. F. 1963. Domestic fuel in primitive society. Roy. Anthrop. Inst. *93*, 186–194.

HEIZER, R. F. 1969. The anthropology of Great Basin human coprolites. *In* Science in Archaeology, 2nd Edition. D. Brothwell and E. Higgs (Editors). Thames and Hudson, London.

HEIZER, R. F., and NAPTON, L. K. 1969. Biological and cultural evidence from prehistoric human coprolites. Science *165*, 563–568.

HELBAEK, H. 1950. Tollund man's last meal. Aarbøger for Nordisk Oldkyndighed og Historie 1950, 311–344. (Norwegian)

HELBAEK, H. 1951. Seeds of weeds as food in the pre-Roman Iron Age. Kuml 1951, Aarhus, 65–71.

HELBAEK, H. 1961. Studying the diet of early man. Archaeol. *14*, 95–101.

HOFFMAN, J. M., and BRUNKER, L. 1976. Studies in California paleopathology. I. A bibliography of California paleopathology. Contr. Archaeol. Res. Fac., Dep. Anthrop., Univ. Calif., Berkeley, Calif. (In press)

HOLMBERG, A. 1950. Nomads of the long bow. Inst. Soc. Anthrop., Smithson. Inst. Publ. *10*., Washington, D. C.

HOWE, P. E. 1939. Can food habits be changed? *In* Food and Life. Yearbook of Agric., U. S. Dep. Agric., Washington, D. C.

HOWELL, F. C. 1965. Early Man. Life Nature Library, Time, Inc., New York.

HOYME, L., and BASS, W. M. 1962. Human Skeletal material remains from Tollifero (Ha-6) and Clarksville (Mc-14) sites, John H. Kerr Reservoir Basin, Virginia. Bur. Am. Ethnol., Smithson. Inst. Bull. *182*, 329–400.
HRDLICKA, A. 1908. Physiological and medical observations among the Indians of Southwestern United States and Northern Mexico. Bur. Am. Ethnol., Smithson. Inst. Bull. *34*.
ISAAC, G. L. 1971. The diet of early man: Aspects of archaeological evidence from Lower and Middle Pleistocene sites in Africa. World Archaeol. *2*, 278–299.
ISAAC, G. L. 1973. Meat eating and human evolution: Aspects of the archaeological evidence from East Africa. Paper presented at the 72nd Annu. Meet. of the Am. Anthrop. Assoc., New Orleans, La.
JAMES, S.R., and GRAZIANI, S. 1975. California Indian warfare. Archaeol. Res. Fac., Dep. Anthrop., Univ. Calif., Berkeley, Calif. Contrib. *8*, 47–109.
JOLLY, C. J. 1970. The seed-eaters: A new model of hominid differentiation based on a baboon analogy. Man *5*, 5–26.
JONES, Q., and EARLE. F. R. 1966. Chemical analyses of seeds. II. Oil and protein content of 759 species. Econ. Bot. *20*, 127–155.
KLIKS, M. 1975. Paleoepidemiological studies on Great Basin coprolites: Estimation of dietary intake and evaluation of the ingestion of anthelmintic plant substances. Archaeol. Res. Fac., Dep. Anthrop., Univ. Calif., Berkeley, Calif.
KLIKS, M. 1976. Paleodietetics: A review of the role of dietary fiber in pre-agricultural human diets. *In* Fiber in Human Nutrition. G. A. Spiller and R. J. Amens (Editors). C. C. Thomas, Springfield, Ill. (In press)
KROEBER, A. L. 1962. The nature of land-holding groups in aboriginal California. Univ. Calif. Archaeol. Surv. Rep. *56*, 19–58.
KROGH, A., and KROGH, M. 1951. A study of the diet and metabolism of Eskimos undertaken in 1908 on an expedition to Greenland. Medd. om Grønland *2*, 1–52.
KUNITZ, S. J., and EULER, R. C. 1972. Aspects of southwestern paleoepidemiology. Prescott Coll. Anthrop. Rep. *2*, Flagstaff, Ariz.
LEE, R. 1968. What hunters do for a living; or how to make out on scarce resources. *In* Man the Hunter. R. Lee and I. DeVore (Editors). Aldine Publishing, Chicago.
LEOPOLD, A. C., and ARDREY, R. 1972A. Toxic substances in plants and the food habits of early man. Science *176*, 512.
LEOPOLD, A. C., and ARDREY, R. 1972B. Early man's food habits. Science *177*, 833–835.
LOWIE, R. H. 1938. Subsistence. *In* General Anthropology. F. Boas (Editor). D. C. Heath, New York.
MC HENRY, H. M. 1975. Fossils and the mosaic nature of human evolution. Science *190*, 425–431.
MC HENRY, H. M., and SCHULZ, P. D. 1975. Harris lines, enamel hypoplasia and subsistence change in prehistoric Central California. Ballena Press Anthrop. Papers, Ramona, Calif. (In press)
MERRIAM, C. H. 1918. The acorn, a possibly neglected source of food. Nat. Geogr. *34*, 129–137.
MOSTNY, G. 1957. The mummy of Cerro el Plomo. Boletin del Museo Nacional de Historia Natural, Santiago, Chile *27*, 1–119. (Spanish)
MOUNTFORD, C. P. 1960. Anthropology and nutrition. Records of the American-Australian Sci. Exped. to Arnhem Land *2*. Melbourne Univ. Press, Melbourne, Australia.
MOVIUS, H. L. 1966. The hearths of the Upper Perigordian and Aurignacian horizon at the Abri Pataud, Les Eyzies (Dordogne) and their possible significance. Am. Anthrop. *68*. 296–325.
MURDOCK, G. P. 1937. Comparative data on division of labor by sex. Social Forces *15*, 551–553.
OAKLEY, K. P. 1956A. Fire as a Paleolithic tool and weapon. Proc. Prehist. Soc. *21*, 36–48.
OAKLEY K. P. 1956B. The earliest tool-makers and the earliest fire-makers. Antiquity *30*, 4–8, 102–107.
PARK, E. A. 1964. The imprinting of nutritional disturbances on the growing bone. Pediatrics *33*, 815–862.
POLUNIN, I. V. 1967. Health and disease in contemporary primitive societies. *In* Diseases in Antiquity. D. Brothwell and A. T. Sandison (Editors). C. C. Thomas, Springfield, Ill.

RIVERA, T. 1949. Diet of a food-gathering people, with chemical analysis of salmon and saskatoons. *In* Indians of the Northwest. M. W. Smith (Editor). Columbia Univ. Contribs. Anthrop. *36*, 19–36.
RONEY J. G. 1959. Paleopathology of a California archaeological site. Bull. Hist. Med. *33*, 97–109.
ROTH, W. E. 1901. Food: Its search, capture and preparation. N. Queensland Ethnog. Bull. *3*, Brisbane, Australia.
RUFFER, M. A. 1921. Studies in the Paleopathology of Egypt. R. L. Moodie (Editor). Univ. Chicago Press, Chicago.
SIMOONS, F. J. 1960. Eat Not This Flesh. Univ. Wisc. Press, Madison, Wisc.
SMITH, C. R., SHIKELTON, M. C., WOLFF, L., and JONES, Q. 1958. Seed protein sources: Amino acid composition and total protein content of various plant seeds. Econ. Bot. *12*, 132–150.
STEFANSSON, V. 1937. Food of the ancient and modern Stone Age man. J. Am. Diet. Assoc. *13*, 102–119.
STEWARD, J. H. 1938. Basin-Plateau aboriginal socio-political groups. Bur. Am. Ethnol., Smithsonian Inst. Bull. *120*.
SULLIVAN, R. J. 1942. The Ten'a food quest. Cath. Univ. of Am., Anthrop. Ser., Washington, D. C. *11*.
SWEENEY, G. 1947. Food supplies of a desert tribe. Oceania *17*, 289–299.
SWEZEY, S. 1975. The energetics of subsistence-assurance ritual in native California. Archaeol. Res. Fac., Dep. Anthrop., Univ. Calif., Berkeley, Calif., Contrib. *23*, 1–46.
VITA-FINZI, C., and HIGGS, E. S. 1970. Prehistoric economy in the Mount Carmel area of Palestine. Proc. Prehist. Soc. *36*, 1–37.
WAKEFIELD, E. G., and DELLINGER, S. C. 1936. Diet of the Bluff Dwellers of the Ozark Mountains and its skeletal effects. Ann. Intern. Med. *9*, 1412–1418.
WASHBURN, S. L., and AVIS, V. 1958. Evolution of human behavior. *In* Behavior and Evolution. A. Roe and G. G. Simpson (Editors). Yale Univ. Press, New Haven, Conn.
WATERMAN, T. T. 1920. Yurok geography. Univ. Calif. Pub. in Am. Archaeol. and Ethnol. *16*, 177–314.
WELLS, C. 1964. Bones, Bodies and Disease. Thames and Hudson, London.
WELLS, C. 1967. A new approach to paleopathology: Harris's lines. *In* Disease in Antiquity. D. Brothwell and A. T. Sandison (Editors). C. C. Thomas, Springfield, Ill.
WHITE, T. E. 1953. A method of calculating the dietary percentage of various food animals utilized by aboriginal peoples. Am. Antiq. *18*, 396–398.
WILKE, P. J., and HALL, H. J. 1975. Analysis of ancient feces: A discussion and annotated bibliography. Archaeol. Res. Fac., Dept. Anthrop., Univ. Calif., Berkeley, Calif.
WILLOUGHBY, N. 1963. Division of labor among the Indians of California. Univ. Calif. Archaeol. Surv. Rep. *60*, 7–79.
WOLF, C. B. 1945. California wild tree crops. Rancho Santa Ana Bot. Garden, Santa Ana, Calif.
YUDKIN, J. 1969. Archaeology and the nutritionist. *In* The Domestication and Exploitation of Plants and Animals. P. J. Ucko and G. W. Dimbleby (Editors). Aldine Publishing, Chicago.

CHAPTER 3

Philip E. L. Smith

Man, The Subsistence Farmer: New Directions in Society and Culture

The archaeologist working on the problem of early agricultural societies, whether in the Old World or the New, feels especially close to nutritionists because there is a central pivot to both fields of study—food and how it interacts with human biology and culture. That is what the so-called Neolithic Revolution comes down to—it was a change in food-getting and in nutrition which eventually transformed the human world and much of the natural world as well.

Here the term "subsistence farmer" is used to mean simple, low-yield agriculturalists whose primary goal is to provide enough food to feed the household until the next harvest, although in more complex or stratified societies they may support some nonfood producers as well.

Recently the authors of a book on human evolution stated that the agricultural revolution of prehistoric times was "the great leap backward" (Tiger and Fox 1971). This statement may surprise some people. What the writers were trying to say is that agriculture returned man to the restrictive drudgery of our primate past as a food-gathering vegetarian, before hunting had developed as a way of life, and was therefore a turning away from the "natural" or "normal" circumstances in which man had developed his peculiar qualities over several million years of evolution during the Pleistocene.

As in most contrived paradoxes, there is a substratum of truth in this statement, but the claim is of course exorbitant because it exaggerates the role of hunting in man's past. Nutritionists and others should be aware that archaeologists have traditionally overemphasized the importance of meat in prehistoric diets because animal bones are usually better preserved than are plant remains. One gets the impression from some authors that certain Paleolithic groups lived entirely on animal protein. Those nutritionists interested in establishing the "natural" or "most suitable" diet for man (Yudkin 1969) should be on their guard against this kind of distortion. Fortunately archaeologists are now more conscious of the refraction caused by uneven sampling or preservation of the materials they study, while recent ethnological studies have emphasized the importance of plant foods among most hunting-gathering peoples of the world.

Nevertheless, the statement quoted above is not entirely wrong. Seen in the long perspective of human evolution, a commitment to food production as the basis for sustenance *is* a kind of aberration. Man was devoted to hunting

27

and gathering for at least several million years—that is, for more than 99% of his career, or at least 100,000 generations. He has been a practicing farmer for just about 10,000 years, which is around 400 generations. So perhaps it is true that man's most basic nature and abilities were built up during the long Paleolithic period in the Old World, that during this time he was "wired" for certain kinds of behavior and reactions, and that there have been no basic changes since then.

But we cannot forget that when he became a subsistence farmer late in his career, he did set into motion a whole series of processes which, given the benefit of hindsight, we can see as a significant divergence from the normal patterns of the Paleolithic. Of course, there is always a danger of exaggerating the differences between the two ways of life, of opposing too simplistically the subsistence farmer and the hunter-gatherer. In fact, there was a considerable degree of continuity, as well as social, economic and technological overlap. And it is even possible, as some prehistorians claim today, that certain Paleolithic people had close man-animal and man-plant relationships that approach what we now call food production (Higgs 1972). In a real sense, then, food production is the culmination of trends that go well back into the Pleistocene.

Thus, many prehistorians object to the expression "Neolithic Revolution" because it seems to downplay the continuities which do exist, or because it contains overtones of explosive change. However, I feel that such qualms are unnecessary. Surely the term is justifiable if we define a revolution as a relatively sudden set of changes leading to a state of affairs which makes a return to the preceding situation virtually impossible. This revolution, occurring some 10,000 years ago, was the most important shift in cultural evolution since the appearance of tool-making homonids several million years before. Of course a great deal happened during those several million years in the biological, mental, social and cultural realms. Nevertheless, I doubt that very many genuinely qualitative changes would have occurred if man had continued as a hunter-gatherer for, say, another million years. I suspect that the limits of this kind of adaptation had just about been reached.

But food production permitted, and may have even required, new forms of cultural and social life to emerge and develop on earth. For better or worse, without the adoption of food production as an economic base, we would be very different creatures today, with thought processes and behavioral patterns we would now find difficult to imagine. So I maintain that the shift to food production marks the great divide or watershed in human history—one which separates us from what might be called, without too much fancy, the infancy of mankind.

WHAT IS FOOD PRODUCTION?

The essence of the change involved in the shift to food production (which is nearly synonymous with agriculture, a term I use here to include horticulture, arboriculture and animal husbandry) is the altered relationship between man on the one hand, and the plant and animal worlds on the other. Food producers occupy an ecological niche which differs in some important ways from that of hunters and gatherers. Although the basic food energy resources remained the same (i.e., plant and animal life), the techniques of *appropriating* these resources—that is, how the food was obtained—were altered, especially by the process familiarly called domestication. Unfortunately, domestication is a very slippery term, and it is difficult to get botanists, zoologists and anthropologists to agree on a definition of it. Let us simply say that it involves a spectrum of close or symbiotic relationships between man, plants and animals, and that it usually includes human interference in the patterns of reproduction and ecological adaptation as artificial selection gradually supplements or replaces natural selection.[1]

Regardless of the precise definition of the word, what man did when he began producing his food was to develop a more productive way of getting at the solar radiant energy stored up in plants. Man had traditionally, from the beginning of his career, exploited this low trophic energy in two ways: directly, by eating edible plants, or indirectly through the animal food chain—especially by eating those herbivores which consume plants (such as most perennials and those containing a high degree of cellulose) that have little food value for humans. (In fact, one kind of specialized food-producer, the pastoral nomad, still lives off the top of the food chain in a sense, although animal products are not necessarily a major part of the diet.)

When man became a food-producer, he merely intensified this process, with a greater emphasis on the base of the food chain in those societies where plants were the staple food. He altered the genetic patterns and distributions of certain plant foods that he could consume directly (especially cereals and root crops), and he controlled the behavior of certain animals (especially herbivores) to make them more efficient converters of plant energy. The result of this coevolution of plants, animals and culture was an agricultural economy, which is nearly always more expandable than hunting-gathering economies. Thus, it allows for increased carrying capacities, much higher levels of food-getting (although usually at the cost of higher labor or capital application), and far more complex forms of cultural and social organization.

In other words, food production served to remove the bottleneck imposed by the hunting and gathering mode of subsistence. With this restriction removed, something new appeared in the world: subsistence farmers, peasants and peasant society. From the time of the Neolithic, this has been the most

---

[1]Of course, we cannot be certain that plants were first encouraged and cultivated for food purposes; and indeed, several geographers have suggested that they were originally cultivated for medicinal reasons (e.g., Harris 1967). Some animals may also have been first brought under control and bred for reasons not directly related to nutrition (Isaac 1970).

numerous and important class in human society, and it remains so today. All of the ancient high civilizations, whether in the Old or New Worlds, rested on the shoulders of the peasant; and except for the most highly industrialized societies, most modern nations are based on the peasant as well.[2]

There is archaeological evidence of populations being transformed by agriculture as early as 10,000 years ago in the Old World (especially in Southwestern Asia) and about 5,000 years ago in the New World (especially in Mesoamerica). By this time, all human populations belonged to the *Homo sapiens sapiens* group and were marked by modern physical form and intellectual capacity. Environmental conditions essentially similar to those of the present were established, and nearly all of the habitable world (apart from the more isolated islands) was occupied by man.

Just where the complex process we call domestication first took place is still a subject of hot archaeological debate, but societies heavily committed to farming probably developed first in the general area of the Near East, where we can confidently speak of subsistence farmers dependent on cereals and animals existing as early as 7000–6000 B. C. It probably took about 2000 or 3000 years for this system to crystallize. Roughly the same amount of time was needed in Mesoamerica (and perhaps also in Peru) to produce permanent communities largely dependent on maize and other edible plants sometime after 2000 B. C. We are not so sure of the transformations in other parts of the world. It had probably taken place in China by 4000 B. C., in Southern Europe by about 6000 B. C., in sub-Saharan Africa by the second millenium B. C., and in North America by 500 A. D. However, much more archeological work is required before we can detail its inception in these latter areas.

Seen from a Paleolithic time perspective, this looks like an explosive change on a global scale. But of course it did not happen overnight. It began in many separate small-scale and sometimes obscure situations, and its earlier phases are often very difficult to recognize archaeologically. Over many generations, various groups sorted out the most advantageous kinds of exploitation and the most acceptable nutritional combinations, while slowly supplementing their hunting and gathering economies with often unlikely foodstuffs that gradually achieved the status of domesticates and cultigens. The movement seems to have been generally unidirectional, although there have been some cases of reversion to hunting-gathering by marginal farmers.

---

[2]Just how complex and large a society can become without an important food-producing base is hard to say. It is usually argued that food production is a necessary, although not a sufficient, condition for the development of permanent urban settlements and states. Probably this is generally true, although there may be some exceptions to the rule; for example, it is now claimed that in coastal Peru between 3000 and 1000 B. C. there were highly developed societies and a genuine urbanism based not on agriculture, but on the extremely abundant marine foods available (Moseley 1975). Nonetheless, this was replaced by food-producing groups, suggesting that the previous situation was unstable and ephemeral in the long term.

In time, food producers took over virtually the entire world, mainly because they could control greater energy and form larger, more permanent groups with more tightly controlled social and political organizations. They also degraded many of the natural resources upon which hunters and gatherers depend. Therefore it is not too surprising that, over the past 10,000 years, such an expansive and predatory form of subsistence should have gradually displaced or eliminated the earlier forms. Only about 30 small groups of hunters and gatherers remain today, and they will probably disappear soon (Murdock 1968).

In the New World, food production was based on cultigens which were mainly tropical or subtropical in origin, especially maize, beans, squash, avocado, manioc, pumpkin, white and sweet potatoes, chili pepper, tomatoes and chocolate. The synergistic combination of beans and maize was a particularly important one, since the beans supplied the amino acid lysine which maize lacks. Only a few animals were domesticated in the New World (llama, alpaca, turkey, guinea pig, Muscovy duck and dog), and they were of little real importance for food. This is in strong contrast to the role of domesticated food animals in many Old World cultures.[3]

There, food production was based on very different combinations of cultigens and domesticated animals that provided meat and dairy products. The main plant foods were such cereals as wheat, barley, rice, millet and sorghum; root crops like yams and taro in the tropics; and various vegetables, legumes, fruits and nuts. Goats, sheep, pigs, cattle, water buffalo, asses, horses, camels and reindeer were domesticated for food and other purposes, although in the Far East fish and plant proteins—especially soya beans—largely took the place of meat and dairy products.

Virtually all the foods on which we depend today were domesticated in Neolithic and equivalent times; no important plants or animals have been domesticated for food purposes since the prehistoric era. The more advanced early civilizations of the Old and New Worlds seem to have been based largely on the cereal crops, with important supplements from root and tree crops in some cases. This is because cereals, in contrast to root crops, are marked by high annual productivity, high nutritional value, ease of storage and a genetic

---

[3]We really do not have a good explanation of why man domesticated animals in the first place. The absence of important food animals in New World cultures shows that domesticated animals are not necessary components of subsistence farming, or of higher civilization based on subsistence farming. Just why many of the Old World groups went in so heavily for raising goats, sheep, pigs and cattle (and for consuming meat, dairy products and blood) is an interesting but unanswered question. Cereals and legumes, supplemented by hunting and fishing, would probably have provided a good diet, just as they did in the New World. While animal husbandry later became extremely important in many areas, it is possible that at the beginning it was a somewhat marginal enterprise which facilitated food production based on plants, and the real purpose was noneconomic in the nutritional sense.

plasticity which permits favorable changes to occur rapidly. The basic, and fascinating, question of why food production happened at all remains essentially unanswered. There are many hypotheses, but not much agreement among prehistorians so far. The question of origins is all the more important when we consider the recent arguments, based on ethnographical and botanical evidence, that hunters and gatherers usually lead lives somewhat closer to *la dolce vita* than we had traditionally believed, at least if they can rely on plant foods (Lee 1968; Harlan 1967).

It has even become fashionable to refer to the Paleolithic as the original "affluent society." After all, if an individual can get by with 12 to 20 hours of work per week, why change to food reproduction, which often requires harder, longer work and is not necessarily more secure? The answer is probably linked to imbalances between population growth and available natural food resources in early Holocene times, with food production gradually emerging as a means of maintaining the enlarged and more sedentary communities which had developed in some areas by that time.

THE CONSEQUENCES

However food production may have begun, we are mainly concerned here with its consequences. Of course, food production modified almost every aspect of human life, including demography, social and political organization, and cognitive or symbolic behavior and attitudes.[4]

Demography

Ultimately, the great increase in the world's population was perhaps the most important consequence of food production. The new subsistence method greatly increased the productivity of those regions where agriculture is possible, and permitted local groups to reach far greater size than can most hunters and gatherers. While there is still no agreement on how many people could have existed at any given time during the Paleolithic, there were probably between five and ten million people alive just before food production began. Today we have about four billion people, and our population is increasing rapidly—a legacy of those first subsistence farmers. In the Near East alone, it is estimated that between 8000 and 4000 B. C. there may have been an increase from about 100,000 people to over five million (Carneiro and Hilse 1966).

Although population was apparently increasing among some hunters and gatherers, food production seems to have caused a real quantum jump. It would seem that, as food production took hold, many of the checks that operate among hunters and gatherers to curb their numbers could now be relaxed. Among these curbs are abortion, infanticide and avoidance of

---

[4]For a more detailed treatment of the various consequences, see Smith (1972, 1976).

intercourse. Less nomadic life patterns probably permitted the more sedentary groups to reduce the interval between children to less than the three year minimum found among modern hunters. There is also some belief that the menarche may occur at a younger age among more sedentary groups and thus permit earlier pregnancies.

Certain dietary changes, especially the use of mushy cereal foods and (later) animal milk in some regions, may have favored infant survival in the critical early years. These dietary substitutes, in turn, would permit a shorter lactation period among mothers and, perhaps, an earlier resumption of ovulation. The lives of some of the older adults (who themselves often function as a "bank" of medical skills) might also have been prolonged by more sedentary conditions and by stores of off-season foods. Finally, we must remember that agriculture often selects for larger families, since there are many tasks (such as weeding and looking after livestock) that can be performed by children.[5]

All of these factors encouraged population growth, and they seem to have more than balanced the effects of various new diseases and nutritional deficiencies that now became effective among the food-producers. While Palaeolithic people certainly had their share of ailments (as shown by the dental abscesses, fractures, and signs of arthritis and rheumatism on their skeletons) it is doubtful that contagious diseases or epidemics were ever very important as long as the hunting-gathering populations were small, dispersed and mobile. There were probably diseases such as malaria and yellow fever, since the pathogens could survive under these conditions.

However, with the more sedentary, crowded and less sanitary conditions following food production, a great many infectious diseases could flourish. These include smallpox, measles, mumps, chickenpox, influenza, polio-myelitis, bubonic plague, leprosy, hookworm and bacillary dysentery. Man has probably had only a few hundred generations to adapt himself to these diseases. Moreover, forest-clearing and irrigation practices probably increased those diseases borne by insects and other organisms, such as malaria, yellow fever, scrub typhus, dengue, sleeping sickness and schis-tosomiasis. Domesticated animals were vehicles for bovine tuberculosis, anthrax, and trypanosomiasis, particularly where they shared living quarters with people.

It is also probable that dietary deficiencies were more common among food-producers than among most hunter-gatherers. The latter, judging by recent examples, generally enjoy better balanced diets than do subsistence farmers who rely heavily on cereal or root crops. The resultant deficiencies often lead to rickets, pellagra and other diseases, while protein malnutrition in

---

[5]Many of the demographic aspects of primitive societies are discussed by the con-tributors to the volume edited by Spooner (1972).

high starch diets produces such diseases as kwashiorkor.[6] The modern !Kung Bushmen of the Kalahari seem to be quite well-nourished in spite of their austere environment, and show no significant vitamin deficiencies, little iron deficiency anemia, and few degenerative diseases of old age such as high blood pressure. It is commonplace for Bushmen to live 60 years, and some apparently even reach 80 (Kolata 1974; Lee 1968).

Thus, it is unlikely that the shift to food production was marked by any general improvement in health, and there is good reason to suspect the opposite was true, especially as agriculture became more intensive. Indeed, one of the interesting lines of evidence archaeologists and physical anthropologists are currently exploring is the degree to which increasing class distinctions in agricultural societies resulted in different degrees of health, as certain groups enjoyed access to better or more abundant food than did others. This seems to be reflected in the skeletons of the Classic Maya of Mesoamerica (Haviland 1967; Saul 1973); there is even some suggestion that disease and malnutrition played a role in the collapse of the Classic Maya civilization about 900 A. D. (Willey and Shimkin 1973).

It is sometimes assumed that the average human life span was prolonged when food production was adopted. However, there is no real evidence for this. The prehistoric skeletal materials from a number of parts of the world suggest that mean life expectancies for Neolithic peoples were about 31–34 years for males, and 28–31 for females (Brothwell and Brothwell 1969); that is not significantly different from those of hunter-gatherers, and perhaps lower in some cases. Frequent survival into middle and late adult age is a comparatively modern phenomenon. Although starvation is not unknown among some hunter-gatherers, it is likely that periodic famines and seasonal hunger with their effects on the mortality rates of the very young and very old, were far more significant for groups dependent on food production. Such hunger periods would reinforce the effects on mortality rates of the diseases and malnutrition mentioned earlier.

Social and Political Organization

Directly linked to the increase in population were the changes in community size and structure, as well as in social and political organization.

---

[6]One wonders if the rate of cannibalism as a dietary supplement increased with food production. Hunters and gatherers eat each other during periods of starvation, or for ritual purposes, and there is some archaeological evidence that this practice goes far back into the Paleolithic. However, for agriculturalists suffering nutritional deficiencies caused by excessive reliance on root crops and some cereals (especially in areas where game was scarce), the human body would be one useful source of protein, vitamins and minerals. Garn and Block (1970) estimate that an adult provides 30 kg of edible muscle mass, or enough to provide one day's protein requirement for about 60 adults. The increased intergroup conflicts which accompanied the intensification of agriculture would have insured a fairly reliable crop of captives and corpses.

Under unusually favorable conditions (as happened in California, where acorns provided a good food source, and on the northwest coast, where fish were abundant), it is possible to find fairly sedentary settlements among hunters, gatherers and fishermen. Such settlements seem to have existed throughout both hemispheres in prehistoric times, but it was not until the formal introduction of food production that they became the norm, expanding both in size and numbers.

The traditional hunting-gathering pattern of seasonal concentration in one place, followed by dispersal according to the availability of wild foods, was modified as domesticated foods were more and more exploited. Important changes in settlement patterns occurred. The earliest subsistence farmers very likely did not remain in one site for the entire year. Moreover, they probably moved their villages or households every few years when productivity declined, as do many modern shifting cultivators. Nevertheless, life in fairly large communities of several hundred or more people within a single wider territory could not be more permanent.

One visible consequence is the great proliferation of durable architectural forms which now appeared in many regions—sizeable houses in mud, brick, stone or wood, often with special facilities for storage or processing of food, as well as for manufacturing and ritual activities. Material possessions and durable goods often seem to increase in quantity and, sometimes, in quality (particularly in such materials as pottery, copper and textiles). There are also increasing numbers of exotic imported items, both utilitarian and luxury. (While pottery is not exclusively associated with food producers, it certainly increased in popularity with food production; it served to enlarge the range of cooking and preserving techniques, and to make edible certain plants—e.g., legumes with pods—which are difficult to digest without boiling.)

It is fairly easy for archaeologists to observe changes in technology among these subsistence farmers. It is much harder to demonstrate changes in social and political organization, in the relations between individuals, or in values and cognitive behavior. Yet there can be no doubt that fundamental changes were taking place in these fields parallel with the more tangible transformations. The very increase in size of many local groupings would enhance the tendency as scale effects occurred. New social mechanisms had to evolve to cope with the new pressures and needs of the communities. The most important of these were related to the manner of producing, processing and sharing of food resources, the adjudication of disputes over land and other matters, and the sexual and age roles of individuals in production and decision making. There also had to be rules governing marriage and the relationships of children to family groupings, since this is at the heart of the recruitment of members to the community. For example, as communities grew larger it is likely that endogamous marriages within the villages increased in importance over exogamous ones.

Some hunting-gathering-fishing peoples can develop quite complex social and political organizations if they are reasonably sedentary and wealthy. Very likely some Upper Paleolithic/Mesolithic groups in the Old World, and Archaic groups in the New, had gone beyond the typical band level of closely linked families with flexible, bilateral, nonterritorial social systems. Some may have attained the tribal level with extended families and lineages. With the advent of food production, however, entirely new kinds of societies could come into being—not only tribes, but also chiefdoms and, eventually, states with marked distinctions in individual rank and status and, usually, some form of writing.[7]

With the gradual intensification of subsistence farming, extended family households and unilineal descent groups probably became more important as means of mobilizing labor, of increasing food production, and of defending property and other rights. The nuclear family may also have lost some of its autonomy as food production developed, with a decreased ability to support itself or to survive outside a more complex structure; indeed, it has been suggested that the return of the nuclear family to primary importance in Western societies since the Industrial Revolution is really the revival of a Paleolithic status that had been greatly modified by the Neolithic Revolution (Dumond 1975).

Kinship groupings might often tend to be supplemented by extra-kin associations such as secret societies, exclusive ceremonial organizations, and age sets. Certain families or lineages might be expected to appropriate for themselves more resources, especially cultivable land, and increase their property and influence by skillful manipulation (somewhat as some large landholders have done in underdeveloped countries since the Green Revolution of recent years). Wealth would increasingly become a marker of social distinction and prestige, as the burials often attest. Status, and often lay or ritual authority, might become hereditary. Leadership became more strongly institutionalized, and was eventually embodied in formal law rather than consensus. Society frequently became inegalitarian and hierarchical, with low-status individuals (including slaves and serfs) required to supply labor and goods to those in authority. Human sacrifice was often practiced. Craft specialization in production and distribution developed, and full-time specialists tended to displace the earlier part-time practitioners in such fields as manufacturing goods, ritual activities and medical services. Intergroup conflict and organized warfare became a regular pattern. Usually some form of writing is developed or borrowed to record and process information re-

---

[7]The question of the origins of states and highly stratified urban societies is another problem about which anthropologists and others have debated a great deal, with no real agreement emerging. I shall only mention here that such societies had appeared in Mesopotamia and Egypt before 3000 B. C., in India by 2500 B. C., in China by 1800 B. C., in Mesoamerica perhaps by 1000 B. C. and in Peru about 200 A. D.

quired to keep the system functioning. More and more centralization of power develops, and large towns or even small cities grow and control larger territories; the formerly independent farming villages and hamlets increasingly become satellites of these larger centers where religious and civil authority is often exercised in large and ostentatious buildings.

As far as the division of labor (or rather, tasks) between the sexes is concerned, this probably did not change significantly with the inception of agriculture. Men probably continued to perform the more strenuous or dangerous tasks—hunting, clearing forests, herding large animals, and fighting outside groups—while women retained those which were more compatible with child care such as collecting, planting, weeding, harvesting and preparing food.

There has been a lot written about the status of women after agriculture began, and much exaggeration about such things as "matriarchal" rule, matrilineal societies, etc. It is a complex question, too difficult to discuss in detail here. However, there was no necessary elevation or depression of female status with the beginning of farming. Female status in hunting-gathering societies can be quite high, especially where they collect much of the food consumed; very likely this did not change in those situations where they made important contributions to the agricultural work, as they do in many horticultural societies today.

With intensive agriculture, however, there is often a tendency for women's status to decline as far as economic and political rights are concerned. This is especially true in plow agriculture, and perhaps irrigation agriculture as well. It is interesting, for instance, that among a recently settled group of !Kung Bushmen, the women seem to be losing their egalitarian status as the importance of their food-collecting role shrinks and male-dominated agriculture is adopted (Kolata 1974); this may have happened, albeit much more gradually, in many prehistoric cases as well. It is even argued that as agriculture developed, women for the first time in cultural evolution dropped out of the mainstream of production and were gradually excluded from central roles in societal institutions (Martin and Voorhies 1975).

Cognitive and Symbolic Attitudes

When the archaeologist talks about changes in such aspects of prehistoric life as religion, mental attitudes, ideology and art, all of which involve a high symbolic content, he is obviously treading on very shaky ground. However, comparative ethnology gives us some clues to look for, and helps avoid excessive speculation. Of course, there may have been no abrupt changes at first, and it probably took many dozens of generations before the transformation of the subsistence base brought about modifications in cognitive systems and expressions.

For example, there do seem to be some differences in personality and world view between peasants (who emphasize security, pragmatism, and work as a fulfillment of divine command) and most hunter-gatherers, who do not seem to value these attitudes highly. While the contrasts between the two groups are not absolute, it is perhaps not illogical to suppose that food production, which involves long-range planning for future needs and much trial-and-error experimentation, should over a long period have selected for a certain range of temperaments and attitudes. Thus, their time perspective might be affected by the long-range processes involved in stock breeding and plant selection, producing an emphasis on the lineality and continuity of the past and future, ancestor worship as a means of validating family and group ownership of resources (especially land), and, incidentally, a need for astronomical and mathematical skills to predict future events related to the agricultural cycle.

How far religious beliefs were altered with the advent of food production is a much debated question, as is the issue of whether a culture based on herd or flock animals induces different religious and cosmological attitudes than one based on cultivated plants. Another question that is not well-explored is whether the coming of agriculture gave new meaning to old ideas about female fertility, "earth" and "mother" goddesses, and rituals of death and resurrection (Issac 1970). But what is clear from the archaeological record is that among many sedentary agriculturalists, there later developed highly formalized religious structures and temple hierarchies which often served also as centers for redistribution of local products, as agents for external trade, and as instruments to reinforce the social and political systems.

Insofar as changes in art are concerned—not only plastic art, but also song, dance and oral literature—the ground is equally slippery for the archaeolgist. Obviously the new range of media available—especially ceramics, metals, textiles and architecture—permitted a whole new spectrum of artistic expression which is highly visible in our excavations. But can we see new and different meaning in this art as the changes inherent in food production infiltrated this domain as well? Again, there is no good answer. The old nineteenth century evolutionist notion that hunter-gatherer art is basically naturalistic while agricultural art is abstract is no longer acceptable. But so far there are very few worthwhile theories to replace it.

However, it might be well to consider the idea that as food production evolved, food itself may have developed into a recognizable art form. As the British social anthropologist, Mary Douglas, recently suggested, the way food is regarded in a society or a social class is governed by certain precise, well-known but usually unwritten rules concerning such things as ingredients and sensory qualities which are integral parts of the social standards of the group, and can even be seen as summations of the symbolic systems of the society concerned (Douglas 1974). In other words, throughout the Neolithic and in later times as well, the growth of more complex social organizations and, perhaps, the increased variety of available foods may have created (or at least enhanced) situations in which food became an art form—that is, where it took on very clear esthetic and symbolic functions above and beyond its nutritional value.

CONCLUSION

It has been suggested that some of the common assumptions about the changes inspired by food production have little foundation. Archaeologists and ethnologists no longer believe that food production guaranteed a more dependable or more nutritious supply of food than did hunting and collecting. It is also probably untrue that subsistence farming involved less work or produced more leisure time and energy for other accomplishments, including the accumulation of food surpluses; in most cases, the opposite is more likely to be true. Farmers are probably harder worked and generally more hungry than most hunters and collectors. It is also doubtful that prehistoric subsistence farmers enjoyed better health or lived longer lives than their predecessors.

Unfortunately, there are other questions that nutritionists might like to ask archaeologists which are still difficult to answer. For instance, did the coming of agriculture widen or narrow the range of foods consumed by the majority of people? There is a general ecological principle that the larger the population, the narrower the range of major food resources used. So it would be quite normal to expect that food production would restrict the resource range by emphasizing a few seed or root crops at the expense of others, or a few kept animals in place of the larger number of species which could be hunted. In the widest sense, this is probably true, but we must be careful to distinguish between the number of domesticated foods potentially available in a large region, once the process of exchange and mixing of local products had accelerated, and the actual situations in specific communities.

Much depends on such factors as the local population density, and the risks of crop failure or herd loss. We know that some hunters and gatherers can be quite choosy in their use of edible foods in their environments, and that subsistence farmers can consume a very wide range of wild plant and animal foods in addition to their domesticates. For example, the Gwembe Tonga of Zambia, who are subsistence farmers in a woodland savannah habitat, consume a wider range of wild plants (in addition to their cultivated millet and sorghum) then do the !Kung Bushmen, who admittedly live in a less diverse environment (Scudder 1971). In the Tehuacan Valley of Mexico the excavations of MacNeish and his colleagues show that between 7000 B.C. and 1540 A.D. there was a gradual trend towards reduction in wild animals and especially wild plants consumed, in favor of domesticated plants and a few domesticated animals; yet the range of foods eaten—wild and domesticated, plant and animal—remained very diverse (MacNeish 1967). Beyond the simple subsistence agriculture level, of course, there probably is a greater tendency towards simplification of the diet, at least among the lower status members of stratified societies.

A second question concerns the degree of resistance or flexibility to changes in eating habits in the past. It has been argued that, prior to food production, people were slow to accept unfamiliar foods. But afterwards, when they had been "released from the tense struggle for basic subsistence" and found themselves with more leisure time, they were much more eclectic and innovative (Smith 1967). However, I am not convinced that this statement holds up as a general rule. At any rate, the topic deserves more serious investigation.

Finally, there is the question of whether the digestive abilities of prehistoric people were similar to those of modern people. We generally assume this to be true, but in fact we don't know. There may well have been some differences (Brothwell and Brothwell 1969). The existence of allergies to animal milk and cereals in some modern populations may indicate that, at least in this case and perhaps in others as well, genetic change and selection have taken place since the beginning of food production. (See Harrison [1975] for a discussion of adult lactase deficiency.)

The human commitment to food production is so recent a phenomenon that a successful adaptation to it has probably not yet been reached. In the realm of biology there is some reason to think that natural selection is still at work in areas of severe nutritional imbalance to permit the survival of segments of the population possessing certain variations in protein metabolism, and in order to compensate for the inadequacies of the defense mechanisms acquired during man's long career as a hunter and gatherer (Stini 1971).

Whether the social and political conflicts with which we live today and the divisions which threaten our existence as a viable species can be resolved so simply is a different problem. Obviously we are still a long way from an ecological or social steady state. What the prehistorian can say, however, is that we are still trying to cope with the consequences of a radical adaptive shift, one which probably began as a means of preserving, rather than undermining, the social and cultural status quo. There is, of course, a certain irony in this, but perhaps it is after all only an illustration of the law of entropy at work—the irreversible transformation of low entropy into high to produce increasing disorder in the universe. This is a law which modern food producers, at least, seem not to have circumvented. Seen as high entropy, perhaps pollution and social conflict are legitimate and inherent components of the game we have been playing for the last 10,000 years.

REFERENCES

BROTHWELL, D. and BROTHWELL, P. 1969. Food in Antiquity: A survey of the diet of early peoples. Thames and Hudson, London.

CARNEIRO, R. L., and HILSE, D. F. 1966. On determining the probable rate of population growth during the Neolithic. Am. Anthrop. *68*, 177–180.

DOUGLAS, M. 1974. Food as an art form. Studio International (London) *188*, 969, 83–88.

DUMOND, D. E. 1975. The limitation of human population: A natural history. Science *187*, 713–721.

GARN, S. M., and BLOCK, W. D. 1970. The limited nutritional value of cannibalism. Am. Anthrop. *72*, 106.

HARLAN, J. R. 1967. A wild wheat harvest in Turkey. Archaeol. *20*, 197–201.

HARRIS, D. R. 1967. New light on plant domestication and the origins of agriculture. Geogr. Rev. *57*, 90–107.

HARRISON, G. G. 1975. Primary adult lactase deficiency: A problem in anthropological genetics. Am. Anthrop. *77*, 812–835.

HAVILAND, W. A. 1967. Stature at Tikal, Guatemala: Implications for ancient Maya demography and social organization. Am. Antiq. *32*, 316–325.

HIGGS, E. S. 1972. Papers in Economic Prehistory. Univ. Press, Cambridge, Eng.

ISSAC, E. 1970. Geography of Domestication. Prentice-Hall, Englewood Cliffs, N.J.

KOLATA, G. B. 1974. !Kung hunter-gatherers: Feminism, diet and birth control. Science *185*, 932–934.

LEE, R. B. 1968. What hunters do for a living, or how to make out on scarce resources. *In* Man the Hunter. R. B. Lee and I. DeVore (Editors). Aldine Publishing Co., Chicago.

MAC NEISH, R. S. 1967. A summary of the subsistence. *In* The Prehistory of the Tehucan Valley, Vol. 1. D. S. Byers (Editor). Univ. Texas Press, Austin, Tex.
Austin, Tex.

MARTIN, M. K., and VOORHIES, R. 1975. Female of the Species. Columbia Univ. Press, New York.

MOSELEY, M. E. 1975. The Maritime Foundations of Andean Civilization. Cummings Publishing Co., Menlo Park, Calif.

MURDOCK, G. P. 1968. The current status of the world's hunting and gathering peoples. *In* Man the Hunter. R. B. Lee and I. Devore (Editors). Aldine Publishing Co., Chicago.

SAUL, F. P. 1973. Disease in the Maya area: The pre-Columbian evidence. *In* The Classic Maya Collapse. T. P. Culbert (Editor). Univ. New Mexico Press, Albuquerque, N.M.

SCUDDER, T. 1971. Gathering among African Woodland Savannah Cultivators. A Case Study: The Gwembe Tonga. Univ. Zambia, Inst. for African Studies, Zambian Papers *5*, Manchester, Eng.

SMITH, C. E., JR. 1967. Plant remains. *In* The Prehistory of the Tehuacan Valley, Vol. 1: Environment and Subsistence. D. S. Byers (Editor). Univ. Texas Press, Austin, Tex.

SMITH, P. E. L. 1972. The Consequences of Food Production. Addison Wesley Modular Publ. in Anthrop. *31*, Reading, Mass.

SMITH, P. E. L. 1976. Food Production and its Consequences. Cummings Publishing Co., Menlo Park, Calif.

SPOONER, B. 1972. Population Growth: Anthropological Implications. M.I.T. Press, Cambridge, Mass.

STINI, W. A. 1971. Evolutionary implications of changing nutritional patterns in human populations. Am. Anthrop. *73*, 1019–1030.

TIGER, L., and FOX. R. 1971. The Imperial Animal. Holt, Rinehart and Winston, New York.

WILLEY, G. R., and SHIMKIN, D. B. 1973. The Classic Maya Collapse: A summary view. *In* The Classic Maya Collapse. T. P. Culbert (Editor). Univ. New Mexico Press, Albuquerque, N.M.

YUDKIN, J. 1969. Archaeology and the nutritionist. *In* The Domestication and Exploitation of Plants and Animals. P. J. Ucko and G. W. Dimbleby (Editors). Aldine Publishing Co., Chicago.

CHAPTER 4

Anthropological Contributions to the Study of Food-Related Cultural Variability

Edward Montgomery

There is now much information, some of it richly descriptive, about eating patterns and food preferences in practice across the world. However, as a composite view of the human diet in present and passing cultures, this information gives an impression of diversity rather than variability. Frankly, very little of it was gotten through research in which variation was an explicit or special concern. (There are some exceptions, e.g., Henry [1951] and Suttles [1960].) In general, cultural and social anthropologists have begun to frame their questions and to phrase their findings in terms of variation only recently (Pelto *et al.* 1975).

Nonetheless, some of what anthropologists have learned about social and cultural differences does relate directly to sources of cultural variability in at least two important ways. First, the body of evidence that social and cultural differences can usually be documented at a large number of separate levels, domains, or units in cultural systems is pertinent here. Second, the knowledge that several different contexts, or features of contexts, may be considered when attempting to explain such documented differences also bears on the variability problem.

The significance of these points can be illustrated in this chapter through a review of major approaches taken in recent decades in studying food use and diets among living peoples.

This orientation to the variability problem requires that the literature of anthropology be selectively reviewed. Several sources not usually held to be important for dietary or nutritional studies merit dicussion here. Some of these are not as yet thought to be part of the literature of nutritional anthropology and nutrition. The reader interested in exploring more of that subfield's contributions is referred to the basic bibliography by C. S. Wilson (1973A) and to the following examples: Mead (1943); Bennett (1946A); Lee (1957); Whiting (1958); Read (1964); Gonzalez (1963, 1964, 1972); Jerome (1969, 1970, 1975); Jerome *et al.* (1972); Gross and Underwood (1971); C. S. Wilson (1973B, 1974, 1976); Arnott (1976); and Haas and Harrison (1977).

ANTHROPOLOGICAL THEORY AND METHODS

A few brief remarks about anthropological theory and methods and their relationships to research findings should be made for the benefit of those approaching this chapter with little or no familiarity with anthropology. To start with, it might be supposed that anthropologists have worked with reference to one body of theory. In fact, major theoretical influences derived from Darwin, Marx, Durkheim and others have been prominent. Anthropology really cannot claim to have had its own theoreticians, but this has not limited debate regarding the borrowed theories.

Positions have varied widely as to the weight which should be given to economic, social and environmental forces which shape human behavior (Harris 1968; Murphy 1971; Kuper 1973; Firth 1975). Viewpoints have also differed markedly on the applicability of canons of science and scientific explanation. For some, given the problem of comprehending meaning in human affairs, the best hope is for an interpretive theory of culture (Geertz 1973). There is also a growing awareness in the debates that questions concerning humanity's future are as much at stake as those of its past and present, since the weightings given to economic, social and environmental factors have broad implications about the changing nature of human society itself. A diversity of variant emphases can be discerned in the studies to be reviewed shortly, and it should be recognized that as yet there appears to be no single major synthesis.

The comparability of findings from anthropological research has to a large extent depended on similarities of method, or—as I would prefer to call them—shared general orientations to research. The following five points may serve to represent those shared orientations which have developed:

(1) The recognition of the necessity to understand people in their own terms;

(2) The maintenance of a healthy suspicion that what people say or believe bears no necessary relationship to what they do;

(3) The recognition that much of "culture" or "cultural behavior" is expressed in nonverbal ways (e.g., gestures, postures, modes of dress, intricate dietary patterns);

(4) The recognition that some of "culture" or "cultural behavior" is "unconscious," in that its existence, performance, or patterning is manifested without the actor's conscious or express awareness; and

(5) The recognition that, in any group of people, significant variations among and within individuals with respect to both beliefs and actions are to be expected.

Some would add a sixth item to this list:

(6) The conviction that valid cross-cultural generalizations can be made. Others, however, would view this item with caution and would prefer to restrict themselves to intra-cultural generalizing.

A practical consequence of these points has been that higher quality research has required greater investments of time, energy and emotion. Careful studies usually have been done only with limited numbers of subjects and for relatively short periods of time (i.e., spans of several months to a few years).

Inevitably, not all aspects of the cultural and social life of a people have been studied by the single researcher or the small team. Invariably, some aspects of the culture have received closer attention and others have been neglected. Thus, theoretical interests have been important in focusing research efforts upon certain aspects of culture. Even the most particular facets of culture have been approached in various ways. Foods and food use are no exceptions.

Five major anthropological approaches to the study of food use are considered in the following sections of this chapter. The review section is essentially chronological, with some earlier contributions being discussed first.

FOODS, NATURAL FACTORS, AND CULTURE AREAS

Perhaps the earliest systematic consideration of foods by anthropologists can be found in the distributional studies which were carried out in the early decades of the twentieth century. Those anthropologists taking this approach looked at foods in relation to the spatial distribution of different cultural groups or cultural traits (Selby 1970). In his 1917 volume, *The American Indian*, Clark Wissler divided the whole of aboriginal North and South America into eight "food areas" which he viewed as having direct relation to the cultures distributed across each of the areas.

The outlook was taken up by A. L. Kroeber and used in his famous 1923 textbook, *Anthropology*, wherein he developed the "culture area" aspect of the approach. The perspective received greatest prominence in his culminating work, *Cultural and Natural Areas of Native North America*, in which he used a subsidiary concept ("subsistence area") to account for dense clusters of native populations at points within cultural areas (Kroeber 1939). However, rather than make bold assertions about major staple foods, Kroeber carefully documented the natural areas with detailed vegetation maps.

Of interest here is the fact that these efforts pointed to units of culture which extended beyond the boundaries of particular cultures. Wissler rather loosely specified these units as "the most tangible and objective of human traits . . . those having to do with food"—that is, hunting, fishing, gathering and agricultural techniques. Kroeber, however, saw "cultures as wholes," and felt that, to an extent, this holism held within his natural and cultural areas. Yet the cultural "elements" or "traits" which he singled out as having distributions across particular culture areas were entities like clan organization, pottery and basketry techniques, as well as calendrical, transportation, and political systems (Kroeber 1923).

As for the context to be considered in explaining these units, Wissler's approach was simple. Food-getting culture was the obvious solution to "one of the eternal problems confronting the several groups of mankind . . . the discovery of practical methods for adapting living forms to dietary requirements." Presumably, ecological aspects of the environment were to be related to particular staple foods which required the application of these "practical methods." Kroeber, in contrast, explicitly looked at both environmental and other cultural factors when seeking to explain each particular case. Though he considered the interaction between the two to be important, he favored explanations in which "culture can be understood primarily only in terms of cultural factors."

FUNCTIONALISM AND NUTRITION

In England during the 1930s, a markedly different approach to foods emerged. Over this period, Bronislaw Malinowski was developing his framework for understanding culture on the basis of a set of basic and derived needs—a viewpoint which came to be labeled "functionalist" or "functionalism" (Kuper 1973). In an effort to counter notions about the primacy of the sex drive in comprehending human behavior, Malinowski directed the attention of some of his students at the London School of Economics to a series of interrelated questions about the social, economic and cultural functions of foods and nutrition. These questions were first clearly framed in Audrey Richards' library-researched monograph, *Hunger and Work in a Savage Tribe, A Functional Study of Nutrition Among the Southern Bantu*, first published in 1932.

Malinowski also emphasized that anthropological problems be investigated through careful "fieldwork"—research in depth while living as a participant-observer in a culture (Wax 1971). Richards next sought to investigate some of these questions in actual fieldwork with the Bemba in 1930-31 and 1933-34. At this time, concern was growing in Britain about the adequacy of diets in the African colonies, and at least two of Malinowski's students (A. I. Richards and R. Firth) were drawn into the study of these issues along with other researchers (Westermann 1936). Thus, the composition of Bemba food items and the chemical composition of the diet for three villages were investigated with the aid of Drs. E. M. Widdowson and R. A. McCance (Richards and Widdowson 1936; Richards 1939).

These efforts are perhaps the first to illustrate the benefits of collaboration between anthropologists and nutritional scientists. Firth's "The Sociological Study of Native Diet" (1934) also emerged from this context, and with it what is probably the first statement concerning the observations which ought to be made when conducting the anthropological portion of a study on food use.

It is clear that results from the consumption studies conducted in Indian villages were then seen to possess research relevance for students of Malinowski. Three useful aspects were perceived: (1) effective quantitative methods had been demonstrated; (2) attention had been paid to internal variation in standards of living within groups; and (3) the inquiries had direct practical issues at heart—poverty, health, land tenure, taxation and governance (Read

1938). Apparently the then growing international concern over the relationships between health and agriculture was another context which found a place in studies of native diets (Orr 1936).

These interests, in combination with the functionalist approach, were implemented to the fullest in Audrey Richards' book on the Bemba study, published in 1939 as *Land, Labour and Diet in Northern Rhodesia*. The volume itself remains monumental, and some of its contents deserve brief mention. The discussions of native views on food, food symbolism, the sharing and distribution of foods, the methods of production and the work diaries can still be read instructively.

The domains or units of food-related culture which were of concern to both Richards and Firth were perhaps best summarized by Firth (1934) as: (1) "the dietetic situation," which was to be viewed as the result of a number of phenomena or steps in a process; and (2) the "social factors" which ". . . at every step in the process . . . enter to condition the result . . . ." The steps in the process were: "a set of natural resources constituting the potential food supply; the selection of certain elements from this range and the conversion of them into a state fit for human consumption; the apportionment and consumption of these products." The list of "social factors" included not only attitudes towards resources through all the steps in the transformation into foods, but also all individuals involved in those transformations: family members, kin, other locals, and outsiders linked through markets, trade, labor and employment relations.

There were two contexts which seemed to receive consideration as explanations for these. First, there was the simple utilitarianism of the functionalist outlook: People were supposedly meeting some sort of needs (social, nutritional or other). And second, the changes brought about by colonialism in Africa were recognized to have led to the deterioration of native diets in a number of situations.

More fully elaborated functionalist studies of food and nutrition never emerged after Richards' contribution. The factors are many. Among those implicated were the coming of World War II, the death of Malinowski, and a shift in emphasis within British social anthropology from functional to structural concerns.

FOOD HABITS RESEARCH IN THE 1940s

Anthropological studies of food use took another turn after the functionalist inquiries. The next burst of interest was in the United States in the early 1940s. The focus was on "food habits," and many of the specific efforts produced under this label were stimulated or organized by the Committee on Food Habits of the National Research Council. This committee was established in late 1940 and was primarily operative over the years 1941 to 1943 (Guthe 1943).

Practical interests formed a guiding orientation for the food habits studies. In the initial phases of the operation of the Committee, there were concerns with equity which had developed in the 1930s under New Deal liberalism, and concerns with the physical readiness of the people of the nation to be involved in the prospective war in Europe (M. L. Wilson 1943A, B). After the United States had entered the war, the issues were how to adequately feed the nation under food rationing, given its diverse ethnic and economic composition, and how to cope with the continuing large numbers of its citizens suffering from malnutrition. In short, the task for all involved in this work was to learn ways to change people's food habits.

Several American anthropologists got into the food habits work, in either of two somewhat different ways. First, after Margaret Mead took up the position of Executive Secretary of the Committee on Food Habits in January 1942, she enlisted the support of a number of colleagues (e.g., Hortense Powdermaker) and students to inquire into the food customs and food habits of American ethnic groups. On the basis of interviews and close work with informants, a number of short reports were prepared by the Committee (see the Committee's list of publications [1943] and its bibliography [1945] for a listing of these mimeographed reports). Some of these reports were presented at a series of national conferences which brought together a great variety of specialists not only from several academic disciplines, but also from government, food industries, advertising and public opinion research.

Second, through W. Lloyd Warner's membership on the committee, some of his colleagues and students in anthropology at the University of Chicago became involved in more extended field research on food habits. Part of this group conducted a series of short projects among Spanish-American and Indian groups in the Southwestern United States in collaboration with Dr. M. Pijoan of Chicago's Committee on Human Development (Eggan and Pijoan 1943; Hawley *et al.* 1943: Redfield 1942). Others became involved in the one large-scale project from this period, the Culture and Foodways Project of Southern Illinois (Bennett 1943A, B, 1946B; Bennett *et al.* 1942; Passin and Bennett 1943). In that study, local variations in diets were examined among ethnic and economic status groups and across time in a region of southern Illinois.

Although both the Mead and Chicago studies were conducted under the same "food habits" rubric, it is of some interest that the specific conceptual frameworks and aims of the two groups contrasted. Mead and her group, clearly following Boasian concerns were interested to learn the "pattern" of the culture expressed in food habits. In this "culture pattern" perspective, the following points were stressed: (1) "culture" was taken to be essentially *the* determinant of behavior; (2) food habits were seen as "a part" of the total culture pattern; (3) change in food habits was thought to involve substituting one culturally standardized set of behaviors for another; and (4) a change in the food habits as part of the total pattern needed to be studied in relation to other parts (e.g., family authority, participation in community life), as they might also be affected by the change. And, of course, in this approach, the locus for the transmission of the cultural pattern was in childrearing (Mead 1943). In sum, this perspective saw the "parts" of the pattern as the units which could vary. Further, "systematically interrelated" parts of the pattern could co-vary. The presence of particular food habits in a particular culture pattern were to be explained by reference to historical context. For example, in the "American food pattern," the importance of white bread was to be related to European peasant concepts; Puritan traditions were to account for the use of foods which were considered dislikable and yet healthful, and for the consumption of delicious foods as rewards for eating the dislikable healthful items.

The Chicago group, on the other hand, sought to investigate a mix of Durkheimian, Weberian and other questions which were then of concern to W. Lloyd Warner and Robert Redfield. Food habits—or "foodways," as the group sometimes called them—were looked upon as indicative of social solidarity, social status, regional society and change within social and economic systems. "Social" and "economic" factors were treated as major determinants of behavior along with "culture," rather then being considered as culture themselves.

Linton's universals/specialties/alternatives classification of cultural elements was converted to a distinction among "core," "secondary core" and "peripheral" to account for stability and variability in the diets of southern Illinois (Passin and Bennett 1943). Changes in these diets were related to a general social and economic shift considered to be "urbanization," which was, in effect, a "folk-urban continuum" applied temporally rather than spatially (Bennett et al. 1942; Passin and Bennett 1943; Bennett 1946B).

For this Chicago group, the domains or units wherein variation could be documented were "habits," "foodways," "uses," "practices," "ideas," "values," "attitudes," "goals," and "social processes." In other words, both units of behavior and belief (and consistency-inconsistency between them) were variable. Presence, function and change for these varying domains were to be explained by reference to the context "social and economic systems," as they were considered to be "integrated" within them (Bennett et al. 1942). Hence, effecting changes in foodways was seen to require changing the social and economic systems. Here, the contrast with Mead's approach was sharpest.

The great majority of the contributions to the food habits work had been made by 1944. As the end of the war approached, most of the anthropologists who had worked in this area turned elsewhere to other problems. The main exception was Margaret Mead, who continued to be involved with cultural aspects of food issues a number of times thereafter (Mead 1964).

ECOLOGICAL APPROACHES

A fourth trend in the anthropological treatment of foods and nutrition has been prominent in the United States for the past 25 years: studies with an ecological orientation. Among the many questions which have been explored in this orientation, three are pertinent here: (1) consideration of food as part of people's environments; (2) consideration of food and nutrition as factors determining people's use of their environments; and (3) consideration of nutrition as an indicator of the quality of people's relations with their environments. Since there are several available accounts of the development of ecology in anthropology (Anderson 1974; Bennett 1976; Helm 1962; Netting 1977; Vayda and Rappaport 1968), this need not be reviewed here. Rather, examples of each of these three ways of considering food and nutrition within an ecological-anthropological framework will illustrate some variability-relevant findings.

First, the adoption of an ecological perspective on human affairs has aided the development of a more systematic understanding of the environment for human groups. Of course, general views of food as part of the environment have been commonplace, but within the past two decades, the analytic use of such ecologic terms as "niche" and "ecosystem" have focused attention more precisely upon the composition of environments. In an early study employing the "niche" concept, Fredrik Barth (1956) sketched how three different ethnic groups residing in a mountain valley in northwestern Pakistan differentially used sectors of the environment. The three groups shared some of the same resources, but their production of certain food items (grain crops and herd animals) at different altitudes apparently had important consequences for quantities produced.

Although neither detailed documentation of resource use, nor evaluation of its consequences in health or nutritional terms, was provided, the study did serve to direct attention to particular microenvironmental features. Geertz's (1963) and Rappaport's (1968) applications of the "ecosystem" concept have been of similar consequence. Perhaps most instructive, however, has been Hardesty's recent demonstration that more careful consideration of food resource quantities, quality, spatial distribution and temporal distribution allows for the measurement of niche shape or niche width for human groups (Hardesty 1975).

As for the units or domains of culture which may vary, these studies are actually less specific than some of those discussed in preceding sections. For Barth's groups in niches, and for Rappaport's and Geertz's groups in ecosystems, virtually all aspects of culture relevant to the occupancy of the niche or ecosystem could be considered as potential variables. A whole series of domains—including relations with outside groups, internal social relations and productive and martial technology—are indicated to be relevant to these groups, whereas Hardesty's concern with niche in a strictly subsistence sense suggests that only subsistence-related components of culture need to be considered as variables.

As for the contexts to be investigated to explain the actual, implied, or potential variability, Barth and Geertz give attention to historical derivations as well as the local functioning of cultural elements, in contrast to Rappaport's and Hardesty's emphasis on the latter. And, as indicated, all are concerned with such functioning in relation to microenvironmental variations of factors such as temperature, moisture and soil properties.

A second stimulating area within the ecologically oriented studies has been the consideration of food and nutrition as factors determining human use of the environment. For example, this implicitly was part of Julian Steward's argument concerning the social and economic basis of primitive bands (Steward 1936). He held that limited availability and dispersion of food resources, in combination with simple subsistence technology, accounted for small social aggregates ("bands") of peoples living in restrictive environments not only in native North America, but also Africa, the Philippines and Australia. For these groups, the band form of social organization was part of their culture (part of the "core culture," as he called it) which had been creatively developed as an adaptation to the environment (Steward 1955, 1968). In consequence, this social form and the simple technology allowed only limited use of the environment and the maintenance of sparse human populations. For Steward (1955), only the elements of the cultural core ("the constellation of features which are most closely related to subsistence and economic arrangements. . .") were those whose variability could be systematically explained in terms of adaptation to the environment.

The beginnings of quantitative efforts to link food production and particular aspects of culture were exemplified by Carneiro's study of Kuikuru settlement patterns (Carneiro 1960). Food energy production estimates in a carrying capacity formula indicated that this group of slash-and-burn agriculturalists in central Brazil could maintain their population on the available land without declining food production or any need to relocate settlements.

More recently, Rappaport (1968) has argued that a series of cultural practices (including an impressive pig-slaughtering ritual) might be linked to the provisioning of scarce protein reserves during times of nutritional stress, and to regulating impacts upon the environment in a region of highland New Guinea. As part of his study, Rappaport weighed the dietary intakes of 16 persons and the foods they rationed to domestic pigs for a span of 246 days. He also tried to estimate quantitatively the full spectrum of foods used by the human population.

This particular study heightened many students' interest in addressing anthropological and ecological questions with more and better quantitative data about human diets and activity patterns. With the use of improved sampling techniques, the several methods for assessing nutritional status and team efforts in research, even more complete studies of questions about the adaptive significance of cultural behaviors are possible (McArthur 1974).

A third outlook on foods and nutrition in ecological studies directs attention to food use and nutrition as indicators of the quality of people's relations with their environment. The best example for illustrating this outlook is R. Brooke Thomas's study of an energy flow system in the high Andes of southern Peru (1973). Thomas studied three aspects of the energy flow system (food energy production, consumption and expenditure), and focused on those relations of the human population with the environment which might be manipulated to improve returns on energy investments. He found that a series of local practices contributed to favorable energy production-expenditure ratios, including the use of energetically efficient crops and domestic animals, interzonal trade for high-energy foods, use of children in production, the temporary and seasonal migrations of some adults, attempts at maximizing fertilities, and the slowing and prolonging of the physical growth pattern.

This set of relations taken together suggested the possibility for stating the relation of the human population to the environment in adaptation terms. Since adaptation in this sense is a sum of favorable relations, it can be interpretively extended to indicate the quality of the group's relations with its environment. And by implication, other human populations with far fewer favorable energy flow relations would presumably be in less advantageous adaptational positions. This outlook requires that one consider virtually all aspects of culture which contribute to energy flow processes, since any of them might vary. The observed variability itself is to be explained in terms of a combination of biobehavioral buffering capacity and energetic efficiency (Thomas 1975).

STRUCTURALIST APPROACHES

During the period when ecological interests were developing, a parallel concern with structuralism emerged among other anthropologists. For many, the structuralist label will bring forth associations with the work of Lévi-Strauss. Although his volumes (*The Raw and The Cooked* and *From Honey to Ashes* in particular) frequently feature food, his position is clearly stated in his well-known phrase to the effect that people hold positive or negative attitudes toward natural species not because they are good to eat, but because they are good to think. Thus, rather than deal with Lévi-Strauss, who has recently come under increasingly severe criticism (e.g., Barth 1975; Friedman 1974; Turner 1975), we might find more instructive material for the present consideration in other variants (which some would label "neostructuralist," e.g., Kuper 1973) that deal with foods.

One provocative structuralist contribution which merits mention here is Edmund Leach's analysis of the problem of food taboos. Leach (1964) asks why the British avoid eating the meat of the horse, cat and dog. He proposes a framework for structuring the social distance between man and pets, farm animals, field animals ("game") and remote wild animals in terms of a parallel framework for an adult male and the following categories of females: sister, cousin, neighbors, and distant strangers. He suggests that the structural proximity between Britishers and their pets renders the pets taboo, just as does the analogous proximity between men and their sisters. And just as there are sanctions against the expression of sexual relations between siblings, so also are there sanctions against the expression of aggression (especially slaughter) toward pets. Thus in England, the Society for the Prevention of Cruelty to Animals and the Anti-Vivisection Society manifest concern, particularly for the welfare of dogs.

Another instructive example of the study of structured ordering in the expression of cultural behavior can be found in Mary Douglas' work on recurring sequences in food consumption. She asks questions like "Why not have dessert first and soup last at dinner?"; or "Why serve drinks to strangers in one's home, but meals to closer acquaintances, friends and family?" (Douglas 1975B). These repetitive orderings, extremely complex and yet largely unexplicated, can be found on a meal-to-meal, daily, weekly, annual and life cycle (e.g., birthdays, weddings) basis.

Some details of the intricacies of such structured sequences have been identified in the results of a recent observational study of four different English working-class families (Douglas 1974). Study of this problem required living with the families simply because asking questions alone could not yield much evidence; detailed observations of the families and the foods were needed. It was found that these families had a sequence of three different kinds of meals: major meals, minor meals and tertiary food events. In the major meal, segregation of liquid foods from solid foods was important, as was the serving of certain foods hot, the changing of dishes and utensils, and giving a central place to potatoes. Nonreversible sequences were found in the order of consumption: Potatoes were eaten before cereals, savouries before sweets and wet foods prior to drier items. The shift from wet to dry was accompanied by a change from forks and spoons to fingers. Further, through the structural sequence of the meal, the visual pattern of the foods acquired an increasing dominance.

Of course, for the structuralists those domains which vary are the "structures." Although frequently the criticism has been raised that the procedures for identifying structures have not been adequately described, attempts are now being made to improve upon the situation (e.g., Leach 1976). As for contexts to be considered when explaining structures. Leach and Douglas would have them understood for their conveyance of cultural information, their creative, social construction of knowledge (cf. Leach 1976; Douglas 1975A).

CONCLUSIONS

These several different approaches to the problem of food and nutrition-related cultural variability suggest five conclusions:

(1) Questions about cultural differences can be rephrased as questions about cultural variability without modifications of existing anthropological methods or theories;

(2) The most useful results have and will probably continue to come from intensive studies in particular cultural settings;

(3) There may be a potential for developing regionally applicable statements about cultural variability, but as yet this topic has barely been examined;

(4) It is not now possible to present globally applicable statements about the food and nutrition-related sphere of cultural variability; and

(5) In general, food and nutrition-related cultural variability cannot be explained on a nutritional basis, since numerous other reasons for food use prevail.

ACKNOWLEDGEMENTS

Thanks are due to John W. Bennett, Allen Johnson, and Christine S. Wilson for their detailed comments and suggestions on this chapter.

REFERENCES

ANDERSON, J. N. 1974. Ecological anthropology and anthropological ecology. *In* Handbook of Social and Cultural Anthropology. J. J. Honigmann (Editor). Rand McNally, Chicago.

ARNOTT, M. L. 1976. Gastronomy: The Anthropology of Food and Food Habits. Aldine Publishing Co., Chicago.

BARTH, F. 1956. Ecologic relationships of ethnic groups in Swat, North Pakistan. Am. Anthrop. *58*, 1079–1089.

BARTH, F. 1975. Ritual and Knowledge among the Baktaman of New Guinea. Yale Univ. Press, New Haven, Conn.

BENNETT, J. W. 1943A. Food and social status in a rural society. Am. Sociol. Rev. *8*, 561–569.

BENNETT, J. W. 1943B. Some problems of status and solidarity in a rural society. Rural Sociol. *8*, 396–408.

BENNETT, J. W. 1946A. An interpretation of the scope and implications of social scientific research in human subsistence. Am. Anthrop. *48*, 553–573.

BENNETT, J. W. 1946B. Subsistence economy and foodways in a rural community: A study of socio-economic and cultural change. Ph.D. Thesis, Univ. Chicago, Chicago.

BENNETT, J. W. 1976. The Ecological Transition: Cultural Anthropology and Human Adaptation. Pergamon Press, New York.

BENNETT, J. W., SMITH, H. L., and PASSIN, H. 1942. Food and culture in southern Illinois— a preliminary report. Am. Sociol. Rev. *7*, 645–660.

CARNEIRO, R. L. 1960. Slash-and-burn agriculture: A closer look at its implications for settlement patterns. *In* Men and Cultures: Selected Papers of the Fifth International Congress of

Anthropological and Ethnological Sciences, September, 1956. Anthony F. C. Wallace (Editor). Univ. Pa. Press, Philadelphia, Pa.

COMMITTEE ON FOOD HABITS. 1943. The Problem of Changing Food Habits. Nat. Res. Counc. Bull. *108.* NAS-NRC, Washington, D. C.

COMMITTEE ON FOOD HABITS. 1945. Manual for the Study of Food Habits. Nat. Res. Counc. Bull. *111.* NAS-NRC, Washington, D. C.

DOUGLAS, M. 1974. Food as an art form. Studio International (London) *188,* 969, 83–88.

DOUGLAS, M. 1975A. Preface. *In* Implicit Meanings. Routledge and Kegan Paul, Boston.

DOUGLAS, M. 1975B. Deciphering a meal. *In* Implicit Meanings. Routledge and Kegan Paul, Boston.

EGGAN, F., and PIJOAN, M. 1943. Some problems in the study of food and nutrition. América Indígena *3,* 9–22.

FIRTH, R. 1934. The sociological study of native diet. Africa *7,* 401–414.

FIRTH, R. 1975. An appraisal of modern social anthropology. Ann. Rev. Anthrop. *4,* 1–25.

FRIEDMAN, J. 1974. Marxism, structuralism, and vulgar materialism. Man (n.s.) *9,* 444–469.

GEERTZ, C. 1963. Agricultural Involution: The Processes of Ecological Change in Indonesia. Univ. Calif. Press, Berkeley, Calif.

GEERTZ, C. 1973. The Interpretation of Cultures. Basic Books, New York.

GONZALEZ, N. L. 1963. Breast-feeding, weaning, and acculturation. J. Pediat. *62,* 577–581.

GONZALEZ, N. L. 1964. Beliefs and practices concerning medicine and nutrition among lower-class urban Guatemalans. Am. J. Pub. Hlth. *54,* 1726–1734.

GONZALEZ, N. L. 1972. Changing dietary patterns of North American Indians. *In* Nutrition, Growth, and Development of North American Indian Children. William M. Moore, Marjorie M. Silverberg and Merrill S. Read (Editors). U. S. Gov. Print. Off., Washington, D. C.

GROSS, D. R., and UNDERWOOD, B. A. 1971. Technological change and caloric costs: Sisal agriculture in northeastern Brazil. Am. Anthrop. *73,* 725–740.

GUTHE, C. E. 1943. History of the Committee on Food Habits. *In* The Problem of Changing Food Habits. Nat. Res. Counc. Bull. *108.* NAS-NRC, Washington, D. C.

HAAS, J., and HARRISON, G. G. 1977. Nutritional anthropology and biological adaptation. Annu. Rev. Anthropol. *6,* 69–101.

HARDESTY, D. L. 1975. The niche concept: Suggestions for its use in human ecology. Hum. Ecol. *3,* 71–85.

HARRIS, M. 1968. The Rise of Anthropological Theory: A History of Theories of Culture. Thomas Y. Crowell Co., New York.

HAWLEY, F., PIJOAN, M., and ELKIN, C. A. 1943. An inquiry into food economy and body economy in Zia Pueblo. Am. Anthrop. *45,* 547–556.

HELM, J. 1962. The ecological approach in anthropology. Am. J. Sociol. *67,* 630–639.

HENRY, J. 1951. The economics of Pilaga food distribution. Am. Anthrop. *53,* 187–219.

JEROME, N. 1969. Northern urbanization and food consumption patterns of Southern-born Negroes. Am. J. Clin. Nutr. *22,* 1667–1669.

JEROME, N. 1970. American culture and food habits. *In* Dimensions of Nutrition. J. Dupont (Editor). Colo. Assoc. Univ. Press, Boulder, Colo.

JEROME, N. 1975. Flavor preferences and food patterns of selected U. S. and Caribbean blacks. Food Technol. *6,* 46–51.

JEROME, N., KISER, B. B., and WEST, E. A. 1972. Infant and child feeding practices in an urban community in the north-central region. *In* Practices of Low-Income Families in Feeding Infants and Small Children, with Particular Attention to Cultural Subgroups. S. J. Fomon and T. A. Anderson (Editors). Maternal and Child Health Service, U. S. Public Health Ser., Rockland, Md.

KROEBER, A. L. 1923. Anthropology. Harcourt, Brace and Co., New York.

KROEBER, A. L. 1939. Cultural and Natural Areas of Native North America. Univ. Calif. Press, Berkeley, Calif.

KUPER, A. 1973. Anthropologists and Anthropology: The British School 1922–1972. Allen Lane, London.

LEACH, E. 1964. Anthropological aspects of language: Animal categories and verbal abuse. *In* New Directions in the Study of Language. E. H. Lenneberg (Editor). MIT Press, Cambridge, Mass.

LEACH, E. 1976. Culture and Communication: The Logic by which Symbols are Connected. Cambridge Univ. Press, London.
LEE, D. 1957. Cultural factors in dietary choice. Am. J. Clin. Nutr. 5, 166–170.
MC ARTHUR, M. 1974. Pigs for the ancestors: A review article. Oceania 45, 87–123.
MEAD, M. 1943. The problem of changing food habits. In The Problem of Changing Food Habits, Nat. Res. Counc. Bull. 108 NAS-NRC, Washington, D. C.
MEAD, M. 1964. Food Habits Research: Problems of the 1960s. NAS-NRC Publ. 1225, Washington, D. C.
MURPHY, R. F. 1971. The Dialectics of Social Life: Alarms and Excursions in Anthropological Theory. Basic Books, New York.
NETTING, R. M. 1977. Cultural Ecology. Cummings Publishing Co., Menlo Park, Calif.
ORR, J. B. 1936. Problems of African native diet: Foreward. Africa 9, 145–146.
PASSIN, H., and BENNETT, J. W. 1943. Social process and dietary change. In The Problem of Changing Food Habits. Nat. Res. Counc. Bull. 108. NAS-NRC, Washington, D. C.
PELTO, P. J. et al. 1975. Intra-cultural variation. Am. Ethnol. 2, 1–206.
RAPPAPORT, R. A. 1968. Pigs for the Ancestors. Yale Univ. Press, New Haven, Conn.
READ, M. 1938. Native standards of living and African culture change. Africa 9, Suppl. to No. 3, 1–64.
READ, M. 1964. The role of the anthropologist. In Changing Food Habits. J. Yudkin and J. C. McKenzie (Editors). Macgibbon and Kee, London.
REDFIELD, R. 1942. Cultural factors in Indian diet. Boletín Indigenista 2, 2, 14–15.
RICHARDS, A. I. 1932. Hunger and Work in a Savage Tribe: A Functional Study of Nutrition among the Southern Bantu. G. Routledge and Sons, London.
RICHARDS, A. I. 1939. Land, Labour, and Diet in Northern Rhodesia: An Economic Study of the Bemba Tribe. Oxford Univ. Press, London.
RICHARDS, A. I., and WIDDOWSON, E. M. 1936. A dietary study in North-Eastern Rhodesia. Africa 9, 166–196.
SELBY, H. A. 1970. Continuities and prospects in anthropological studies. In Current Directions in Anthropology. A. Fischer (Editor). Bull. Am. Anthrop. Assoc. 3, No. 3, Part 2, 35–53.
STEWARD J. H. 1936. The economic and social basis of primitive bands. In Essays in Anthropology Presented to A. L. Kroeber. R. H. Lowie (Editor). Univ. Calif. Press, Berkeley, Calif.
STEWARD, J. H. 1955. The concept and method of cultural ecology. In Theory of Culture Change. Univ. Ill. Press. Urbana, Ill.
STEWARD, J. H. 1968. Cultural ecology. Intl. Encycl. Soc. Sci. 4, 337–344.
SUTTLES, W. 1960. Affinal ties, subsistence, and prestige among the Coast Salish. Am. Anthrop. 62, 296–305.
THOMAS R. B. 1973. Human Adaptation to a High Andean Energy Flow System. Occas. Pap. in Anthropol. 7. Dep. Anthrop., Penn. State Univ., University Park, Pa.
THOMAS, R. B. 1975. The ecology of work. In Physiological Anthropology. A. Damon (Editor). Oxford Univ. Press, New York.
TURNER, V. 1975. Symbolic studies. Ann. Rev. Anthrop. 4, 145–161.
VAYDA, A. P., and RAPPAPORT, R. A. 1968. Ecology: Cultural and noncultural. In Introduction to Cultural Anthropology. J. A. Clifton (Editor). Houghton Mifflin, Boston.
WAX, R. H. 1971. A historical sketch of fieldwork. In Doing Fieldwork: Warnings and Advice. Univ. Chicago Press, Chicago.
WESTERMANN, D. 1936. Problems of African native diet: A note on the general situation. Africa 9, 146–149.
WHITING, M. G. 1958. A cross-cultural nutrition survey of 118 societies representing the major cultural areas of the world. D. Sc. Thesis, Harvard Univ., Boston.
WILSON, C. S. 1973A. Food habits: A selected annotated bibliography. J. Nutr. Educ. 5, Suppl. 1 to No. 1, 38–72.
WILSON, C. S. 1973B. Food taboos of childbirth: The Malay example. Ecol. Food Nutr. 2, 267–274.
WILSON, C. S. 1974. Child following: A technic for learning food and nutrient intakes. J. Trop. Pediat. Environ. Child Hlth. 20, 9–14.
WILSON, C. S. 1976. Nutrition in two cultures: Mexican-American and Malay ways with food. In Gastronomy: The Anthropology of Food and Food Habits. M. L. Arnott (Editor). Aldine Publishing Co. Chicago.

WILSON, M. L. 1943A. Nutrition, food attitudes, and food supply. *In* Postwar Economic Problems. S. E. Harris (Editor). McGraw-Hill Book Co., New York.
WILSON, M. L. 1943B. Preface. *In* The Problem of Changing Food Habits. Nat. Res. Counc. Bull. *108.* NAS-NRC, Washington, D. C.
WISSLER, C. 1917. The American Indian. Douglas C. McMurtrie, New York.

POSTSCRIPT

The interested reader will find some more recent developments in anthropological studies of food and nutrition discussed in the following: MONTGOMERY, E., and BENNETT, J. W. 1978. Anthropological studies of food and nutrition: The 1940s and the 1970s. *In* The Uses of Anthropology. W. W. Goldschmidt (Editor). Am. Anthropol. Assoc., Washington, D. C.

CHAPTER 5

Brian Hayden

Section Review and Analysis

In large measure, the preceding papers constitute a series of data summaries pertaining to hunting-gathering groups, horticultural groups, agricultural groups and contemporary groups. I would like to provide a contextual overview from my own perspective, beginning with a classification of those groups and then discussing their general characteristics and some of the evolutionary implications for the present time. The tendency throughout these anthropological papers is to pit hunting-gathering groups against agricultural groups. This, I think, is too simplistic an approach. While there are many ways in which these groups can be classified, I would like to adopt a point of view which will, I hope, make considerable evolutionary sense.

My division of these groups (bearing in mind that there are transitional levels) is the following:

(1) Simple hunters-gatherers characterized by comparatively low consumption, low density resources and an inability or unwillingness to produce food;

(2) Technologically complex and environmentally rich hunter-gatherers marked by relatively high consumption, but unable or unwilling to produce food;

(3) Simple food producers with comparable consumption to technologically complex hunter-gatherers in rich environments; and

(4) High-level food producers who are extremely productive and utilize true agriculture.

The characteristics of each of these levels require elaboration.

At the lowest level, that of the simple hunting-gathering groups, we find several characteristics among contemporary hunter-gatherers which seem to pertain as well to the majority of groups in the Paleolithic. Such groups appear to have been relatively stable both nutritionally and demographically. Their populations did not fluctuate rapidly, nor did they attempt to alter their environment. On the contrary, changes in the environment often created serious pressures on populations.

The role of population pressure was discussed earlier and I would like to emphasize that there have been severe and dramatic changes in climate throughout the past two or three million years. As a result, hunting-gathering groups were often forced out of areas or had new territories opened up to them. One example might be that of the Near East, in the area around Shanidar Cave in Iraq, which seems to have been completely abandoned at some point between Mousterian times and the Upper Paleolithic. Similar events occurred in Europe when enormous ice floes came down and covered large areas of land.

But while these changes in population pressure occurred throughout the ice ages, they do not seem to have had much effect on the nature of cultural adaptations. Rather than invent new methods of coping with a changed environment, man largely chose to move on to a more suitable habitat. In some cases, perhaps, they died out. Dr. Heizer indicated that the limiting factor on population was some sort of minimum resource pool experienced every generation. This notion, however, is highly controversial; while it seems to be one of the more likely options, it is still speculative. Thus, throughout the ice ages there seems to have been little impetus toward improvements in technological efficiency in the exploitation of food or resources, and such occurrences were extremely sporadic.

Simple hunter-gatherers, then, form a somewhat paradoxical picture. The group sizes were small, the people seem to have been fairly well-satisfied with what they had. Resource shortages *did* occur at times—perhaps once every generation, perhaps at longer or shorter intervals. But when these shortages occurred, the people did not involve themselves with technological elaboration.

Why this disinterest in technology? The answer, I think, rests with the most important factor in the socioecology of the simple hunter-gatherer: That given an already heavy exploitation of limited resources, any increase in the level of that exploitation is more likely to destroy the resource base than to benefit the group in the long run. This fact, coupled with the relatively infrequent occurrence and generally brief duration of these episodes of deprivation, made it preferable for the people involved to simply move out of the area, rather than try to devise some new technological solution which would carry them through these stress periods.

The fact that exploiting limited resources more intensively tends to destroy them leads us to another important characteristic of these simple hunter-gatherers, which is their tendency to discourage competition. Because competition over resources can lead to their destruction, hunting-gathering groups at this level are essentially cooperative. When resource shortages occur among one group, they borrow from a neighboring group that is somewhat better off. Groups in Australia, for example, have characteristically accepted other groups as guests for the duration of a famine. Thus, food sharing and cooperation are both characteristic and highly adaptive for those people who have limited resources and no potential for increasing them.

Another effect of such relationships is that individual ownership of resources (which embodies rivalry and competition) is rare except in some marginal cases involving nonessential resources. Sources of conflict over resources are tightly controlled and monitored. This is not to say that conflict did not occur in the Paleolithic (as it still does among the vast majority of hunter-gatherers), but that conflict was nearly always over women or to revenge a previous death. Only rarely were conflicts directly over resources.

Yet another effect of living under such low-production conditions with *limited* resources is a lowered birth rate. It makes little sense, after all, for parents to have a large number of children to help support them when they become old. More children at a simple hunter-gatherer level simply means a greater exploitation of the already limited resources and might well lead to their depletion. The potentially destructive effect of children, combined with an essentially cooperative social structure, leads to very little increase in population.

In spite of all this stability, cooperation and contentment, however, changes in the shape of very infrequent technological innovations did occur. And there were occasional periods of hardship. These sporadic episodes of stress may have been the ultimate driving force behind the slow movement toward increased technological complexity which we see occurring throughout the Paleolithic. It is perhaps a tribute to the efficacy and general standard of living of Paleolithic man that his culture has continued over the past two million years with so little essential change.

In the next classification, we find technologically complex hunting-gathering groups with relatively high production. Advanced hunter-gatherers learned to exploit resources very effectively through complex technology. Probably without exception, such groups required, in addition to that technology, an area rich in natural resources. and I would argue that this combination came about fairly late in the archaeological record. Given a rich environment and a technology capable of *consistently* culling enormous amounts of food from it, people could exploit their resources *from a single location* almost indefinitely without planting or utilizing any other method of food production. Natives on the California and British Columbian Northwest coasts provide one example of such groups, and the prehistoric wild wheat gatherers of the Near East provide another. (As Harlan's experiments have demonstrated, one acre of cereal can provide enormous energy returns. However, a relatively complex gathering and processing technology is required to make use of this abundant resource.)

Given the conditions of complex technology in resource-rich areas, we begin to see a fairly high degree of sedentism, which in turn makes the accumulation of wealth possible. With the advent of complex technology, groups could extract vast quantities of food from some environments. Sedentism made the storage of wealth feasible, so it was no longer maladaptive in chosen environments to compete over resources. As a result, we perceive, in archaeological terms, the first material signs of status achievement and—by inference—competition.

Another, and perhaps crucial, factor which made resources seem inexhaustible at this level (and which mitigated the maladaptiveness of competition ove resources) was a change in the nature of the resources which were being exploited. This change is characterized by a shift from the consumption of relatively large food items with a large energy return per unit of energy expended to an increasing reliance on relatively small food items with very low energy returns. . . unless technological gadgets are used to harvest and process them *en masse*. There are two important ecological effects of this change. First, the larger the food items are, the lower their density, so that an absolute quantity of small resources has the potential to surpass the energy yield per hectare of large item resources. Second, and most important, there is a direct relationship between the size of a food item and the ease with which it can be driven to local extinction by over exploitation.

Larger items are not only less dense and fewer in number (therefore making them easier to eliminate), but they also tend to take more time to reproduce and mature; thus, they are much more susceptible to extinction at the hands of an overexploiting band. On the other hand, small resources are generally so numerous and reproduce at such brief and frequent intervals that they are almost impossible to eliminate, or even appreciably affect (as every gardener knows), on a yearly basis. Because small food items are more abundant, an emphasis on such food in prime areas creates a reproductively inexhaustible resource base—*if* the appropriate technology is available.

This increased investment in technology represents the first step toward labor-intensive food collecting. While it is true that some small resources were utilized by simple hunter-gatherers, it was probably not until the end of the Paleolithic that adequate technology was available to make this type of resource dominant in the subsistence regimen of favored areas. This development made sedentism possible, and competition over resources lost its stigma in terms of survival. With the advent of competition, we observe a breakdown of all of those advantages which accrued from not competing over resources. There was an expansion of population, as well as the beginnings of real warfare.

Moving on to the food producer, it is important to distinguish between those groups which are essentially competitive and those which are not. As far as I know, this point has not really been stressed before. I would cite the previously mentioned Kuikuru as a prime example of the noncompetitive group. They have enormous amounts of available land, they produce more than enough food, and they are not oriented toward expansion. R. L. Carneiro reports that they are essentially slash-and-burn horticulturalists who overproduce considerably in the event of famine, destruction or other disaster. In fact, he reports that one group was utterly unperturbed when a whole month's supply of powdered manioc went up in flames—they simply harvested more of the readily available manioc and continued to subsist quite comfortably.

While it has often been assumed that food producers have less leisure time then do hunter-gatherers, this is not substantiated in the case of the Kuikuru, who spend 2 to 5 hours daily working for food—the same number of hours as most hunter-gatherers. Famine is relatively infrequent, and their nutrition seems to be adequate. Exactly why these low-level food-producing societies are not more competitive over resources is problematic, as is the reason they so often leave large amounts of land vacant. One of the logical possibilities is that specialized but necessary aspects of subsistence (such as protein in tropical rain forests) may be limiting factors; such a notion, in fact, has recently been argued—and quite competently—for the case of the Amazon basin.

At a still higher level, we see the beginnings of true agriculture. It is at this point, I would argue, that we find the most intensive forms of competition; or, rather, we find intense competition resulting in agriculture. And I would also argue that it is the advent of competitive systems which has produced many cases of starvation, overuse of the land and all of the other problems we associate with agriculture.

Unlike the hunter-gatherers, who often exhaust their resources by investing additional work in subsistence collecting, the food producers can increase their food resources through a greater investment of labor. This increased output can be achieved either by an increase in the intensity of labor within a single area, or by simply increasing the amount of land under cultivation. As a result, the food producer has an almost unlimited resource base—although it remains to be seen how much longer this situation can continue. Agricultural groups tend to be larger than hunter-gatherer societies, and I would maintain that population pressure at this level is actually a result of competition, as are the various advances in technology.

Taking an overall view of these evolutionary stages, we can see that, throughout prehistory and into contemporary society, man has consistently tried to increase the reliability of his resource base so as to avoid those situations in which famine occurs. Nomadic groups, for example, are often forced to leave behind the old, the young and the sick whenever periods of stress occur. Clearly this is an undesirable solution wherever bonds of affection exist. Thus, one of man's prime motivations in the effort to increase his technological repertory and bring more foodstuffs into his network of consumption has probably been an attempt to avoid stress, whether nutritional, pathological or emotional.

In the hunting-and-gathering era, these changes occurred infrequently, and technological progress affecting food potential was very slow. Nevertheless, it was continuous and unidirectional. According to ecological theory, the most important way to increase resource reliability is to increase resource diversity, thereby lessening the change of total resource failure. In this sense, resource specialization in an unstable environment presents a strong risk in terms of survival, since it provides no safeguard against the failure of the primary resource.

If we were to graph the progress of resource variety over time (Fig. 5.1), we would probably find that the level of diversity in the Lower Paleolithic remained relatively stable for a very long time, since it was tied to local ecological limitations and to what could be easily gotten with simple tech-

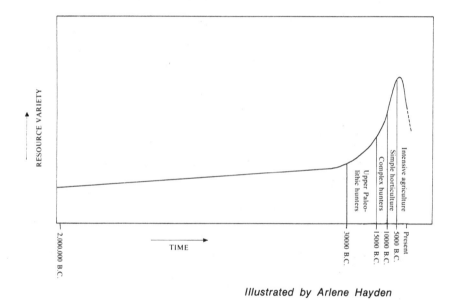

Illustrated by Arlene Hayden

FIG. 5.1. SCHEMATIC REPRESENTATION OF THE CHANGE IN THE VARIETY OF
RESOURCES EXPLOITED BY DOMINANT CULTURE TYPES AT VARIOUS POINTS IN
CULTURAL EVOLUTION

nology. Throughout the Pleistocene, the level of resource diversity rose very slightly, but it was a unidirectional trend. While exceedingly slow for more than two million years, the trend was nonetheless consistent.

By the time we arrive at what is usually referred to as the Mesolithic (a period equivalent to the Jomon in Japan, the Archaic in North America and the Mesolithic in Europe), we suddenly find a wide range of technological complexity. Given these new techniques—the incorporation of seeds, the harvest of fish, the discovery of plants with removable toxins, the development of new processing techniques like grinding and boiling, and other relatively late subsistence additions—we find a much wider range of resources which could be exploited to insure survival.

This variety in resources increases rather markedly around the time of the Upper Paleolithic (some 30,000 years ago), reaching a hunting-gathering peak in the Mesolithic. What I would like to suggest is that the movement from hunting-and-gathering strategies to food production was in many ways a normal and logical consequence of this trend. That is, instead of merely relying on *wild* foods at the end of the Paleolithic, people continued to increase both the variety and the reliability of their resource base by *planting* foods. By supplementing the wild foods with planted crops, they increased the stability of their economy—something they had been trying to do for the past two million years.

(It is not true, by the way, that primitive horticulturalists and agriculturalists specialized in just a few items. In fact, the greatest diversity of local food resources in the world occurs at this level. Incredibly, Freeman records several thousand plant species used for food by the Iban. And if we look at early horticultural occurrences, such as Iron Age remains in Europe or early sites in the Near East, we find that domestic plants and animals account for only 20–30% of the entire food intake.)

With the advent of competitive agricultural societies, we find a reversal in this trend toward diversity. In competitive groups, we find people trying to monopolize land, to acquire territory and to control other people. Under these conditions, there is a rapid expansion in population and a reduction in the variety of available resources. That is, we find a concentration on a few primary, starchy agricultural products—those which are most productive and which will nourish the greatest number of people, irrespective of the quality of their diet. Other logical consequences of such a system are fairly frequent famines and high levels of morbidity and starvation due to malnutrition.

It seems that simple, noncompetitive food producers have been replaced in most areas of the world by complex, overspecialized, competitive agriculturalists, and the trend continues up to the present time. Enormous areas are now given over to the production of a single type of crop. With the advent of intensive competition there has been a significant reduction in resource variability. Despite the fact that we have developed transportation and communication systems (which are even more fragile than natural ecosystems) to compensate for the loss in local resource variability, the total variability has markedly decreased. This trend has continued to such a point that some botanists now fear that genetically viable crops might be lost and have begun to establish genetic banks for plants. However, this is a rather feeble response to the dominating pressure of competition. The outlook for diversified natural foods is indeed bleak.

In summary, the unidirectional trend toward greater resource reliability was unaffected up until the Mesolithic. Competition was viewed as destructive to the individual and to his environment. Society was essentially noncompetitive, and maintained a balanced relationship with the environment. The desire for increased resource reliability created a critical threshhold in the Mesolithic when, through technological improvement, it made possible the first appearances of sedentism, the accumulation of wealth, intense competition and a seemingly inexhaustible supply of food in favorable areas.

This combination of factors, I would argue, has been the principal driving force behind the incredibly rapid evolution of culture in the past 10,000 years, during which we have moved from the Paleolithic to the moon. And it seems to me that these forces will continue to operate as long as we maintain sufficient resources. These trends have not shown any signs of stabilization, and therefore may be projected into the future.

In this sense, man can be seen as a creature carving out his own ecological niche, beginning over two million years ago. Instead of exploiting a single type of plant, he has used cultural means to exploit as many as possible. He has reached the point where he has no strong competition from any single biological or zoological source. And until recently, he has had a seemingly infinite supply of nutrition. But he has become so involuted in his exploitation (a process which led to food production and competition) that he has now become encapsulated within a limited system. He is now trying to increase his resource reliability by maintaining a constant environment via technological means.

If we project this out to situations on other planets, such as the moon or Mars, we find that the logical consequence of this trend is the encapsulation of culture within strict, limited boundaries in order to maintain a viable environment. In this respect, cultural evolution is recapitulating many of the early biological and evolutionary events.

Finally, Edward Montgomery takes a somewhat different perspective: One of his most important points is that what people say and what they actually do are seldom the same thing. Anyone dealing with a nutritional problem should be thoroughly aware of this fact—that there are often unstated and unconscious reasons for doing things. His last point was extremely well-made, that is, that we are dealing with a very complex socioeconomic phenomenon in which feasting activities are highly important. I could not help but be reminded of the many feasting complexes throughout the Third World which have definite functions in regard to the redistribution of food, and have a survival value in those terms. These are fairly widespread throughout the world, but they are too often ignored in contemporary contexts as nutritional and power-centralizing institutions.

SECTION II

THE EFFECTS OF MAN'S CULTURAL AND BIOLOGICAL INTERACTIONS AND VARIABILITY ON NUTRITION

CHAPTER 6

Derrick B. Jelliffe
E.F.P. Jelliffe

Food Habits and Taboos: How Have They Protected Man in His Evolution?

It is perhaps unnecessary to emphasize the fact that food habits are one of the most significant and deeply held aspects of man's cultural pattern in any part of the world. Nor should we have to stress the idea that a community's cultural pattern (including its food habits) consists of behavior which is learned from parents, siblings and others in the community who, in turn, have learned from *their* elders and ancestors.

In practice, the term "food habits" can cover a smaller or a larger segment of life. It can include different methods of obtaining foods (such as hunting and foraging) or producing them (such as agriculture or animal husbandry). Also involved are the various means of harvesting, storing, preparing and cooking food, and, of course, the very act of eating food, including the implements used, the etiquette regarded as important, and the pattern of interfamilial food distribution.

As with any other aspect of culture, all of these are really interrelated, forming part of a continuum of interacting forces and patterns of behavior. Therefore, it is artificial to consider food habits by themselves, ignoring other aspects of the cultural pattern—up to and including its fundamental values or life goals.

The purpose of this presentation is to consider whether the food patterns of men in different communities, both in the past and in the present, have been related mainly to (1) the ecology in which he finds himself—that is, his physical environment and the potential for food production of that particular area—or (2) the cultural patterns which he has created for himself. Are food habits protective, or are they harmful? Are they merely arbitrary, or do they serve a purpose?

All over the world, people select the foods which make up their dietary pattern for two main reasons: physical and cultural-symbolic.

PHYSICAL FACTORS

In looking at the physical factors, it is useful to transport oneself back many hundreds of thousands of years to the time when man was a hunter-gatherer. In view of the fact that man has spent most of his time on this planet as a hunter-gatherer, we must realize that present-day food habits are more closely related to conditions in those ancient times than is generally appreciated. The time scale is significant—of man's 1,000,000 years of existence, the keeping of milk animals only dates back 10,000 years.

One of the principal physical factors is what might be termed "primary physiological urges." There is, first of all, the influence of the taste buds, of which there are four main types: two can be classified as "rejectors," and are situated toward the back of the tongue; the other two are "acceptors," and are located near the front. The "rejectors" screen for bitter and sour tastes, presumably as a defense against swallowing foods which fall into these categories. The "acceptor" taste buds select for sweetness and saltiness, two dominant flavors. The primary physiological urge of the taste buds toward sweetness and saltiness may be very relevant to the way man's food habits have evolved in the past and continue to operate in the present.

Other primary physiological urges are perhaps directed toward the softness of food. Certainly so far as fruit is concerned, softness and sweetness signify ripeness. In addition, there may be responses in our atavistic memory toward attributes of other foods which gained appeal during man's period as hunter-gatherer. During those vast eons of time, prehistoric man must have come to enjoy the "crunchiness" of bones and uncooked foods in particular. It is not too fanciful to suggest that such organoleptic "mouth-feel" may play a part in the appeal of certain foods today.

Another primary physiological urge dating from some 50,000 years ago is gluttony. Eating all that was available as soon as possible was a desirable practice. Indeed, it was *necessary*, for two reasons: first, to store up fat in order to make good the calorie shortage during the hungry season or other period when food was in short supply; and second, as a means of portage, or carrying food. In a community which lives by hunting, transporting the killed game is a major problem. The easiest way to carry it and to store it is to eat it; in this sense, Mother Nature's "deep freeze" is the alimentary canal. Gluttony, then, is perhaps a physiological or basic drive.

A second group of physical factors can be called "food availability"—in other words, the foods which are most readily available in the community in terms of hunting or agriculture or marketing.

Third, ill effects (whether real or coincidental) may lead to the restriction of certain foods. For example, lactase deficiency may be an ancient genetic anomaly, and ill effects from milk drinking would undoubtedly lead to its avoidance. Similarly, various fruits and berries in different parts of the world are poisonous. Once a few members of the group had died after eating a certain food, man (like other animals) would eventually recognize these substances and exclude them from his diet. At the same time, unplanned experiments were undoubtedly made in certain communities, as a result of which methods were discovered for removing the toxic principles in some foods (cassava is a good example).

Another factor might be an *apparently* harmful effect—a coincidental linking of an episode of illness with the intake of a certain food.

CULTURAL-SYMBOLIC FACTORS

In addition to the physical factors which have guided man throughout history in selecting his diet, there are important cultural-symbolic factors. Coincidence appears to have been very important in the development of some of these factors. If, for example, a person in a particular community happens to eat a certain type of food and then, quite coincidentally, develops a recognized form of illness, or perhaps breaks a leg, there is a very great possibility that these events will be linked as cause and effect by the rest of the community.

The symbolism of food is a major attribute which differentiates man from his fellow creatures, reflecting an ability to think, to categorize, and to seek explanations. Symbolism is largely concerned with deriving explanations for events, such as why hurricanes and other natural disasters occur, or why a wild animal did or did not attack. Symbolism is also related to man's attempt to control events and to keep the hierarchy in a particular community just as it is. Food selection in a community seems to be made up from a blend of physical and symbolic considerations. The symbolic considerations may be based on coincidence, status, or religious and ultra-human associations.

FIVE MAJOR ECOLOGIES

Man has always lived (and still lives) in a changing culture based on one of five major ecologies: the hunter-gatherer, the agriculturalist, the herdsman, the townsman and the modern urban dweller. Plainly, there have been great changes in ecology and food patterns during this time. Nevertheless, many of the threads from man's ancient past still influence space-age food habits.

Talking about food habits in general is a difficult task because there are so many different types in so many different forms from so many different cultures, all of which have varied throughout the past and into the present. For example, these ecologies constantly change in response to climate, migration and, more recently, the introduction of modern technology.

In varying degrees, each of the five types of ecology can be found at the present time, all in the process of change, some of them dwindling while others increase. There are representatives of each form in contemporary East Africa, where studies were recently undertaken in different communities to discover how the people had adapted to the difficult, sometimes extremely hostile, environments in which they live. These studies were part of a series of investigations into child health and were not confined to nutrition, because nutrition cannot be divorced from other aspects of life (including the infective burden a child may bear at any particular time).

Hunters and Gatherers

One such study was undertaken among the Hadza people, a hunting-gathering community in rural Tanzania (Jelliffe *et al.* 1962). A small group, they were still living just as they had for thousands of years. The classic differentiation in work (and hence, in dietary opportunities) between men and women were in effect. The men hunted, using powerful bows and poisoned arrows. Because they were the ones who tracked, shot and obtained the meat, they automatically received a much larger share. (As mentioned before, carrying large amounts of meat back to the camp is difficult without a means of transportation.) Primarily for this reason, the male diet in this community differed from that of the females, who were responsible for looking after the camps and the children. From a dietary point of view, women were concerned with two types of food: human milk, and gathered foods (such as wild roots, berries and eggs). As with other hunter-gatherers, the division of labor meant that most of the meat would go to the men, and the gathered foods to the women.

The method of infant feeding under these circumstances is extremely interesting. In brief, this begins with biological breast-feeding, with its child-spacing effect due to the lactation amenorrhea. Other foods were introduced during the second six months of life, all of which were "homogenized" by the mother—that is, she prechewed the meat and fed it to the child by means of finger or tongue. Another excellent soft food often used for feeding these young children was bone marrow. During this one survey, there was very little evidence of malnutrition among the children, and certainly no incidence of kwashiorkor. However, one has to be very cautious in drawing conclusions which may be too sweeping. The study was conducted during a short period of time at one season of one particular year.

The Hadza live under great difficulty, constantly on the move in search of water, game, berries, fruit and wild honey. Under these circumstances, one would think that nearly everything that was available would be eaten. This is not so, however. There are certain foods which have special symbolism and meaning, and which were reserved for or denied to certain groups within the community. One of these restrictions is particularly interesting. It involves a category of food which the Hadza call *epeme*—that is, meat which is forbidden to women. The meat was principally that from the animal's omentum, and was reserved exclusively for the men. From a nutritional point of view, it represents a calorie-rich part of the diet. Some of these food attitudes are difficult to understand; others are easy. Among the latter is the prohibition against eating those animals, such as the vulture and the maribou stork, which feed on carrion. Again, this may have a symbolic significance.

Agriculturalists

As an example of an agricultural community in East Africa, one might mention the Baganda people of Uganda (Jelliffe 1968). As with most agriculturalists, the Baganda linked themselves with a main staple—a cultural superfood—which dominated their lives, and around which their history and mythology centered. This superfood is plantain, which when cooked in a special way looks rather like brown mashed potatoes (*matoke*). In this *matoke*-centered culture, life revolves around the plantain; their customs and habits are closely related to what can or cannot be done with it. Whenever a baby is born, for example, the placenta is buried under a certain plantain tree. The local beer is fermented from plantain.

The nature of the superfood in such agricultural communities is critical. It is much easier to survive and thrive if the cultural superfood is a relatively high protein cereal grain. Plantain, however, is high in water and cellulose. In the northern part of Uganda, where people are not so "developed," the cultural superfood is a form of millet. As a result, there is much less kwashiorkor in the north than in the *matoke*-dominated, more highly developed south.

Herdsmen

There are many types of herdsmen in Uganda, such as the Karamajory (Jelliffe *et al.* 1964). The people in this culture are cattle-centered and have evolved a vast number of ideas, habits and mores concerning their herds, which mean much more to them than a mere source of milk, blood and occasional meat. Even though cattle are available to produce milk, the culture surrounding the cattle, the way they are perceived, is totally different from that found in Westernized countries. From a rational or scientific point of view, it would seem logical that the milk go to certain disadvantaged, highly vulnerable groups within the society. But this may not be the case in many cultures because of differing attitudes toward and ideas concerning the symbolism of milk and cattle, as well as differing views of people in varying stages of life. In some cultures, for example, milk may be principally reserved for elderly males.

Urban Dwellers

The townsmen and city dwellers inhabit increasingly important ecologies. Indeed, it is this group (and especially the newly arrived townsman) which is presently afflicted with the greatest nutritional problems (Jelliffe and Jelliffe 1970). First, the physical availability of their food has changed from the traditional foods available in their homelands to those "urbanized" foods which are more easily transported and stored. Moreover, they have switched from foods which were grown to those which have to be bought. And finally, their cultural attitudes are in a state of flux as they try to adapt to the new ecology.

Nutritional problems related to the physical lack of availability or to cultural-symbolic factors occur in traditional urban societies. However, it is the new shantytown dwellers, moving from a well-defined culture to something between a vacuum and cultural chaos, who are highly at risk. They do not know what foods to eat, and they usually lack the skills needed to find employment so that they can buy food at all. Nutritionists ought to be concerned with the forces at work upon those urban townspeople who are trying to adjust to a totally new, strange and often frightening ecology.

PROTECTIVE OR HARMFUL FOOD HABITS

Food habits can be either protective or harmful, but any categorization should be considered in terms of three overlapping aspects: *physical protection* gained from appropriate food habits, *social protection* and, since man does not live by beta-carotene alone, *spiritual protection*.

Physical Protection

Westernized people automatically tend to think that the best foods in a community ought to go to young children and pregnant women. In most traditional societies, however, the best foods usually go to the men, and particularly to the elders. If, on the other hand, one looks at the physiologically vulnerable groups (pregnant or lactating women and young children), one can learn a number of interesting lessons, as well as encounter a number of real conundrums.

The only rational, biological way to view the feeding of pregnant or lactating women and young children is to follow Bostock's theory (1962), which holds that the human fetus takes 18 months to develop; but because the head is large and the birth canal small, the fetus is pushed out when it is only half mature. For the first 6 to 9 months of life, then, a baby is best regarded as an "exterogestate fetus." After this period, the baby enters a "transitional" stage in which it moves from a milk diet to adult foods; there are also immunological and psychological transitions involved.

Using these three stages (fetal, exterogestate and transitional), we can make a number of interesting generalizations about traditional societies. Very frequently, the nutrition of the pregnant woman—and therefore of the fetus—is more harmed than protected by food restrictions. By contrast, the exterogestate fetus is at a tremendous advantage in traditional societies, where infant feeding is generally more biological than in most Westernized countries. This advantage is enhanced by various practices during the perinatal period (especially after birth). Such a practice is the presence of a *doula* (Raphael 1973), a culturally defined member of the family (usually a woman) who assists the mother during pregnancy and in the puerperium, offering both physical and emotional support which makes lactation easier. (This is in marked contrast to most Westernized countries, where lactation is often made more difficult by cultural practices surrounding maternity.) One result of the generally high incidence of breast-feeding in traditional societies is that the children often reach a lifetime nutritional peak during these first few months.

In contrast, the customs related to the feeding of a young transitional (the so-called "weaning" period) seem to be more harmful than protective. Perhaps this is due to changes in various parts of the world since studies have been reported; that is, within the last 50 years. What seems to be true is that dietary practices related to the pregnant woman, the fetus and the transitional infant seem to be more harmful than protective. If this indeed the case, the question is—why?

Three reasons may be considered. As suggested above, it may simply be that the situation has changed in recent years. Or perhaps it is due to the fact that during these periods of life (pregnancy, childbirth and weaning), people are more likely to be sick from a variety of infections, etc.; because of this, various food habits may have been intended to protect individuals during what are recognized as dangerous phases of life. A third possibility is that this continues the pattern laid down in early hunting-gathering societies, where the best food (especially meat) was automatically channeled to those present at the kill; thus, the prized foods still go to the dominant members of the family—the men and the elders.

From the group's point of view, is this such a bad way of doing things? We might understand better if we could step back and view the situation as it was 500,000 years ago. Then, the essential concern was the physical protection and survival of the *group*, not of the small child, who was fairly easily replaced and rather likely to die anyway. Since men, as hunters and defenders, were essential to the survival of the group, they naturally got the best foods. So far as the elders were concerned, they might get better food because they were not regarded (as is often the case in Westernized societies) as useless social outcasts, but as living biological data banks filled with invaluable knowledge garnered throughout their lifetimes.

Social Protection

Since man is a social creature, many of his food habits are designed to protect the social group. It is well-recognized that group identification is closely related to dietary customs. But the reverse is also true—food may serve to emphasize divisions between groups. Insults in many parts of the world are related to the foods used by another community—Germans are krauts, the French are frogs, the British limeys and so on. These group identifications often have a religious basis. It is likely that, in the years after Europe was Christianized, the horse became a forbidden food not because it was disliked, but because it had been identified with the worship of the pagan god Wotan.

Many other aspects of diet are related to group relationships, social rank and social cohesion, and these factors often mitigate against a nutritionally equitable mode of food distribution. In New Guinea, for example, there is little food of animal origin. The pig is kept in these communities, but in much the way dogs are kept in Western nations—it is a first-class citizen, close to the family, and indeed, at one time actually breast-fed by the women. Yet on certain occasions, pigs are exchanged throughout the country, and hundreds of them are roasted and eaten in large feasts. From a nutritional point of view, this is an absurd use of pork. But its role in terms of social protection is to cement social relationships and promote reciprocity among various people in the community.

Spiritual Protection

In regard to spiritual protection, we might note that man has a tremendous imagination and potential for abstract thought. He strives for understanding, explanation and a basis for hope. By following various food practices, he may feel that he can intervene with the ultrahuman forces he thinks influence his life, thereby averting disaster.

As an example of physical factors blending with cultural symbolism, we might consider the cow in Hindu society. To the Indian, the cow has many different attributes. From a physical point of view, the cow supplies milk, a valuable food in an otherwise vegetarian community. In social terms, the refusal to eat the cow promotes social identification as an orthodox Hindu and fosters group cohesion. Spiritually, the cow is important because of the role it plays in the Hindu conception of the creation of the world.

SUMMARY

Do these considerations make any difference in the modern world? It would seem so, particularly in regard to *cultural changes* and their effect on nutrition. In the resource-rich industrialized countries, the "primary physiological urges" which were so important to ancestral man—the drives for sugar, for fat, for crunchiness and for gluttony—may no longer be a form of protective selection, but may actually promote the *harmful* selection of foods. In the towns, the cultural confusion in regard to food habits is extremely important. For the resource-rich countries, there is a great danger that physical and cultural factors which operated in the past are no longer appropriate. This leads to something between cultural chaos and cultural vacuum.

If this is indeed the case, we must ask who is filling this vacuum? The role seems to have gone to commercial interests, which leads to almost inevitable clashes (or conflicts of interest) between nutrition and profit. Thus, it is important for nutritionists to realize that present-day food habits in Westernized, resource-rich countries are in a state of flux. The methods tested over thousands of years in different societies are no longer pristine. Westernized man can eat as much sugar as he wants to, or as much fat. He can overeat, but to his disadvantage because there is no "hungry season" to deplete his body stores.

Moreover, these ancient urges can be—and *are*—reinforced and exploited by people who are more concerned with selling a product than with the nutritional end result. We obviously need more nutritional education, and some sort of compromise to temper commercial persuasion.

We find a similar situation in resource-poor countries. Here, people have come to the towns, the slums, the *favellas* and the shantytowns, and cultural confusion is once again the result. The protection afforded by the ancient cultural patterns of a community may have been flawed in respect to the pregnant woman, the fetus or the transitional child, but on the whole, it was attuned, albeit in different degrees, to the ecology of the region, and quite remarkably adapted to the available foods. But once in the towns, even that protection is lost. Food is bought instead of grown, and familiar items may not be available on the market. And there is the ever increasing pressure of advertising, which has had a particularly disastrous effect on breast-feeding and, therefore, on the nutritional health of the exterogestate fetus.

In every part of the world, dietary patterns and food habits are based on physical availability and cultural symbolism. What we ought to do is to examine the methods of food selection in traditional societies and realize that there is much wisdom to be found along with the unwisdom. We ought to realize as well that populations in urbanized societies find themselves in situations where the available foods differ from those of previous times. Conditions in Kampala are far different than those in rural Uganda. A supermarket in Los Angeles is a far cry from the rural United States just a few years ago.

Not only has the physical availability of food changed, but the cultural pattern has been altered—especially since it is no longer the sole property of the community. Instead, it is molded by commercial interests. One of the most important issues facing an urban society, whether the country be resource-rich or resource-poor, is the effort to create an adequate supply of nutritious food and to devise a cultural pattern which will not be over-exploited. To do this, we must use not only the best of modern scientific knowledge, but also the wisdom and experience of man's vast biological and cultural heritage.

REFERENCES

BOSTOCK, J. 1962. Evolutionary approaches to infant care. Lancet *1*, 1033–1035.
JELLIFFE, D.B. 1968. Infant Nutrition in the Subtropics and Tropics, 2nd Edition. WHO Monograph *2*, Geneva, Switzerland.
JELLIFFE, D.B., and JELLIFFE, E.F.P. 1970. The urban avalanche. J. Am. Dietet. Assoc. *57*, 115–118.
JELLIFFE, D.B., WOODBURN, J., BENNETT, F.J., and JELLIFFE, E.F.P. 1962. The children of the Hadza hunters. J. Pediatr. *50*, 907–912.
JELLIFFE, D.B., BENNETT, F.J., JELLIFFE, E.F.P., and WHITE, R.H.R. 1964. The ecology of childhealth among the Karamajory of Uganda. Arch. Env. Hlth. *9*, 25–30.
RAPHAEL, D. 1973. The role of breast feeding in the bottle feeding world. Ecol. Food Nutr. *12*, 121–124.

CHAPTER 7

Osamu Sinoda

Rice: How It Defined the Life Pattern Among Asian Races

GENERAL REMARKS

Rice as a Cereal Crop

Rice yields an excellent harvest, since it is a summer crop which can utilize the full energy of the tropical and subtropical sunshine of eastern Asia. Moreover, it is constantly irrigated and thereby fertilized throughout its cultivation by dissolved minerals in the water.

At the same time, a rice crop involves a high risk of famine, since it contains a high concentration of starch, as compared with fat or protein. Therefore, those components of the soil associated with starch synthesis are quickly used up, which may result in crop failures. But even if the crops did not fail, sole reliance on rice for food can lead to malnutrition. (A somewhat similar phenomenon was observed in the potato famine of Ireland, when crops did fail.)

Rice as a Food Crop

As seen in Table 7.1, the biological value of rice is relatively high (the lysine level is known to be low); thus, it can provide an adequate protein quality with the addition of side dishes. This greatly benefits poor people. On the other hand, rice is low in total protein, very low in fat, and contains too little calcium and a rather high level of magnesium.

Further, if one were to attempt to satisfy his daily protein demands with rice alone, far too much starch would be consumed in the process, leading to dilation of the stomach and hemorrhoids. (As the Germans say, *Kein Bauer nicht fressen.* A Chinese proverb holds that nine out of ten people suffer from hemorrhoids.)

Table 7.2 illustrates the fact that the arginine content of rice is much like that of meat, that is, a rich source. Arginine is known to be the main component of nucleoprotein (Table 7.3) in which sperm cells happen to be particularly rich. Thus, rice protein causes premature growth of the gonads (especially in the male). This fact may explain why rice-eating peoples tend to be so prolific. (In Iwate Prefecture at the northeastern border of Japan proper, it is reported that poor farming couples at age 35 generally have sexual relations seven times a week. According to the Kinsey report, the figure for Americans is 2.5 to 3.5 times a week.)

TABLE 7.1

BIOLOGICAL VALUES OF SOME PROTEINS

Beef	100	Pea	56
Rice	88	Maize	30
Wheat	40	Fish	95
Milk	96-100	Bread	35

TABLE 7.2

ARGININE CONTENT OF SOME PROTEINS

Beef	7.2%	Flour	3.7%
Milk	4.3%	Rice	7.4%
Fish	7.4%	Maize	4.0%

TABLE 7.3

AMINO ACID COMPOSITION OF CLUPEIN, A NUCLEOPROTEIN

Alanine	3%	Arginine	89%
Proline	11%	Serine	3%
Varine	6%		

ETHNOLOGICAL REMARKS

Patriarchy

In those areas where patriarchal systems still predominate, their effects upon nutrition are easily documented. Take, for example, the *ani-meshi*, or "heir's meal." In the northern mountain region of Kyoto Prefecture, only the head of the family and his heir were allowed to eat polished rice meal (the so-called "silver meal"). The wife and other members of the family ate a mixture of rice and barley. This practice continued for some years after the close of World War II.

Old farmers (and particularly the women) have a very slight bridge to the nose. Rarely able to afford dining in restaurants, these people generally ate rice meal and pickles at home. The resulting calcium deficiency produced the low nose bridge. After the war, boys and girls were fed equally in school lunch programs, and no differences in the nose can be observed.

In Matsue City, Shimane Prefecture, I tested about 50 university women and male teachers in regard to their choice of vinegars. The men preferred brewed vinegar to the imitation (a synthesized mixture of pure acetic acid and various condiments). This is due to the fact that men often dine at restaurants and are familiar with the taste of brewed vinegar; women, on the other hand, are confined at home and are more accustomed to the irritant aroma of pure acetic acid.

Suicide is thought to be most prevalent among younger people, but in those regions still dominated by patriarchal systems, it occurs very often among the elderly. When they were masters of the home, these old men and women were absolute tyrants. But once they were forced to retire (because of illness or other reasons) or became widowed, all rights fell into the hands of their heirs and daughters-in-law, often to such a degree that even their daily meal allotments are rigidly controlled. This situation is often so depressing for the elderly that they are driven to suicide.

During the feudal period under the Tokugawa Shogunate, the effects of famine were far more severe than they are today. Each *daimyo* closed its borders and ceased the exportation of rice and other foodstuffs. As a result, many people in small villages surrounded by *daimyos* other than their own died of starvation.

Malnutrition (The Effect of a Pure Rice Diet)

In the northern part of Shiga Prefecture, there are three villages, each twelve kilometers apart: Maibara, a railroad junction with a large factory; Tara, a purely farming community; and Iso, a fishing village on Lake Biwa. The physical constitution of school children is best at Iso and worst at Tara, and can be traced to the diet available.

According to Professor T. Kanazeki, the height of Japanese people was greatest during the Yayoi Period (ca. 300 B.C.) and least during the late Yedo Period, a phenomenon he explains as the consequence of social prematurity. At any rate, prematurity and low birth weight babies may be an effect of a pure rice diet.

In 1918, the mountain aborigines of Formosa (all hunters, or even head-hunters) were tall, slender and extremely manly. When I visited them again in 1973, I was astonished to find that they were all short and slight. An "old man" of 45 told me that when he was a boy, he knew two men who were nine feet tall and regularly dined on raw deer meat. He claimed that his people lost their stature when they stopped hunting. (The mountain Taiyals are all farmers now, and chiefly cultivate millet, corn, beans and temperate fruits. These crops are sold to the Chinese in the plains region, and rice is bought in their stead.)

In the region between Osaka, Nara and Wakayama Prefectures, the men eat or sip rice gruel in place of ordinary rice meal. This gruel is extremely thin and consumed several times a day, causing dilatation of the stomach. Gastric cancer is very prevalent in this region, and it is significant to note that a high rice diet has been implicated in the etiology of gastric carcinomas.

This brief discussion is meant to illustrate how a high rice diet may lead to poverty and prolificacy among people whose diet consists principally of this grain.

CHAPTER 8

Cultures in Conflict: When Does Man's Cultural Heritage No Longer Act as a Protective Device?

Richard Orraca-Tetteh

For the present subject, culture is defined as the way of life of a people. Clearly, then, culture involves many facets of life and does not remain static; in fact, change and adaptation are often necessary to revitalize a particular culture. But it is when these changes are imported that we find the conflict of cultures becoming evident. Those who would simply "borrow" aspects of another culture often fail to recognize the fact that the environmental conditions and demands in their homeland may be very different from those of the culture they seek to emulate. Judicious selection is required in order to insure that what is borrowed actually suits the needs of any particular culture.

THE TRADITIONAL SCENE

In most developing parts of the world, the influence of culture on family life is very strong. In African countries, for example, the home surroundings are such as to allow interaction between family members. The houses are built in a compound, with several units surrounding an open space (or compound) in the center. The compound itself is used for various family functions, such as "outdooring" a newborn baby, holding family meetings or celebrating festivals.

In such home surroundings, the influence of the head of the household upon other members of the family is very strong; he determines, for example, how the children are to be raised and introduced to the customs and traditions of their people. Often this takes the form of ritual, as with the "outdooring" custom of the Ga people of Ghana: Early on the morning of the eighth day following the birth of a child, the baby is brought outdoors to be named. Three times the infant is raised to the sky and then placed on the bare ground, each time with various ritual pronouncements. After being placed on the ground the third time, the baby is given a drink brewed from maize, the principal food utilized by this group.

CARE OF THE YOUNG

The feeding of children is greatly influenced by culture. Normally, an infant is breast-fed for as long as possible (usually a year or more). In the traditional pattern, relatives encourage the young mother to breast-feed her child. Usually it is the maternal grandmother who supervises the activities of the young mother. Supplementary foods are introduced after the first six months of breast-feeding. Weaning foods differ according to area: in the south of Ghana, it is maize porridge; in northern Ghana, millet porridge is used (Orraca-Tetteh 1961). East Africans wean their children on cereals and starchy foods; in Uganda, for example, the weaning mixture is bananas and plantain.

Traditionally, very few protein foods are given to infants under the age of one year. Most mothers will explain this by saying that foods rich in protein are too heavy and too difficult for the child to digest, and children fed such foods develop diarrhea. The avoidance of protein-rich foods can also be explained by their high cost.

THE TRADITIONAL FOOD SUPPLY SYSTEM

The size of most farms is small, usually one or two hectares. This small size is dictated by the fact that the traditional hoe and cutlass are used for clearing land and for cultivation. In the customary farming system, relatives and neighbors all work together in clearing and cultivating the farms. On the days a farm is to be cleared, the owner prepares food and alcoholic beverages for his neighbors, to be consumed by everyone once the work has been completed. The same communal pattern is manifested during the harvest season.

Clearly the use of manual labor for all farming activities limits both the size of the farm and its yield. However, food production was generally sufficient to support the small populations. The limitations of space and time fostered the cultivation of tree crops and perennials. (In Ghana, for example, the system led to the production of cocoa.)

The villages are the utilization centers for the food produced on the farms, and age-old methods are used for storage and preservation. Cereals, such as maize, are stored in raised barns open to the weather. Fresh vegetables are carried to markets which are within easy distance of the farm. Root crops, like cassava, are normally dug up when needed on specific market days. Fish, whether taken from the river or the sea, are preserved by drying in the sun, smoking or salting.

INTRODUCTION OF INDUSTRIAL CULTURE

In most parts of the developing world, culture has been changing, a trend influenced by contact with other peoples. But the greatest changes in culture have come about as a result of industrialization. The adoption of industry is not simply a technological change, but a cultural one as well, since industry affects the way people live. In the developed world, these radical changes took place over a long stretch of time, during the period known as the Industrial Revolution. But however drastic these changes may have been, they cannot compare with what is currently happening in most developing countries.

Countries in the developing world are becoming industrialized at a much more rapid pace, and their way of life is being driven farther and farther from traditional patterns. Therefore, the traditional culture must be modified if it is to keep pace with the new way of life. This clash or conflict of cultures is evident in most developing countries, since the old culture cannot protect itself against the introduction of the new.

INCREASING URBANIZATION

The most glaring evidence of this new industrial culture in developing countries is increased urbanization. Towns and cities are springing up around industrial centers, and large numbers of people gravitate to these cities in search of employment. Most of these workers have left the traditional form of family life, and are forced to maintain their new homes in very unfamiliar surroundings. The gathering of populations in these urban centers has brought about various social and economic problems. Rebellion against established traditions has increased because the traditional sanctions against certain forms of behavior are no longer in force. Women in the cities, for example, marry at a much younger age.

URBAN FOOD SUPPLY

This shift of population from rural farming areas to urban industrial towns has created a number of problems. Most of these rural immigrants are employed in steel mills, construction companies, textile factories, oil refineries or commercial businesses; as a result, their income is much higher than it would have been if they had remained in the villages. Thus a new class has arisen within the population, with money readily available to meet its needs.

This new class has caused problems with food supply, since it has increased the demand for food by increasing the population. But the supply of food has not increased. In their haste to industrialize, most developing countries have neglected to modernize their food production systems, leaving agriculture in the hands of the old culture with its hoe and cutlass. The farms cannot satisfy the needs of the urban centers. The flow of young people from the farms to the cities only makes matters worse, increasing the number of food consumers and depleting further the ranks of food producers. Clearly, the amount of food produced under the present system with its limited technology cannot keep pace with the needs of the population.

As a result, food prices are soaring and the urban worker spends an ever increasing percentage of his salary on food. Since the other amenities of life, such as housing and transportation, are more costly in the cities, the urban worker's food budget is even further reduced. Thus the worker is unable to buy enough food to meet the needs of his family, and what he does buy is usually of poor quality.

MECHANIZED FARMING

To meet this high demand for food, new farming techniques—largely those involving the use of machinery and fertilizers—have been introduced into many developing countries. Large areas of land have been cleared and planted with such crops as maize, yams, rice, cassava and sugar cane. But this large-scale cultivation further interferes with traditional practice.

Take, for example, the case of yam growing. In the traditional pattern, the newly harvested yams cannot be used until the yam festival has been celebrated. The yam festival is a harvest ritual involving a number of celebrations; the new yams are eaten by the people during ceremonies conducted by the traditional authorities in the village. But the large-scale yam grower has no time for such ceremonies; he cannot hold up a crop which is urgently needed by an ever increasing urban population until the yam festival has been conducted. As a result, most large-scale yam farmers have abandoned the traditional practices.

A further effort to increase food supply involves the introduction of large boats for deep-sea fishing, since the traditional canoe cannot provide enough fish to meet the demand. Here, too, we find cultural conflict. In Ghana, for example, the Ga people celebrate a harvest festival called *Homowo*. The food used in this celebration is steamed maize dough and a palm nut soup which also contains a special type of fish called breem. Traditionally, this fish cannot be caught for several months prior to the festival—that is, until the breem fishing ceremony has been performed by the traditional authorities. After the ceremony has been completed, the breem can be brought ashore. Clearly, however, the large fishing companies with huge investments at stake find it difficult, if not impossible, to conform to such cultural practices.

FOOD IMPORTATION

The continued introduction of mechanized agriculture has led to some increase in the amount of available food. But with continued urbanization and increasing population, the food supply in most developing countries is still inadequate. One way to reduce the disparity between supply and demand is by importing food, and many African nations have greatly increased the amount of their food imports.

Some of these imported items include wheat flour, canned fish and meat, sugar, milk and milk products. Some legumes, such as baked beans and frozen peas, are also imported. In many developing countries, these imported foods tend to be status symbols, and are replacing the traditional foods. In those urban areas which have seen a new social stratification, the consumption of imported food items among middle and high income groups has achieved a prestige value which often outstrips nutritional value.

One of these prestige items is imported alcoholic beverages. Moreover, a number of breweries and distilleries have been established, some of which merely import their alcohol from the developed countries and bottle it for the home market. With this increase in availability, alcoholism has become an increasing problem in the towns and cities. And since alcoholics tend to eat poorly, the incidence of alcohol-related malnutrition is also on the rise.

The ready availability of imported foods has led to changes in food habits. In Ghana, for example, the importation of wheat flour has increased over the years, with much of it being used in the preparation of breads, cakes and other wheat flour products. With the increasing consumption of bread, a number of wheat milling operations have been established, milling imported wheat for the local market. The number of bakeries operating both in towns and villages has also grown. Thus we see a great acceptance of wheat products in a culture where wheat is not grown.

CASH CROP PRODUCTION

In order to pay for the importation of food and other commodities needed for further development, a viable means of foreign exchange is required. In many developing countries, this is accomplished through the export of cash crops. The main source of foreign exchange capital in Ghana is cocoa, and cocoa production has received a good deal of government stimulus. But while the production of cocoa has increased, the price on the world market has not been favorable.

Many African nations are experiencing the same problem. Kenya, for example, produces one of the finest coffees, while Nigeria and Senegal produce huge quantities of groundnuts—in both cases, these are cash crops which were encouraged during the period prior to independence. These same cash crops were expected to form the basis for foreign exchange earnings once national independence had been achieved. But while the production of such cash crops as rubber, groundnuts, cocoa, copra, coffee, tea, palm oil and timber has increased, the prices paid for such commodities have not; in fact, in some cases, the price has decreased. The problem is aggravated by the fact that many developing countries have turned to synthetic products, thereby reducing the market for some of these cash crops and disturbing the economy of various developing nations.

The irony is this: During the colonial period, these countries were encouraged to produce cash crops at the expense of food crops. The prices commanded by these crops were good. After independence, however, the situation declined drastically, to the detriment of both food crop and cash crop production. The cash crop culture of the developing world seems to be involved in a head-on collision with the foreign exchange earning culture.

Another aspect of the cash crop situation is that it forces the developing nations to export large quantities of protein-rich crops to the developed world, despite the fact that these same developing nations themselves have a shortage of protein nutrition. A company has been established in Ghana to catch and export tuna fish to developing countries to earn foreign exchange capital. Thus it seems that the new industrial culture is in conflict with the self-interest of the people.

THE EFFECTS OF THE SAHELIAN DROUGHT

The Sahelian zone in Africa provides us with an example of how cultural heritage can fail to protect a population. The inhabitants of the Sahel are small farmers in the hoe and cutlass tradition. They have always depended on the vagaries of nature to provide them with enough water for cultivation, as well as for human and animal needs. Food production is low, usually only enough to last for one farming season. Any excess would probably be wasted, since extensive food stores are not part of their culture.

Thus the effects of the recent Sahelian drought, one of the worst in its history, were far-reaching. Whole areas were devastated, with a great loss of human and animal life. Communities were uprooted and moved into the urban areas. As yet, the full effect of this drought on the culture of the Sahel has not been appreciated. The culture of these nomadic people ought to be carefully examined so that necessary changes in their way of life can be made in the hope of safeguarding them from future calamities of this nature.

THE FAMILY IN THE CHANGING ENVIRONMENT

The movement of people from rural areas to urban centers has led to changes in cultural behavior. In the traditional setting, women are urged by their relatives—and particularly by their grandmothers—to have as many children as possible. Children, it is said, are gifts, and they must be produced as often as possible for as long as possible. Thus, families of eight or more children are common. In terms of their usefulness in agriculture and other activities, great numbers of children are an advantage. On the other hand, the proper feeding of large, poorly spaced families is a problem. Children are often fed on carbohydrate foods and deprived of protein; many children therefore suffer from malnutrition.

In urban areas, raising large families imposes a great financial strain on the parents, due to the high costs of food and shelter. As a result, many families have begun to limit the number of children they have, and the provision of family planning services in urban areas seems to be welcome. In this case, a modification of culture is working to the advantage of the people.

Breast-feeding of infants and children is waning in the urban areas. The rural woman who is now living in a city is attracted by the various infant food mixtures she sees advertised. Since she sees these methods being used by members of the upper class, she adopts them for herself. The result is often bottle-feeding with unhygienic and poorly prepared mixtures, which aids the development of malnutrition. A second factor leading to the decline of breast-feeding is that many women must leave the home in order to work.

"NEW" CULTURAL INFLUENCES IN DEVELOPED COUNTRIES

At present, there is a movement in many developed countries to break away from established cultural patterns. Small numbers of people are joining together in communes, sharing common facilities. Some of these communes are even trying to raise their own food in backyard gardens. The movement toward organically grown food has steadily increased, and its effects are widely known.

In addition to these communes, a number of new religious sects have sprung up in developed countries. Many of these cults originate in the developing nations, where they have long been a part of the culture. Obviously, these cultural introductions have affected the behavior of such practitioners, and this in turn affects their children. For example, the food habits in such communes and religious cults often differ radically from those of the majority culture. The imposition of these new food habits on children can be detrimental to proper nutrition (Robson et al. 1974). It is important to take note of such occurences in developed countries where a cultural backlash from the developing countries is taking place.

The conflict of cultures is the starting point for change in human societies. Throughout the ages, cultures have been modified in response to the introduction of elements drawn from other cultures, thereby enriching the human experience. Such changes and modifications are needed if we are to achieve any harmony between cultures.

In October 1975, the Ministers of Culture from many African governments held a conference in Ghana to stress the importance of culture in the development of African nations. In the field of food and nutrition, it seems obvious that great weight should be given to the influence of cultural practices on nutrition within various population groups.

REFERENCES

ORRACA-TETTEH. R. 1961. The place of food science and technology in the campaign against malnutrition: Problems and some solutions in Ghana. Proc. Nutr. Soc. 20, 109–112.
ROBSON. J. R. K., KONLANDE, J. E., LARKIN, F. A., and O'CONNOR, P. A. 1974. Zen macrobiotic dietary problems in infancy. Pediatrics 53, 326–329.

SECTION III

BIOLOGICAL VARIABLES IN HUMAN
NUTRITION: HUMAN ADAPTABILITY TO
NUTRITIONAL VARIABLES

CHAPTER 9

Josef Brožek

Introduction: Biological
Variability in Human Nutrition

The variability of organisms has two aspects: (1) interindividual and intergroup variability (e.g., differences in thiamine excretion of individuals maintained on identical intakes of thiamine, and differences in the mean serum cholesterol levels of different populations); and (2) intraindividual variability (e.g., age-related changes in physical activity or body composition). In this classification, adaptation of an individual to high altitude is an example of intraindividual variability.

Several years ago at a meeting on The Biology of Human Variation (Brožek 1966) sponsored by the New York Academy of Sciences, attention was directed toward the implications of the concept for nutrition, including variability in nutritional requirements (Thirumurthi and Longenecker 1966). The presence and relevance of individual differences is clearly acknowledged in the usual practice of taking into account body size and age in estimating the calorie needs of various populations (Consolazio 1966). The biological roots of individual differences need further exploration and interpretation in the context of nutritional research. In introducing the topic, I shall briefly consider individual differences in behavior toward food under conditions of thiamine deprivation.

In reviewing Russian work on nutrition and "higher nervous activity," I was struck by the large differences in the behavioral response of dogs maintained on identical diets, free of thiamine. In that particular study, the onset of partial refusal to eat was reported to vary from 12 to 94 days, while the onset of total refusal to eat ranged from 30 to 150 days (Brožek 1962; Shekun 1960). These are remarkable differences and call for a clarification of the underlying factors.

The Russians related the time differences in the development of behavioral manifestations of dietary deficiencies to "typological characteristics" of the central nervous system (C.N.S.) of the experimental animals (cf. Brožek 1962). It is difficult to interpret with confidence the Russian literature on the subject, but the issue of individual differences in C.N.S. function and their nutritional implications is important enough to call for a critical reexamination of the problem.

Our own investigations, from about the same era, were carried out in adult male volunteers (Brožek 1957). Among individuals maintained on diets essentially free of thiamine, we observed large differences in the timing of the appearance of symptoms of thiamine deficiency, with first vomiting occuring as early as the 5th day of acute thiamine deprivation and as late as the 22nd day. In 2 of our 10 experimental subjects, vomiting did not occur at all during the 27-day period on the thiamine-free diet.

In this experiment, the differential response of the individuals can be interpreted largely in terms of their prior thiamine intake. During the 6-month period preceding the removal of thiamine from the diet of 3 moderately active young men, the total daily intakes of thiamine were 0.6, 1.0 and 1.8 mg. In the subsequent period, during which all subjects were maintained on a thiamine-free diet, the average time of onset of severe nausea in these three groups was 5, 12 and 18 days respectively.

The phenomena of biological variability (Keys 1949), considered alone and in interaction with cultural factors, is a fascinating area of study.

REFERENCES

BROŽEK, J. 1957. Psychological effects of thiamine restriction and deprivation in normal young men. *In* Symposium on Nutrition and Behavior. J. Brožek (Editor). National Vitamin Foundation, New York; also Am. J. Clin. Nutr. *5*, 109–120.
BROŽEK, J. 1962. Soviet studies on nutrition and higher nervous activity. Ann. N.Y. Acad. Sci. *93*, 665–714.
BROŽEK, J. 1966. The Biology of Human Variation. Ann. *134*. N.Y. Acad. Sci., New York.
CONSOLAZIO, C. F. 1966. Nutritional variation in world populations and performance potential. *In* The Biology of Human Variation. J. Brožek (Editor). N.Y. Acad. Sci.. New York.
KEYS, A. 1949. The physiology of the individual as an approach to a more quantitative biology of man. Fed. Proc. *8*, 523–529.
SHEKUN, L. A. 1960. Changes in food intake under conditions of experimental thiamine deficiency and subsequent vitamin therapy in dogs. Vopr. Pitan. *19*, 56–61. (Russian)
THIRUMURTHI, H. R., and LONGENECKER, J. B. 1966. Nutritional considerations of biological variation. *In* The Biology of Human Variation. J. Brožek (Editor). N.Y. Acad. Sci., New York.

CHAPTER 10

Roberta M. Palmour

Multifactorial Components in Cultural-Biological Interactions

This paper will review some contemporary findings in human genetics of particular relevance to multifactorial inheritance, with additional comments on the relationship between multifactoral inheritance and the cultural aspects of the nutritional dilemma currently facing us. A consideration of multifactorial inheritance is, in many ways, an ideal bridging mechanism between environmental factors on the one hand and biological factors on the other.

As many investigators have pointed out, we now have a great deal of knowledge about the genetics and biochemistry of diseases inherited in a simple Mendelian fashion. McKusick's catalogue of Mendelian inheritance lists some 1500 single gene disorders; in about 8-10% of these cases, a specific enzyme deficiency has been identified (McKusick 1975). Individually, however, the incidence of each enzyme deficiency is rare; even the more common metabolic diseases affect only 1/500 to 1/10,000 live births. Some enzyme deficiencies are more common among specific populations, a point to which we will return later. By contrast, diseases such as diabetes, gout, schizophrenia, ischemic heart disease and rheumatoid arthritis each affect more than 10 individuals per 1000; diabetes alone affects 1-2% of the population (Cavalli-Sforza and Bodmer 1969). Collectively, these diseases involve a sizeable portion of the population. For each of these examples, and for many other common disorders, there is inescapable evidence of genetic involvement, but the etiology of these diseases cannot be traced to single Mendelian genes. In each case, there is a long anecdotal history that the disease "runs in families," but the transmission does not fit any simple mode of inheritance.

The specific example of diabetes may be illustrative of this point. There is a very long and confusing literature attempting to study the genetic transmission of diabetes; virtually every mode of inheritance has been implicated, but no single mode fits all cases. There is no doubt, however, that a strong genetic component contributes to the expression of diabetes. Classical evidence for a heritable component in diabetes rests primarily upon the observations of a three-fold increase in the risk of diabetes among first degree relatives of known diabetics, and upon a 48% concordance for diabetes among monozygotic twins (Rimoin and Schimke 1971). Autosomal recessive inheritance has been suggested by many investigators, but the low incidence (5–50%) of clinical diabetes among offspring of conjugal diabetics is inconsistent with simple recessive transmission (Cooke *et al.* 1966; Kahn *et al.* 1969). Other investigators have suggested that diabetes is in fact controlled by an autosomal dominant gene with reduced penetrance, and in some few multigenerational families, segregation consistent with autosomal dominant inheritance and reliable parent to child transmission has indeed been observed (Barbosa and Dow 1975; Tattersall and Fajans 1975). Many geneticists simply state that diabetes is a polygenically inherited trait; that is, that several distinct genes contribute to the diabetic genotype (Simpson 1964; Falconer 1967; Neel 1969). More recent observations suggest that the term *multifactoral inheritance* is more appropriate.

Multifactorial inheritance may most simply be described as a situation in which the clinical expression of a disease state is dependent upon the interaction of a particular genetic predisposition with a particular constellation of environmental factors. The precise nature of the genetic component and of the environmental agents is difficult to specify in most cases; both the genetic and the environmental components may be multiple. There are some few instances, however, for which we have been able to identify both a Mendelian gene and an environmental insult involved in disease expression; generally these are far simpler cases than that of diabetes.

One approach commonly used in differentiating multifactorial or polygenic disorders from simple Mendelian traits is to study the distribution of a particular clinical variable in the total population (Falconer 1965). In the most extreme cases, Mendelian traits show bimodality; two populations of individuals—those who manifest the trait and those who do not—can be clearly differentiated from one another. In the specific case of phenylketonuria, the plasma concentration of phenylalanine in normal adults ranges from 0.04 to 0.24 μM/ml while in affected persons, the phenylalanine concentration ranges from 1.18 to 1.96 μM/ml (Fig. 10.1). The two dis-

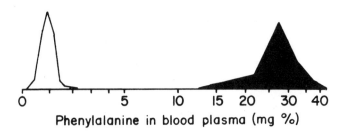

Phenylalanine in blood plasma (mg %)

From Harris (1955)

FIG. 10.1. FREQUENCY DISTRIBUTION LEVELS OF PHENYLALANINE IN BLOOD PLASMA IN PHENLYKETONURIC PATIENTS (RIGHT) AND IN CONTROL POPULATION (LEFT)

tributions are clearly separated from one another and do not overlap. Heterozygotic individuals have serum phenylalanine levels ranging from 0.075 to 0.254, well toward the normal end of the scale (Berry *et al.* 1957; Knox and Messinger 1958). By contrast, the clinically significant factors for diagnosis of many multifactorial disorders display a unimodal distribution in the population as a whole. The distribution of blood glucose (the diagnostic criterion for diabetes) and that of serum uric acid (the diagnostic criterion for gout) are both unimodal, though somewhat skewed from Gaussian distributions (Fig. 10.2). Consequently, some physicians hold the notion that elevated blood glucose or serum uric acid is simply one end of a normal distribution, and is therefore unremarkable in the absence of other symptoms (Renold *et al.* 1972; Wyngaarden and Kelly 1972).

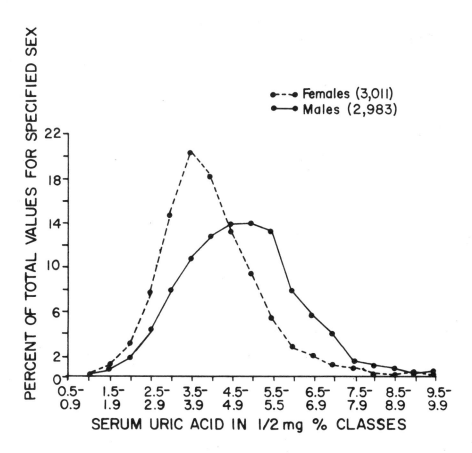

From Mikkelsen, Dodge, and Valkenburgh (1965)

FIG. 10.2. DISTRIBUTIONS OF SERUM URATE VALUES IN MALE AND FEMALE
POPULATION OF TECUMSEH, MICHIGAN, 1959-1960

The diagnostic utilization of a parameter displaying unimodality, whatever that parameter may be, imposes certain limitations both in clinical practice and upon scientific investigation. For example, it is not possible to say unequivocally what the dividing line is between normality and disease. Secondly, the task of identifying underlying genetic causes becomes much more difficult, as it is not possible to partition similar groups of patients on any basis other than that of familial identity. Furthermore, in the case of nonspecific physiological parameters, such as serum uric acid or blood glucose, clinical manifestations may be very far removed from the primary genetic defect. Finally, the identification of clinically unaffected but genetically predisposed individuals becomes almost impossible; the identification of such persons would facilitate a variety of prospective and controlled studies not presently feasible.

One brief word of caution is in order with regard to unimodal and bimodal distributions. If the activity of the red cell enzyme acid phosphatase is determined in a random population, it turns out that the values are unimodally distributed without clear discontinuities in distribution (Fig. 10.3). Biochemical analysis and genetic studies show, however, that each individual has two alleles at single red cell acid phosphatase locus; there are three common alleles, each of which has a specific, but different, mean activity. Thus the unimodal distribution in this case simply represents the summation of a series of separate but overlapping activity distributions (Spencer *et al.* 1964). The general point to consider here is that only when

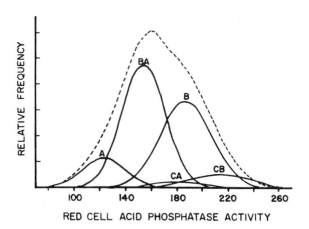

RED CELL ACID PHOSPHATASE ACTIVITY

From Harris (1975)

FIG. 10.3. DISTRIBUTION OF RED CELL PHOSPHATASE ACTIVITIES IN THE GENERAL POPULATION (BROKEN LINE) AND IN THE SEPARATE PHENOTYPES, USING THE FREQUENCIES OF THE DIFFERENT PHENOTYPES AS FOUND IN THE ENGLISH POPULATION

you have a clearly defined biochemical marker with a known genetic basis can you be certain of an interpretation.

With regard to the more common multifactorial disorders, for all the reasons detailed previously, our knowledge has not proceeded to this degree of sophistication. There are, however, several generalizations which can serve as a guide to present understanding and to future investigations. I should simply like to draw your attention to these generalizations, and then to refer to them periodically as I consider genetic components and environmental components in more detail.

(1) Multifactorial disorders are characterized by the interaction of genetic and environmental factors; however, in virtually no case can we assess the relative contributions of the two components.

(2) In multifactorial inheritance, the genetic component itself is heterogeneous; in each well-characterized instance, there are multiple separate genes, which may themselves act individually, additively or interactionally.

(3) In a large number of cases, the environmental component is likewise heterogeneous, and a combination of environmental agents may be additive.

(4) Clinical manifestation of the disease only occurs when an individual with a specific genetic predisposition encounters the appropriate environmental trigger; the intensity of the genetic predisposition and the requisite exposure to an environmental agent may vary from person to person, and probably vary inversely with respect to one another.

Let me now move to a specific consideration of the sorts of genetic components we find operating in multifactorial inheritance. In the simplest case—one which technically falls outside the category of multifactorial inheritance—there is the interaction between a single Mendelian gene and a specified class of environmental agent. In man, there is an enzyme called serum pseudocholinesterase for which there are genetic variants separable by kinetic analysis and family studies. This enzyme is related to acetylcholinesterase, which is found primarily in nervous tissue; serum pseudocholinesterase hydrolyzes a variety of substrates chemically related to acetylcholine. Following administration of suxamethonium (succinyl dicholine), a muscle relaxant, one can identify susceptible individuals who remain anesthetized for an unusually long time. In the European population, the incidence of susceptible individuals is about 1/2000. It turns out that the pseudocholinesterase activity is very low in these people; they appear to be homozygotic for a deficient allele at the pseudocholinesterase locus. If the total population is screened for activity of pseudocholinesterase, the various genotypes cannot be clearly delineated; the distribution of enzymatic activities is fairly continuous. However, if physicochemical studies are performed, one can clearly distinguish both homozygotes and heterozygotes for the sensitive allele, as well as for other alleles at that same locus. In all cases, individuals with the sensitive genotype react adversely to administration of the drug, but would have no symptoms at all unless exposed to drugs of this type (Davies *et al.* 1960; Harris *et al.* 1960). The point here is twofold—that in some cases adverse reactions to an environmental component can be predicted on the basis of genotype, and secondly, that a sensitive genotype may in some cases only be identified when an environmental challenge is encountered.

A somewhat more complicated example is provided by the case of multiple, but separately acting, genes; recent studies on the genetic basis of gout demonstrate this type of interaction. The association between gout and diet has long been established; classically, gout was a disease of the wealthy and was attributed to excessive indulgence in rich foods and wines. Clinically, gout is identified with overproduction of uric acid, leading to hyperuricemia, deposition of uric acid crystals, arthritis and inflammatory attacks. Hyperuricemia, however, also occurs in asymptomatic individuals, and particularly in relatives of gouty patients. If uric acid values—the diagnostic criterion for gout—are monitored for a total population, a continuous distribution of values with no clear bimodality is observed (Fig. 10.2). Beginning in about 1955, the biosynthesis of uric acid was elucidated and an understanding of purine metabolism quickly followed. It is now known that purine biosynthesis may proceed by either of two pathways, a *de novo* synthetic pathway or a salvage pathway. *De novo* synthesis of purines is catalyzed by ten consecutive enzymes, with the rate of synthesis being controlled by the first enzyme in the pathway, PRPP amidotransferase. The activity of this enzyme is inhibited by high intracellular concentrations of purines. Salvage recovery of purines is likewise enzymatically catalyzed, with the critical enzyme in this case being hypoxanthine phosphoribosyltransferase (HPRT). The rate-limiting factor for both pathways is the availability of PRPP (Holmes *et al.* 1973; Wood *et al.* 1973). It is now clear that at least four separate enzyme alterations may result in clinical gout without other clinical findings. The specific enzyme alterations are:

(1) PRPP amidotransferase with altered feedback inhibition, such that purines continue to be synthesized even when high levels of purine are already present. Excess purine is then catabolized to yield excessive amounts of uric acid (Henderson *et al.* 1968).

(2) Partial HPRT deficiency, such that there is decreased PRPP utilization by the salvage pathway. Excess PRPP is then available for the *de novo* pathway, leading to excessive synthesis of purines and to excess uric acid (Kelly *et al.* 1967).

(3) Increased activity of glutathionine reductase, leading to increased PRPP production and the same consequences described above (Long 1967).

(4) Increased activity of PRPP synthetase, likewise leading to increased

availability of PRPP and the same physiological consequences described above (Becker *et al.* 1973).

Finally, there are two severe metabolic diseases (complete HRPT deficiency and glucose-6-phosphatase deficiency) which include severe gout among their stigmata (Seegmiller *et al.* 1967; Alepa *et al.* 1967). Each of these mechanisms individually accounts for only a small proportion of the total number of gouty patients; furthermore, most cases of gout undoubtedly have a more complex etiology. However, the example of gout makes two important points: (1) common disorders with a polygenic component are in fact genetically heterogeneous; and (2) separate gene alterations in biochemically related pathways might possibly interact to produce a clinically recognizable phenotype.

This last point— that genes or gene products may interact to produce a given phenotype—leads us directly to a still more complicated type of polygenic model. One could envision a situation in which a series of very small enzymatic alterations, each of which would be individually negligible, might in combination lead to diseases with just the sort of complicated genetic predisposition and environmental compounding that we see in gout and diabetes. Unfortunately, molecular substantiation of this type of hypothesis may be very difficult, as identification of small alterations will necessitate extremely sensitive techniques. At the level of epidemiological and quantitative studies of the inheritance of common traits, however, such models have been studied both in human populations and in animal and plant experimental populations. It has been suggested, for example, that the distribution of liability to such diseases as cleft lip and palate in human populations follows a Gaussian mode, as shown in Fig. 10.4, and that only individuals whose genotypes place them above a certain threshold T run an appreciable risk of manifesting the disorder (Falconer 1965; Carter 1973). According to at least one statement of this hypothesis, exposure of liable individuals to precipitating environmental agents leads to clinical manifestation of the disease (Carter 1973). An important prediction of this model is that first degree relatives of affected individuals have a risk of disease which is increased above the general populational risk; the specific increase in risk can be calculated if one knows the incidence of the particular disorder in the general population. Second and third degree relatives likewise have an increased and predictable risk of developing the disease under study. As it turns out, the actual population data for increased incidence of both cleft lip and palate and diabetes among monozygotic twins and first and second degree relatives of affected individuals fit the values predicted by a threshold model quite well (Cavalli-Sforza 1969). As a variety of investigators have noted, a threshold model is conceptually consistent with both polygenic and multifactorial inheritance.

A more direct approach to the study of additive or interacting genes is

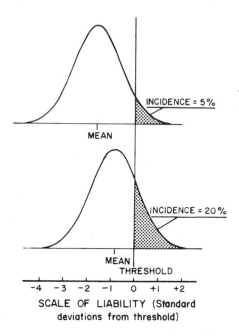

From Falconer (1965)

FIG. 10.4. ILLUSTRATIONS OF TWO POPULATIONS OR GROUPS WITH DIFFERENT
MEAN LIABILITIES.

The liability is normally distributed, with the same variance in the two groups. The
groups are compared by reference to a fixed threshold. The stippled portions are the
affected individuals with the incidences shown.

possible with plant or animal experimental systems. Here the environment
may be kept virtually constant, so that one may attribute all observed
variance to genetic differences; or conversely, the genotype may be held
constant, so that all observed variance may be attributed to environmental
factors. If the assumption is made that each gene contributes equally to the
expression of phenotype, it is then possible to (1) calculate the number of
genes involved in the production of a given phenotype and (2) specify the
environmental factors which will precipitate the expression of disease in a
genetically susceptible individual. Several studies of this type have been
carried out with laboratory animals which do and do not develop diabetes
in their natural environment. The findings of these studies are too numerous to discuss; in a particularly striking series of experiments, however,
Gerritsen and his associates conducted a series of matings between different
inbred strains of nondiabetic Chinese hamsters, and attempted to predict
the incidence of diabetes among offspring derived from these matings. They
found their data to be consistent with a model in which four separate,

autosomal recessive loci contributed to a genetic predisposition for the diabetes state (Gerritsen *et al.* 1970). In other animal models, it is clear that additional and different factors are involved. In summary, then, the genetic contributions to multifactorial inheritance may be single, may be multiple but separately acting, or may be multiple and act additively or inter-actionally.

Just as the genetic components in multifactorial situations are hetero-geneous, so are the environmental components multiple. The role of diet, for example, in the development and exacerbation of gout and diabetes is well-known. In the case of diabetes, general obesity, excessive intake of carbohydrates and increased level of stress have each been suggested as important (and in some cases, exclusive) precipitating factors in the clinical manifestation of the disease state (Cohen 1961; Rimoin and Schimke 1971). We have already mentioned a case in which a chemical compound (suxa-methonium) is the triggering factor in the development of a disease state. The recent description of a genetically based differential sensitivity to the hydrocarbons found in tobacco smoke adds an additional example of chemically mediated disease (Kellerman *et al.* 1973). As more and more carcinogenic compounds are identified, more differentially susceptible gen-otypes will probably be found. In addition to diet and chemicals, it now appears that viruses may be involved in the clinical manifestation of certain multifactorial disorders. Studies of mouse mammary tumors, for example, clearly demonstrate the interaction between specific viruses and genetically susceptible animals. Recent research suggests that acute juvenile diabetes may most frequently result from viral infection of genetically susceptible youngsters (Maugh 1975). An exhaustive enumeration of possible environ-mental agents contributing to multifactorial disorders would include many additional categories; diet, chemical compounds and viruses are simply illustrative and perhaps the most cogent examples.

I would now like to turn to a brief consideration of the interaction between genetic and environmental factors, by returning to the example of diabetes. In attempting to explain the high populational incidence of diabetes, Neel (1962) proposed that the diabetic phenotype was in fact an evolutionary relic of a "thrifty" genotype which, under conditions of nutri-tional scarcity, would have increased survival value. Certain of the bio-chemical foundations upon which Need bases his arguments may no longer be valid, but the general concept remains a useful model from which to work. Briefly, he suggests that a genotype which is maximally responsive to changes in blood glucose level might be able to make optimum use of stored food substances, and thus might have an increased survival potential in terms of relative insufficiency of food. In primitive conditions, where periods of plenty alternate with periods of starvation, and where intense physical activity was required as a condition of survival, a responsive genotype would be a definite asset. By contrast, in modern society, where food is constantly available and where increased stress is not commonly accompanied by increased physical activity, such a genotype would be disadvantageous. In civilized societies, there is an increased incidence in diabetes associated with increased obesity and paralleled by (or associated with?) increased stress. Neel suggests that if present resources continue to dwindle, the "thrifty" genotype may once again possess a selective advantage. Unfortunately, a molecular understanding of the genetic-environmental interactions for diabetes, and indeed for most multifactorial disorders, is almost nonexistent at the present time.

Finally, we might ask what the relationship between multifactorial inheritance and our present world nutritional dilemma is. First, in attempting to solve nutritional problems for the total human population, it is useful to remember that subpopulations differ from one another genetically and biochemically; one might even speak of the biochemical individuality of a particular human population. Thus there may be distinct biological constraints on the appropriate nutrients for a given individual, as well as cultural constraints on the types of nutrients which are palatable to a particular person. If we remember this sort of constraint, we should be able to avoid the dilemma of starvation on the one hand versus inappropriate nutrition on the other. Secondly, it may be useful to note that the particular sort of "over-nutrition" characteristic of some civilized societies may in itself be disease-producing, and that health may best be served by somewhat greater nutritional restraint. The goal, it seems to me, is not maximal quantity of nutritional resources, but appropriate distribution of quality resources.

REFERENCES

ALEPA, F. P., HOWELL, R. R., KLINENBERG, J. R., and SEEGMILLER, J. E. 1967. Relationship between glycogen storage disease and tophaceous gout. Am. J. Med. *42*, 58.
BARBOSA, J., and DOW, R. P. 1975. Autosomal dominant inheritance of juvenile onset, non-insulin dependent diabetes mellitus. Diabetes *24*, 402.
BECKER, M. A., MEYER, L. J., WOOD, A. W., and SEEGMILLER, J. E. 1973. Purine overproduction in man associated with increased phosphoribosylpyrophosphate synthetase activity. Science *179*, 1123.
BERRY, H., SUTHERLAND, B. S., and GUEST, G. M. 1957. Phenylalanine tolerance tests on relatives of phenylketonuric children. Am. J. Hum. Genet. *9*, 310.
CARTER, C. O. 1969. Genetics of common disorders. Br. Med. Bull. *25*, 52.
CARTER, C. O. 1973. Multifactorial genetic disease. *In* Medical Genetics. V. A. McKusick and R. Claiborne (Editors). HP Publishing Co., New York.
CAVALLI-SFORZA, L. L., and BODMER, W. F. 1969. The Genetics of Human Populations. W. H. Freeman, San Francisco.
COHEN, A. M. 1961. Prevalence of diabetes among different ethnic Jewish groups in Israel. Metabolism *10*, 50.
COOKE, A. M., FITZGERALD, M. G., MALINS, J. M., and PYKE, D. A. 1966. Diabetes in children of diabetic couples. Br. Med. J. *2*, 674.

DAVIES, R. O., MARTON, A. V., and KALOW, W. 1960. The action of normal and atypical cholinesterase of human serum upon a series of esters of choline. Can. J. Biochem. Physiol. *38*, 545.

FALCONER, D. S. 1965. The inheritance of liability to certain diseases, estimated from the incidence among relatives. Ann. Hum. Genet. *29*, 51.

FALCONER, D. S. 1967. The inheritance of liability to diseases with variable age of onset with particular reference to diabetes mellitus. Ann. Hum. Genet. *31*, 1.

GERRITSEN, G. C., NEEDHAM, L. B., SCHMIDT, F. L., and DULIN, W. E. 1970. Studies on the prediction and development of diabetes in offspring of diabetic Chinese hamsters. Diabetologia *6*, 158.

HARRIS, H., WHITTAKER, M., LEHMANN, H., and SILK, E. 1960. The pseudocholinesterase variants. Esterase levels and dibucaine numbers in families seleted through suxamethonium sensitive individuals. Acta. Genet. Stat. Med. *10*, 1.

HENDERSON, J. F., ROSENBLOOM, F. M., KELLY, W. N., and SEEGMILLER, J. E. 1968. Variations in purine metabolism of cultured skin fibroblasts from patients with gout. J. Clin. Invest. *47*, 1511.

HOLMES, E. W., WYNGAARDEN, J. B., and KELLEY, W. N. 1973. Human glutamine phosphoribosyl pyrophosphate amidotransferase: Two molecular forms interconvertible by purine nucleotides and phosphoribosylpyrophosphate. J. Biol. Chem. *248*, 6035.

KAHN, C. B., SOELDNER, J. S., GLEASON, R. E., ROJAS, L., CAMERINI-DAVALOS, R. A., and MARBLE, A. 1969. Clinical and chemical diabetes in offspring of diabetic couples. New Eng. J. Med. *281*, 343.

KELLERMAN, G., LUYTEN-KELLERMAN, M., and SHAW, C. R. 1973. Genetic variation of aryl hydrocarbon hydroxylase in human lymphocytes. Am. J. Hum. Genet. *25*, 327.

KELLEY, W. N., ROSENBLOOM, F. M., HENDERSON, J. F., and SEEGMILLER, J. E. 1967. A specific enzyme defect in gout associated with overproduction of uric acid. Proc. Nat. Acad. Sci. USA *57*, 1735.

KNOX, W. E., and MESSINGER, E. 1958. The detection of the metabolic effects of the recessive gene for phenylketonuria. Am. J. Hum. Genet. *10*, 53.

LONG, W. K. 1967. Glutathione reductase in red blood cells: Variant association with gout. Science *155*, 712.

MAUGH, T. 1975. Diabetes III (Research News), Science *188*, 920.

MC KUSICK, V. A. 1975. Mendelian Inheritance in Man, 4th Edition. Johns Hopkins Univ. Press, Baltimore, Md.

NEEL, J. V. 1962. Diabetes mellitus: A "thrifty" genotype rendered detrimental by "progress"? Am. J. Hum. Genet. *14*, 353.

NEEL, J. V. 1969. Current concepts of the genetic basis of diabetes mellitus and the biological significance of the diabetic predisposition. Excerpta Medica *72S*, 68.

RENOLD, A. E., STAUFFACHER, W., and CAHILL, G. F. 1972. Diabetes mellitus, *In* The Metabolic Basis of Inherited Disease. J. B. Stanbury, J. B. Wyngaarden and D. S. Frederickson (Editors). McGraw Hill, New York.

RIMOIN, D. L., and SCHIMKE, N. 1971. Genetic Disorders of the Endocrine Glands. C. V. Mosby Co., St. Louis, Mo.

SEEGMILLER, J. E., ROSENBLOOM, F. M., and KELLEY, W. N. 1967. Enzyme defect associated with a sex-linked human neurological disorder and excessive purine synthesis. Science *155*, 1682.

SIMPSON, N. E. 1964. Multifactorial inheritance: A possible hypothesis for diabetes. Diabetes *11*, 56.

SPENCER, N., HOPKINSON, D. A., and HARRIS, H. 1964. Quantitative differences and gene dosage in the human red cell acid phosphatase polymorphism. Nature *201*, 299.

TATTERSALL, R. B., and FAJANS, S. S. 1975. A difference between the inheritance of classical juvenile-onset and maturity-onset type diabetes of young people. Diabetes *24*, 44.

WOOD, A. W., BECKER, M. A., and SEEGMILLER, J. E. 1973. Purine nucleotide synthesis in lymphoblasts cultured from normal subjects and a patient with Lesch-Nyhan syndrome. Biochem. Genet. *9*, 261.

WYNGAARDEN, J. B., and KELLEY, W. N. 1972. Gout. *In* The Metabolic Basis of Inherited Disease. J. B. Stanbury, J. B. Wyngaarden and D. S. Frederickson (Editors). McGraw Hill, New York.

CHAPTER 11

Nevin S. Scrimshaw
Vernon R. Young

Biological Variability and Nutrient Needs

The recommended safe allowances for the essential nutrients, as developed by various FAO/WHO Expert Committees (1975), are intended to apply to all healthy populations of the world, and most national recommended allowances are derived from them. Yet, almost without exception, they are based on limited available data from small and unrepresentative numbers of persons. Most commonly, these have been healthy young Caucasian adults studied under protected and favorable circumstances. In fact, the available data are not adequate for assessing the nature and extent of variability in the requirements among individuals for any of the known essential nutrients.

Appropriate minimum physiological allowances cannot be formulated for population groups until the variation in requirements among apparently similar individuals has been studied in a systematic and critical way by valid criteria. Persons with complicating physical conditions or who give results which appear anomalous are generally eliminated from these studies. The latter may need to be omitted until it is determined whether they represent biological variation or experimental errors of various sorts, but such follow-up is rarely done or reported.

In this discussion we emphasize the multiple factors contributing to individual variations in nutrient requirements and then illustrate their specific application to dietary requirements for iron and for protein. The requirements for these two nutrients are of far more than just academic interest, since on a global basis more than 460 million persons have been estimated to be suffering from serious protein-calorie malnutrition (NAS 1975), and iron deficiency is the most widespread nutritional deficiency in industrialized countries (Kessner and Kalk 1973) and common throughout the world (WHO 1968).

GENERAL PRINCIPLES

The first component of variation in requirements is that introduced by genetic differences. The numerous inborn errors of metabolism are extreme examples of genetic variation in humans, and many of these have important nutritional implications. Examples are the high vitamin B-6 requirement of individuals with deficient activity of cystathionine synthase (Mudd et al. 1970), and the need to restrict phenylalanine and branched

102

chain amino acids in patients suffering from deficiencies in phenylalanine hydroxylase and branched chain ketoacid decarboxylase respectively (Scriver and Rosenberg 1973). Any biochemical value offers an example of the so-called normal variation. Figure 11.1 shows the distribution in plasma alanine aminotransferase and asparate aminotransferase activity for a population of 12,682 healthy people of various ages (Siest *et al*. 1975), although some part of this variation is due to nongenetic factors, including age, environmental and methodological variables. The same cannot be said, however, of the anatomical variation in normal stomachs, shown pictorially in Fig. 11.2, although this variation could be influenced by external factors affecting the intrauterine environment.

The universality of biological variation is well-recognized and accepted, although insufficient attention has been given to the extent to which the expression of genes is influenced by environmental factors. In the practice of nutrition, the variation of importance is the actual expression of genes in

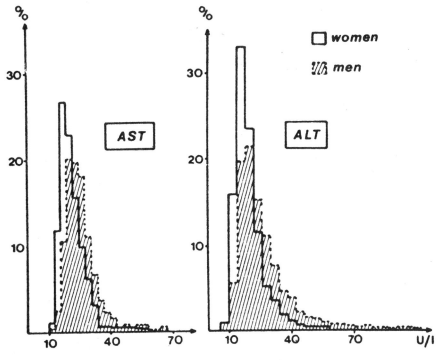

From Siest et al. (1975)

FIG. 11.1. HISTOGRAMS OF PLASMA ASPARATE AMINOTRANSFERASE AND ALANINE AMINOTRANFERASE ACTIVITIES IN STUDY POPULATION OF 12,682 HEALTHY PEOPLE

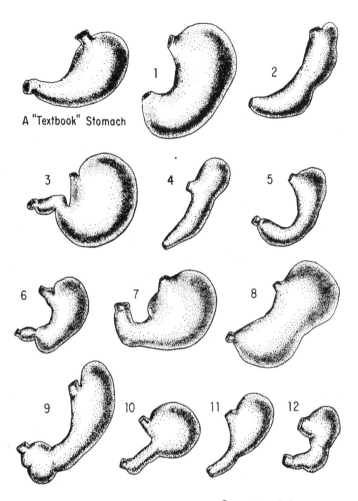

A "Textbook" Stomach

Courtesy of Anson

FIG. 11.2. GROSS ANATOMICAL VARIATIONS IN HUMAN STOMACHS

The figures are drawn from actual specimens by B. J. Anson.

the individual, not their inherent potential alone. Thus, it is the *phenotype*, rather than the genotype, with which an assessment of nutrient requirements and allowances is chiefly concerned.

Genes for tallness will not give rise to a tall individual if malnutrition during pregnancy and early childhood limits growth. Some individuals reared in favorable circumstances will be short for genetic reasons, and others in underprivileged circumstances may be of equal stature for environmental reasons. The latter then become for this characteristic a phenocopy of the former. When individuals who are short in stature for environmental, rather than genetic, reasons become exposed to favorable conditions, stature is increased, as exemplified by the secular trends in height of Japanese adults, with a greater proportion of the full genetic potential being expressed (Kimura 1967). Other striking examples are the studies of Walton and Hammond (1938), which showed the marked influences of the maternal environment on the growth and development of large and small breeds of horses.

Frequently, differences in body size are dismissed as unimportant for the individual or society. When they are due to genetic differences, this is so. But when differences in growth, development, and body size are due to nutritional and other environmental factors, they cannot be disregarded. There is abundant evidence that under these conditions impaired growth is associated with increased susceptibility to infection (Scrimshaw et al. 1968), decreased performance on various tests of learning and behavior (Scrimshaw and Gordon 1968), and other undesirable functional qualities. Limited growth may represent successful physical and metabolic adaptation to inadequate nutrition, but it may only be achieved at a social cost that is unacceptable in today's world. Man's future survival will depend far more on his capacity to achieve social adaptation than directly on his ability to adjust metabolically and physiologically to environmental changes.

Nutrient requirements depend on a variety of environmental and host factors (Table 11.1). Those host factors which are associated with inherent genetic variation and with sex, growth and development, pregnancy and lactation are generally taken into account in the formulation of recom-

TABLE 11.1

A LISTING OF HOST AND ENVIRONMENTAL FACTORS IN
RELATION TO NUTRIENT REQUIREMENTS

Host Factors	Environmental Factors
Age	Physical
Sex	Biological
Genetic	Social (Cultural,
Physiological states	Economic, Political)
Growth	
Pregnancy	
Lactation	
Aging	
Pathological states	
Metabolic	
Traumatic	
Infectious	
Other Stress	
Neoplastic	

mended allowances for nutrients, but age considerations are usually limited to the growth period. Subsequent revisions of national and international allowances will need to pay more attention to the special nutritional problems of the elderly, since their numbers are increasing in the populations of North America and Europe. It is unrealistic to propose allowances intended only for the healthy elderly person if an important proportion of older individuals suffer from a variety of chronic pathologies that increase their nutritional needs.

In addition, differences in the frequency of stressful stimuli, such as infection and other pathological factors among the general population, have not been taken sufficiently into account in arriving at estimates of population allowances for essential nutrients. Nevertheless, they cannot be ignored without risk to the health of individuals in the regions of the world where these factors are of general public health significance.

Most host factors are influenced by environmental factors that may be physical (such as ambient temperature), biological (such as the presence of parasites and other infectious organisms) and/or social (such as physical activity, the wearing of clothes and other patterns of behavior). Environmental factors influence nutritional status through their effects on the production and availability of food and on the actual consumption of food, as well as their effect on nutrient requirements, which is the focus of our interest here. These principles can be illustrated more specifically by examining variation in iron requirements.

VARIATION IN IRON REQUIREMENTS

The epidemiological factors that contribute to variation in the dietary needs for iron and in iron nutritional status among individuals are shown in Fig. 11.3. Dietary iron requirements are influenced not only by growth, by physiological status, and by pathologies that lead to acute or chronic blood loss or interfere with the absorption and utilization of dietary iron, but also by iron nutritional status *per se*, since intestinal absorption of iron is greater in individuals with evidence of reduced iron reserves (Turnbull 1974). Even in well-nourished Swedish adults whose iron status is considered to be normal, there is wide variation in the efficiency of dietary iron absorption (Fig. 11.4). Under conditions where iron deficiency is common, as in the studies carried out in Caracas, the variation in iron absorption is even greater. Although studies show that there is a general relationship between iron nutritional status and the efficiency of dietary iron absorption, a relatively small proportion of the variability in iron absorption among individuals appears to be explained by differences in iron status *per se*, as currently assessed (see Hegsted 1972). The relatively low efficiency of iron absorption is a major factor in the determination of iron allowances, and it is important that the basis for the variation in iron absorption among healthy individuals be better understood.

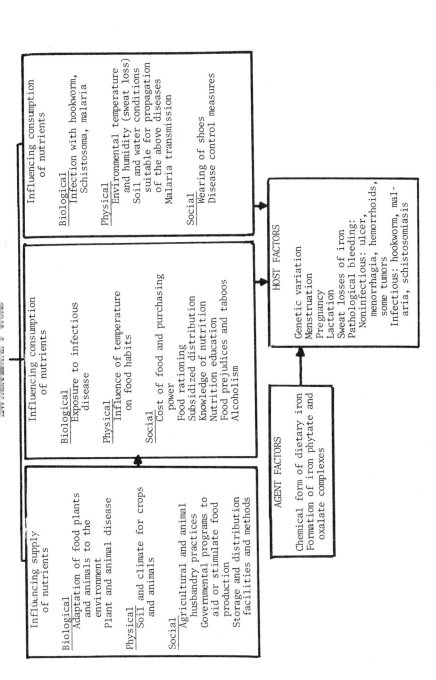

FIG. 11.3. A SCHEMATIC REPRESENTATION OF ENVIRONMENTAL, HOST AND AGENT FACTORS INFLUENCING IRON INTAKE, UTILIZATION AND REQUIREMENTS

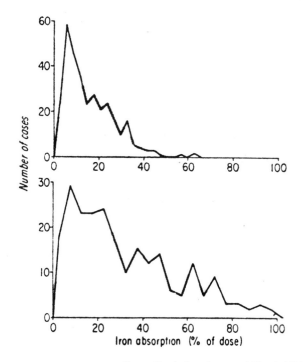

From Cook, Layrisse and Finch (1969)

FIG. 11.4. IRON ABSORPTION, EXPRESSED AS % OF ADMINISTERED DOSE, IN
320 HEALTHY SWEDISH (UPPER FIGURE) AND 234 VENEZUELAN (LOWER FIGURE)
SUBJECTS

Environmental influences in iron requirements are multiple. For iron requirements, as for those of most nutrients, the physical environment is the least important external influence, although enhanced sweating at high environmental temperatures might increase body iron loss in the tropics (Consolazio *et al.* 1963; Venkatachalem 1968; Green *et al.* 1968).

The infections arising out of the biological environment are potentially of great importance, especially the intestinal blood losses associated with hookworm and visceral schistosomiasis, urinary blood loss with schistosomiasis of the bladder, and the sequestering of iron in malaria pigment (Scrimshaw 1968; Beaton 1974). Similarly, the availability of plants with high phytate and oxalate content leads to decreased iron absorption (Turnbull 1974).

In the same sense that a microorganism is the agent of infectious disease, a dietary shortage of the nutrient may be considered as the agent of nutritional disease. However, in the epidemiological sense, disease is rarely caused by the agent alone; rather, it is the result of the complex interaction of environmental, host and agent factors. The same is true for nutritional disease and nutrient requirements. Therefore, appropriate dietary allowances will be determined by the interplay among these various factors for a given population group.

Agent factors for iron deficiency are also listed in Fig. 11.3. Reduced iron—that is, iron in the ferrous state as in ferrous sulfate or finely divided elemental iron—is more effectively absorbed than ferric iron, such as ferric chloride or iron pyrophosphate (Scrimshaw 1968). However, as stated

TABLE 11.2

1973 FAO/WHO APPROACH TO THE FACTORIAL ESTIMATION OF
HUMAN PROTEIN REQUIREMENTS AND ALLOWANCES

(1) Total obligatory N losses (O_N)	=	Obligatory urinary N + obligatory fecal N + skin N + miscellaneous N
(2) Other N requirements:		Growth (G_N) Pregnancy (P_N) Lactation (L_N)
(3) Total minimum N requirements for maintenance or growth	=	$O_N + G_N$
(4) Nitrogen requirement adjusted for efficiency N utilization (R_N)	=	$(O_N + G_N) \times 1.3$
(5) Safe practical allowance, adjusting for individual variability (SPA)	=	$R_N \times 1.3$
(6) Allowance for pregnancy or lactation	=	$SPA + [(P_N \text{ or } L_N)(1.3)] \times 1.3$

Note: The safe practical allowance for nitrogen is converted to a protein allowance by multiplying with the factor 6.25.

earlier, the absorption of ferrous iron is modified when ingested in combination with phytates and oxalates, found naturally in spinach and other green leaves (Beaton 1974). The whole grain, unleavened bread in North Africa and the Middle East is also high in these factors, potentially reducing the availability of iron, zinc and probably other mineral elements. Other inhibitory factors may also contribute to the low absorption of iron for diets typical of lower socioeconomic segments of populations in Southeast Asia (Hallberg et al. 1974). Conversely, the heme iron found in meat is much better absorbed than iron of vegetable origin. In general, iron is poorly absorbed from diets without some heme iron, and small amounts of red meat improve the overall absorption of dietary iron (Cook and Monsen 1975).

The extent to which the diet is high in phytates and oxalates and low in heme iron from meat depends primarily on social, economic and cultural factors, such as economic status, governmental policies, food beliefs and practices, to mention only a few. This is also true for the occurrence of infections influencing iron requirements. Hookworm occurrence depends on favorable temperature and soil conditions, but also on defecation habits and the wearing of shoes. The prevalence of schistosomiasis is associated with irrigation, bathing and washing practices.

From these considerations, it would clearly be inappropriate, as a basis for estimating safe iron intakes for all of the populations of the world, to study only a small group of Caucasian U. S. university students who are free of all identifiable disease, and whose diet contains a generous amount of meat protein. It is equally inappropriate to similarly limit the experimental studies for assessing protein allowances.

VARIATION IN PROTEIN REQUIREMENTS

The factorial approach to protein requirements was first used in the 1965 joint FAO/WHO Expert Committee Report on Protein Requirements (FAO/WHO 1965). This approach, represented in Table 11.2 was subsequently utilized by the 1971 FAO/WHO Expert Group on Energy and Protein Requirements (FAO/WHO 1973). This procedure is based on the assumption that maintenance protein needs in adult man should be related to the sum of the minimum or obligatory nitrogen losses, i.e., losses which occur when the body is subjected to conditions of maximum adaptation induced by ingestion of a diet low in protein. Thus, these nitrogen losses were determined after subjects consumed a protein-free, but otherwise fully adequate, diet for about one or two weeks. Estimations of nitrogen retained during growth and pregnancy, as well as the protein and amino acid nitrogen excreted in breast milk during lactation, are added to these summated losses to arrive at allowances for infants, children and adolescents, and for pregnant and lactating women. Some of the methodological and physiological inadequacies of this approach have been discussed earlier by us (Young et al. 1973, Young and Scrimshaw 1977), but they are worth considering here in the context of variability in nutrient requirements.

For normal distribution, the mean total obligatory nitrogen loss plus 1 standard deviation (S.D.) covers approximately two-thirds of the populations, and the mean plus 2 S.D. approximately 97.5%. This concept, on the population distribution of nutrient requirements, is schematically depicted in Fig. 11.5.

When individual MIT students were given a very low protein or protein-free diet (Fig. 11.6), they responded differently with respect to the time taken to adjust to a new level of urinary nitrogen output, as well as in the level achieved (Scrimshaw et al. 1972; Rand et al. 1976). The actual dis-

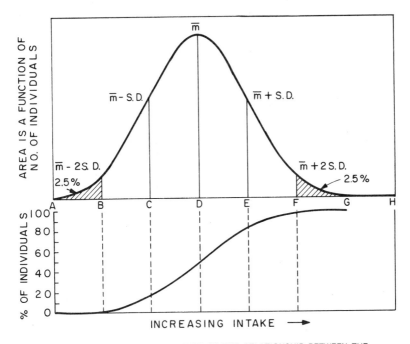

tribution of obligatory nitrogen values for 83 Caucasian male MIT students
during the last 5 days of a 14-day protein-free diet period, during which the
dietary energy intake was generous, is given in Fig. 11.7. The standard
deviation of this distribution corresponds to about 15% of the mean value.
The mean plus 30% should account for the obligatory urinary loss of about
97.5% of this population.

Figure 11.8 shows how well this population fits the normal curve for this
parameter. The straight line is the theoretical Caucasian distribution, and
the points for obligatory urinary nitrogen losses all fall almost precisely on
this line. These are the only adequate existing data on the nature of the
distribution of nitrogen requirements within a population group, assuming
that obligatory urinary nitrogen losses bear a predictable relationship to
the individual's actual protein needs. However, this assumption has not
been sufficiently tested experimentally.

When this study on the obligatory urinary nitrogen losses was repeated
in an essentially identical manner on university students in Taiwan National University (Huang *et al.* 1972), the distribution of obligatory nitrogen
values proved to be quite different (Fig. 11.7). We do not know how much

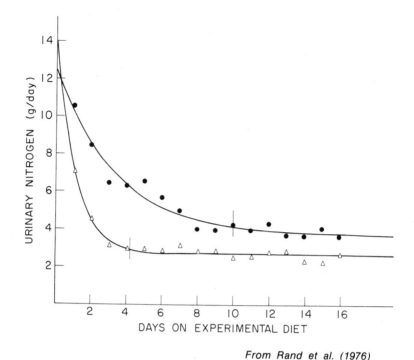

From Rand et al. (1976)

FIG. 11.6. DATA AND PLOTS OF THE SINGLE EXPONENTIAL EQUATION FITS OF
URINARY NITROGEN EXCRETION FOR TWO YOUNG MEN CONSUMING A VERY
LOW PROTEIN DIET

The solid lines represent the fitted equation for each subject, and the vertical lines at
4.2 and 10 days represent estimated time to achieve stability in urinary N output.

of these differences in host response are due to genetic influences, and how
much to adaptive phenotypic alterations in the metabolism and utilization
of amino acids for maintenance of body protein. The possibility cannot be
ruled out that prior protein intake—represented by a dependence for generations, or even a lifetime, on rice as a major source of protein—has
resulted in the development of efficient mechanisms for conservation when
the dietary supply is low in essential amino acids. This problem is somewhat analogous to the marked differences in the amount of calcium required to meet maintenance requirements in adult subjects, depending on
their habitual calcium and protein intakes (Irwin and Kienholz 1973).

The matter is far more complicated than expected since, as shown in
Table 11.3, a reexamination of some of these same individuals during the
hot season of the year gave still lower values for total obligatory nitrogen
losses (Huang et al. 1972). More important than variation in obligatory
urinary nitrogen losses, however, are the intakes of protein required for

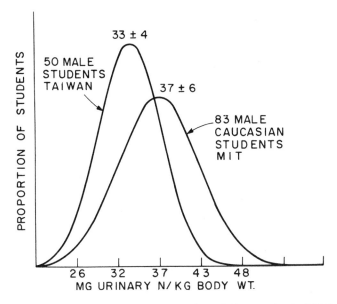

Adapted from Scrimshaw et al. and Huang et. al. (1972)

FIG. 11.7. DISTRIBUTION OF OBLIGATORY URINARY NITROGEN LOSSES IN A
POPULATION OF 83 MALE MIT STUDENTS, AND IN A POPULATION OF 50 MALE
STUDENTS AT THE TAIWAN NATIONAL UNIVERSITY

normal maintenance among individuals. For this, many additional factors
need to be considered.

Figure 11.9 shows the poorer absorption of protein by children recovered
from kwashiorkor in Guatemala than by MIT students (Scrimshaw 1963).
Differences between the two groups are presumably not simply due to an
age factor, since well-nourished infants and children show high apparent
nitrogen absorption comparable to that for healthy adults.

Figure 11.10 shows that, despite the generally good absorption of egg
protein by normal MIT students, there may be marked variation even
within a small group, with one subject absorbing only 55–60%. There
appears to be even greater individual variation in the apparent absorption
of nitrogen in young men consuming a single-cell protein source (Fig.
11.11).

It should be pointed out here that all of these studies only suggest the
extent of individual variation in nitrogen utilization because we do not
know the accuracy of the methods utilized. At the very least, repeated
observations within the same subjects at different times are needed. This
poses major practical and financial problems because of the difficulty and
the cost of human metabolic balance studies.

It is well-recognized that requirements are not basically for protein, but

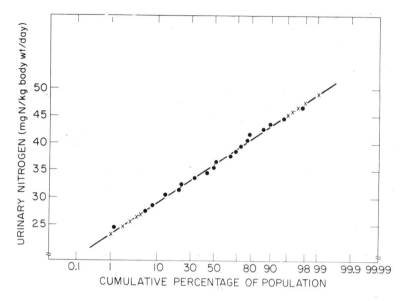

From Scrimshaw et al. (1972)

FIG. 11.8. PROBABILITY PLOT OF OBLIGATORY N LOSSES IN 83 YOUNG MIT
STUDENTS. SOLID DOTS ARE ACTUAL VALUES AND CROSSES INDICATE ESTI-
MATES OF HIGHEST AND LOWEST PERCENTILES

for essential amino acid in appropriate proportions and a source of nonspecific nitrogen. This aspect of protein nutrition need not be discussed
here. It is worth noting, however, that present estimates of adult amino
acid requirements are based mainly on metabolic balance studies with small
numbers of midwestern university students, studied about 25–30 years ago
(Rose 1957). Differences of over 100% among individuals with lowest and
highest requirements were often observed for some of the essential amino
acids. This has been a common finding in more recent studies (Holt and

TABLE 11.3

EFFECT OF ENVIRONMENTAL TEMPERATURE ON
OBLIGATORY URINARY NITROGEN LOSSES IN
NINE YOUNG MEN

Season	Temp (°C)	Urinary N (mg/day)
Hot	28.2	1717 ± 293[1]
Cooler	17.1	1948 ± 189

Calculated from data of Huang et al. (1972).
[1]Mean ± S.D. for 9 subjects. Difference between the two seasons was statistically significant
(P < 0.01).

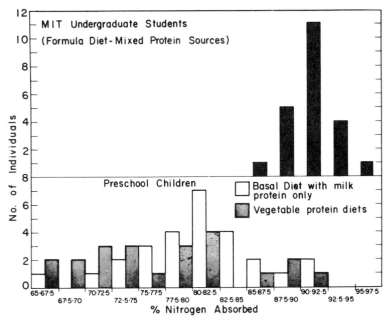

INDIVIDUAL VARIATION IN % OF DIETARY N INTAKE ABSORBED

Adapted from Scrimshaw (1963)

FIG. 11.9. COMPARISON OF DIETARY N ABSORPTION IN HEALTHY YOUNG MIT
STUDENTS AND IN PRE-SCHOOL CHILDREN WHO HAD RECOVERED FROM
KWASHIORKOR

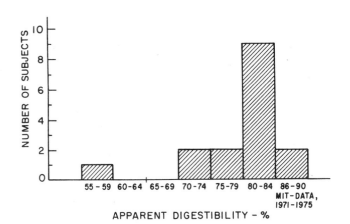

Adapted from Young et al. (1973)

FIG. 11.10. INDIVIDUAL VARIATION IN DIGESTIBILITY OF EGG PROTEIN, WITHIN
THE SUBMAINTENANCE RANGE IN PROTEIN INTAKE, IN YOUNG MEN

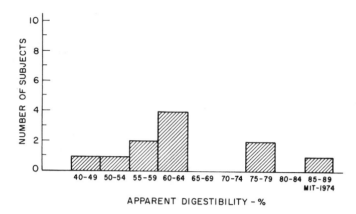

From unpublished MIT results

FIG. 11.11   INDIVIDUAL VARIATION IN DIGESTIBILITY OF A FUNGAL SOURCE OF SINGLE CELL PROTEIN (SCP) IN YOUNG ADULT MEN

Snyderman 1965; Leverton *et al.* 1956A, B, C; Hegsted 1963) concerned with estimation of individual essential amino acid requirements, including the studies of the tryptophan and leucine requirements of adult subjects which are summarized in Table 11.4

In addition to the variation in requirements among individuals in a single experiment, this table shows that the dietary condition and criteria used to judge the requirements have varied both among and within laboratories. This makes it impossible to utilize the aggregate data to develop even an approximation of the variation in requirements for any of the essential amino acids, as we have discussed previously (Young and Scrimshaw 1977).

As illustrated in Table 11.5, foods also differ markedly in their concentration of essential amino acids relative to total protein (FAO/WHO 1965), the so-called E/T ratio, with foods of animal origin generally being higher in essential amino acid concentration. The possible nutritional significance of E/T ratios for the individual can be tested by feeding a diet constant in protein and energy and progressively replacing some of the protein with a nonspecific nitrogen source, such as a mixture of glycine and diammonium citrate or a mixture of nonessential amino acids. Under these conditions, a change in urinary nitrogen excretion with such replacements (dilution) would indicate that the efficiency of utilization of the ingested nitrogen was altered.

The data shown in Fig. 11.12 indicate that, for the conditions tested, a young male university student could utilize egg protein diluted with 30% nonspecific nitrogen with no loss in efficiency of utilization; but with 40%

TABLE 11.4

A PARTIAL SUMMARY OF ESTIMATES OF THE ISOLEUCINE, LEUCINE, VALINE AND TRYPTOPHAN REQUIREMENTS IN ADULT SUBJECTS

Amino Acid	No. of Subjects	Sex	Estimated Requirement (mg/day)	(mg/kg/day)	Dietary Conditions EAAN[1]	TN[1]	Tryptophan (mg/day)	Amino Acid Pattern	Reference
Isoleucine	4	M	650–700	9–13	~1.7	10	300	Rat[2]	Rose et al. (1955)
	7	F	250–450	4–8	~1.0	6 or 7	150	Egg[3]	Swendseid & Dunn (1956)
	8	F	>422	7.5	0.7	6 or 10	320	Human[4]	Linkswiler et al. (1960)
Leucine	5	M	500–1100	7–14	1.2	10	300	Rat	Rose et al. (1955)
	13	F	170–710	3–12	~1.1	9.5	300	Egg	Leverton et al. (1956)
	19	F	40–150	0.7–3	0.7	5	320	Rose	Fisher et al. (1971)
Valine	5	M	400–800	7–13	1.3	10	500	Rat	Rose et al. (1955B)
	7	F	465–650	8–10	1.1	9	300	Egg	Leverton et al. (1956B)
	7	F	230–480	4–8	0.7	10	273	Human	Linkswiler et al (1958)
	9	F	100–200	2	0.7	5	320	Rose	Fisher et al. (1971)
Tryptophan	3	M	150–250	2–4	3.5	7–10	–	Rat	Rose et al. (1954)
	5	M	<225	3	?	7	–	Casein	Baldwin & Berg (1949)
	12	M	144–187	3	2.2	5.5	–	Egg	Young et al. (1971)
	8	F	82–157	1.5–3	1.2	10	–	Egg	Leverton et al. (1956C)
	5	F	50 or <	0.9 or <	0.7	5	–	Rose	Fisher et al. (1969)

[1]g/day

2, 3, 4 Patterned after rat amino acid requirement, egg protein and human requirement, respectively.

TABLE 11.5

RATIO OF TOTAL ESSENTIAL AMINO ACIDS TO TOTAL NITROGEN
IN SELECTED FOODSTUFFS AND IN THE FAO PROVISIONAL
PATTERN

Protein Sources	E/T Ratio (g/g)
Cassein	3.25
Egg, hen's	3.22
Milk, cow's	3.20
Milk, human	3.13
Beef liver	2.94
Beef heart	2.85
Beef muscle	2.79
Navy bean	2.79
Corn meal	2.78
Millet (Eleusine coracana)	2.75
Sweet potato	2.70
Pork tenderloin	2.67
Fish	2.66
Rice	2.61
Peas	2.59
Soya flour	2.58
Spinach	2.50
Sesame seed	2.47
Oats	2.30
Rye	2.17
Cotton seed	2.15
Sunflower seed	2.11
Peanut flour	2.08
White wheat flour	2.02
1957 FAO Pattern	2.02
Wheat gluten	1.99
Cassava	1.31
Gelatin	1.05

Source: FAO/ WHO (1965).

replacement with nonspecific nitrogen, urinary nitrogen excretion increased, reflecting a decrease in nitrogen utilization (Scrimshaw *et al.* 1966A). In the present context, an important point is that individuals varied greatly in this respect. In a group of 8 young men, one could not tolerate a replacement of more than 20%. For 3, the limit was 30% with 4, it was 40%, and one had not reached the limit at 50%. How this relates to man as either a carnivore or a vegetarian we leave to the speculation of anthropologists.

Figure 11.13 reveals another important variable in this respect: An individual who normally could tolerate 25% replacement of beef protein showed a marked increase in urinary nitrogen excretion at a lower (20%) replacement during a mild infection (Huang *et al.* 1966). An environmental

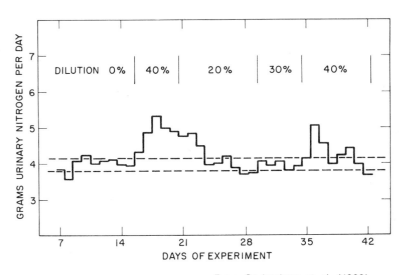

From Scrimshaw et al. (1966)

FIG. 11.12. EFFECT OF VARYING LEVELS OF ISONITROGENOUS REPLACEMENT (DILUTIN) OF EGG PROTEIN WITH A NON-SPECIFIC URINARY NITROGEN EXCRETION IN A YOUNG MALE MIT STUDENT CONSUMING A DIET PROVIDING 0.4G PROTEIN/KG/DAY

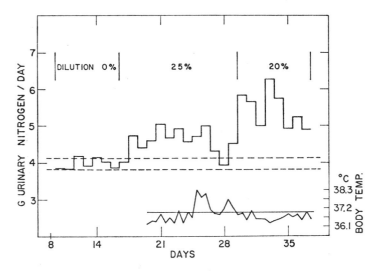

From Huang et al. (1966)

FIG. 11.13. EFFECTS OF A MILD, SPONTANEOUS INFECTION ON URINARY NITRO-GEN EXCRETION IN A YOUNG MALE STUDENT BEING STUDIED FOR THE IN-FLUENCE OF AN ISONITROGENOUS REPLACEMENT OF BEEF PROTEIN WITH NON-SPECIFIC NITROGEN

factor of major significance for individual protein needs and requirements for most other nutrients is the occurrence of infection. Any infection, no matter how mild or subclinical, has potentially adverse consequences whose significance depends on the previous nutritional status of the individual, the nature, severity, and duration of the infection, and the diet during and after the infectious episode.

During even mild infections, appetite is reduced and urinary nitrogen excretion is increased, as illustrated in Fig. 11.14, which shows nitrogen balance in adult men subjected to experimental tularemia (Beisel 1966).

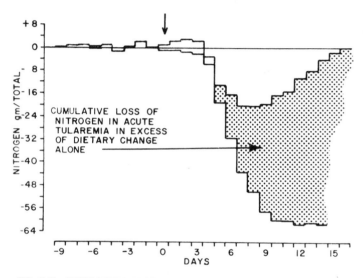

FIG. 11.14. CUMULATIVE NITROGEN LOSS IN ADULT SUBJECTS WITH TYPICAL TULUREMIA AND NON-EXPOSED MEN WHOSE DIETARY INTAKE WAS ADJUSTED TO MATCH THE CHANGES IN CONSUMPTION OBSERVED DURING ILLNESS

Where fever and/or diarrhea is present, particularly in young children, solid food tends to be withdrawn in favor of watery gruels. This social behavior adds to the adverse biological consequences of infection. Figure 11.15 illustrates the very high incidence of infection in children during the first 3 years of age in a Guatemalan village (Mata 1975). Because young children in developing countries have a high frequency of acute respiratory, diarrheal and other infections, the effects of infections on increases in the variability of individual needs for protein and other nutrients, as well as for dietary energy, are of great significance for public health programs and agricultural and food policies.

Other sources of stress can also result in increased nitrogen excretion, and therefore modify protein requirements. This is shown in Fig. 11.16,

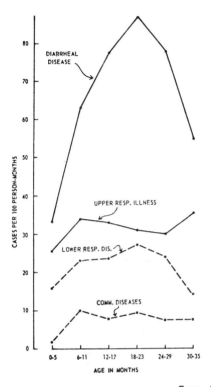

From Mata (1975)

FIG. 11.15. MORBIDITY RATES OF INFECTIOUS DISEASES BY AGE FOR 45
COHORT CHILDREN OBSERVED BETWEEN BIRTH AND THREE YEARS IN A GUATE-
MALAN VILLAGE

which demonstrates the effect of severe pain on nitrogen balance (Masek 1959). Also, we previously observed increasing negative nitrogen balance in a male high school student receiving protein sufficient to support nitrogen balance, but suffering acute anxiety about the study. As shown in Fig. 11.17, when this subject was transferred to a normal diet, the marked loss of body nitrogen was arrested. However, a return to the liquid formula diet again brought on anxiety and a further loss of body nitrogen. Similar effects on body nitrogen loss were seen in young men during metabolic balance studies carried out prior to and during final examinations, with about one-third of the MIT students responding with marked increases in daily urinary nitrogen output (Scrimshaw *et al.* 1966B).

Sweat loss during heavy physical exercise, as shown in Table 11.6 for nitrogen losses, is another possible source of variation in requirements for some nutrients, and one of potential importance for tropical countries.

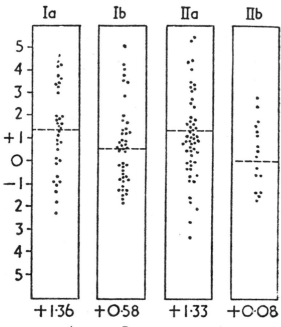

ACTION OF PHARMACOLOGICAL ANALGESIA
ON N BALANCE DURING PAIN

From Masek (1959)

FIG. 11.16. EFFECTS OF PAIN ON NITROGEN BALANCE IN ADULT HUMAN
SUBJECTS

Ia=days without pain; Ib=days when patients suffered from pain; IIa=days when pain was
alleviated by analgesics; IIb=days when pain was not relaxed after analgesics

However, discussion of the extent of possible adaptation to high environmental temperatures and sweat rates is beyond the scope of this paper.

Profound changes in physiological and biochemical parameters occur
during progression of the adult years, and an increased incidence of disease
is characteristic of old age (Strehler 1962). A neglected area of human
nutrient requirements concerns the effects of aging and of old age. Figure
11.18 illustrates the decrease in body cell mass with age, as estimated from
whole body potassium. In Table 11.7, the amount of body nitrogen has
been estimated for various stages of life. Changes in the amount and metabolic activity of the body cell mass with progressive aging probably affect
nutrient requirements, but again there is little adequate evidence to expand
upon this point (Young *et al.* 1976; Winterer *et al.* 1976).

In order to explore the metabolic basis and requirements for dietary

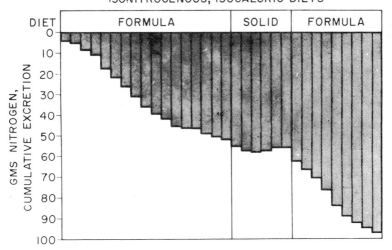

FIG. 11.17. CUMULATIVE N BALANCE IN A SINGLE MALE SUBJECT WHO DE-
VELOPED ACUTE ANXIETY WHILE PARTICIPATING IN A METABOLIC BALANCE
STUDY WHICH WAS BASED ON THE USE OF A LIQUID FORMULA DIET SUPPLYING
ADEQUATE PROTEIN AND ENERGY.

To eliminate the subject's concern, he was transferred for a period to an isonitrogenous,
isocaloric diet based on solid food. Each bar represents one day.

TABLE 11.6

INCREASE IN SWEAT NITROGEN LOSSES (MG N) IN UNTRAINED
YOUNG MEN, ADAPTED TO LOW LEVELS OF DIETARY PROTEIN
INTAKE, DURING A 30-MINUTE EXERCISE PERIOD

| Subject | Dietary Protein Intake (g/kg/day) | |
No.	0	0.3
	(mg N loss during exercise)	
1	302	395
2	359	279
3	253	267
4	126	163
5	243	-

Source: Unpublished results of Bourges, MIT Ph.D. Thesis (1968).
Note: Treadmill exercise at 4 m.p.h. and 10% grade, for 30 minutes under comfortable indoor
conditions.

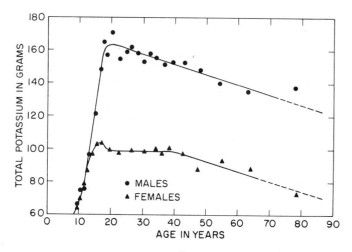

From Allen et al. (1960)

FIG. 11.18. TOTAL BODY POTASSIUM AS A FUNCTION OF AGE

protein in the elderly, we have measured obligatory nitrogen loss in older women and have compared the results with young adult men and women studied under essentially comparable experimental conditions (Table 11.8). The obligatory urinary nitrogen loss per kg body weight is similar in young and elderly women. From our preliminary evidence, however, it appears that ingested nitrogen may be used less efficiently in elderly women at nitrogen intakes of egg protein which are approximately double the total obligatory nitrogen losses.

TABLE 11.7

AN ESTIMATE OF TOTAL BODY NITROGEN
CONTENT IN MALE HUMANS AT VARIOUS TIMES OF LIFE

Stage of Life	g	g/kg body wt
Newborn (full term)[1]	66	19
Infant - 1 month[2]	64	15
Child - 8 years[3]	499	22
Teenager - 15 years[3]	1225	20
Young adult - 25 years[3]	1339	18
Elderly - 65 to 70 years[3]	1066	15

[1]From Widdowson and Dickerson (1964).
[2,3]Infant data calculated from those of Novak et al. (1970) and for older age groups from Forbes and Reina (1970) and Forbes (1972). Estimates of body nitrogen made from whole body potassium measurements assuming 68.1 mEq K per kg lean body mass and that 3 mEq K equivalent to 1 g nitrogen.

TABLE 11.8

OBLIGATORY NITROGEN LOSSES IN ELDERLY WOMEN, COMPARED
WITH PREVIOUS ESTIMATES IN YOUNG WOMEN AND YOUNG MEN[1]

Daily N Losses	Elderly Women[1]	Young Women[2]	Young Men[3]
Urinary			
g	1.52 ± 0.29	1.45 ± 0.20	2.69 ± 0.48
mg/kg body wt	24.4 ± 5.2	25.2 ± 3.3	37.2 ± 5.5
mg/basal kcal	1.44 ± 0.14[4]	1.14 ± 0.11	1.77 ± 0.30
g/g creatinine	2.11 ± 0.28	1.49 ± 0.02	1.58 ± 0.22
mg/kg BCM	89.5 ± 17.1	62 ± 10[5]	76.8 ± 12.5
Fecal			
g	0.61 ± 0.16	0.50 ± 0.08	0.63 ± 0.15
mg/kg body wt	9.8 ± 2.7	8.7 ± 2.5	8.8 ± 2.1
mg/basal kcal	0.59 ± 0.17[3]	0.40 ± 0.07	0.42 ± 0.11
Total (fecal & urinary)			
g	2.13 ± 0.36	1.96 ± 0.19	3.33 ± 0.54
mg/kg body wt	34.2 ± 6.3	33.9 ± 4.2	46.0 ± 6.0
mg/basal kcal	2.03 ± 0.24	1.54 ± 0.14	2.19 ± 0.34
g/g creatinine	2.96 ± 0.32	2.01 ± 0.14	1.94 ± 0.24

[1]From Scrimshaw et al. (1976).
[2]From Bricker and Smith (1951).
[3]From Scrimshaw et al. (1972).
[4]Based on data from 7 subjects.
[5]For comparative purposes, BCM was estimated from Forbes (1974).

Since most elderly people are not as healthy as those selected for our studies, the adequacy of the present FAO/WHO protein allowance, based on studies in young adults, is highly doubtful. More comparative studies in young adult and elderly subjects will be necessary before this aspect of protein nutrition in the elderly is satisfactorily resolved. Nevertheless, it seems likely from available data that individual variation is greater in this age group, even when the subjects have been selected for their apparent good health.

A final factor influencing variability in protein requirements is the effect of energy intake. It is an extremely important one, although frequently misunderstood and scientifically controversial. Energy requirements themselves vary widely among individuals, and are dependent upon the various environmental and host factors already discussed. Physical activity is a most important and well-recognized variable, but others are undoubtedly important as well. There are wide differences in the efficiency of utilization of energy for purposes of supporting tissue and organ functions (those involving the generation and subsequent utilization of high energy phosphate compounds such as ATP). The possible nutritional significance of this factor for man has not been sufficiently considered, despite the differing efficiencies of nutrient and energy utilization among breeds of farm livestock animals (NAS 1975B) and lines of mice (Bakker 1974). It is tempting to speculate that the variation in protein requirements among individuals may be determined, in part, by variations in the efficiency of energy utilization for protein synthetic functions.

In the past, considerable emphasis has been placed on the poorer utilization of dietary protein when dietary energy intake is deficient. But so often when this appears to be the case (from comparison of dietary intakes with FAO/WHO estimated caloric requirements), the energy intake is, in fact, not functionally inadequate because survival requires the individual to reduce his physical activity to the point where a balance between energy intake and expenditure is achieved. If this does not occur, the individual will waste away and eventually die. However, it is important to recognize that physiological adaptation to reduced energy intake may only be achieved at a social cost, and that the adaptation may still compromise the utilization of dietary protein.

Previous and current estimations of human protein requirements have paid little attention to the fact that excesses of energy intake decrease protein needs. The diets employed in short-term balance studies have usually been designed to prevent weight loss and maximize dietary protein utilization. The effect of this is that long-term protein requirements at usual caloric intakes have been underestimated.

This has been clearly demonstrated by the studies of Inoue et al. (1973); their results are summarized in Table 11.9. When usual energy intakes are maintained, more protein is needed for nitrogen balance than when excess energy is consumed. Furthermore, Calloway (1975) has shown that young men receiving 115% of the normal dietary energy requirements daily, plus 12 gm nitrogen from egg protein, lose less nitrogen in the urine than those

TABLE 11.9

EFFECT OF EXCESS ENERGY INTAKE ON THE UTILIZATION AND REQUIREMENTS FOR EGG AND RICE PROTEINS IN YOUNG MEN[1]

Protein Source	Energy	Efficiency of N Utilization[2] (%)	Mean Requirement Nitrogen (mg/kg)	Mean Requirement Conventional Protein (g/kg)
Egg	Excess	54	67	0.42
	Maintenance	41	90	0.56
Rice	Excess	47	82	0.51
	Maintenance	27	119	0.74

[1]From Inoue et al. (1973). Excess energy = 57 ± 2 kcal/kg. Maintenance energy = 45 ± 2 kcal/g.
[2]Value obtained from slope of regression of N balance on N intake.

receiving 100% or 85% of the estimated energy needs. Recently, Nageswara Rao *et al.* (1975) at the National Nutrition Institute in Hyderabad, India, described a similar inverse relationship between the level of energy intake and daily output of urinary nitrogen when dietary protein intake was held constant. Our own studies (Garza *et al.* 1976) confirm these observations and show (Fig. 11.19) that an approximately 9–20% energy intake in excess of estimated energy needs is required in order to achieve nitrogen balance or equilibrium in young men consuming the 1973 FAO/WHO "safe practical allowance" for egg protein.

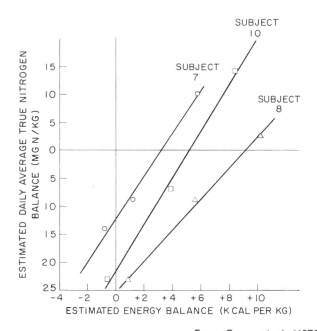

From Garza et al. (1976)

FIG. 11.19.   AN ESTIMATE OF THE EFFECT ON N BALANCE OF INCREMENTS IN ENERGY INTAKE ABOVE ESTIMATED ENERGY NEEDS IN THREE YOUNG MEN GIVEN EGG PROTEIN AT A LEVEL OF 0.57 G/KG/DAY

Energy balance was estimated by assuming that body weight change in excess of that predicted from the N retention represented fat deposition equivalent to 7800 Kcals.

Even more significant, our studies reveal that, when nitrogen balance is achieved only by excess energy intake, the resulting protein nutritional status may be inadequate, as detected by increases in the activity of serum alanine and aspartate aminotransferases, indicating deterioration in liver function (Garza *et al.* 1976). These results once again underscore the fact that metabolic interactions significantly influence the dietary requirements for nutrients, and introduce an additional level of complexity into the assessment of variability in nutrient requirements among individuals.

In summary, the multiple factors associated with the host and environment, plus the chemical form and availability of individual nutrients, result in a variability in nutrient requirements which is undoubtedly beyond that observed in controlled laboratory studies of select groups of healthy young adult subjects in industrialized countries. It is a sad commentary that we do not know the precise nature and extent of the individual variation in requirements for any of the essential nutrients, nor the quantitative importance of the host, agent and environmental factors which affect them.

With the increasingly precarious balance between population and food supply, it is important to determine, far more precisely that at present, the range of human nutritional requirements for adequate health. This will require the development of improved methodology, and the conduct of long-term studies in a wide range of population groups to cover differences in age, sex, physiological status and environmental factors. It is for this reason that one of the four priority areas of the Malnutrition Program of the U.S.-Japan Cooperative Medical Sciences Program stresses the urgent need for studies of the nutrient requirements of individuals living under the conditions prevailing in developing countries.

ACKNOWLEDGEMENTS

This is publication No. 2850 from the Department of Nutrition and Food Science, Massachusetts Institute of Technology. Unpublished studies by the authors referred to in this paper were supported by the MIT Health Sciences Fund and NIH grants AG00475 and AM15856.

REFERENCES

ALLEN, T. H., ANDERSON, E. C., and LANGHAM, W. H. 1960. Total body potassium and gross body composition in relation to age. J. Gerontol. *15*, 348.

BAKKER, H. 1974. Effect of selection for relative growth rate and body weight of mice on rate, composition and efficiency of growth. Meded. Landbouwhogeschool Wageningen *78*, 8, 1.

BALDWIN, H. R., and BERG, C. P. 1949. The influence of optical isomerism and acetylation upon the availability of tryptophan for maintenance in man. J. Nutr. *39*, 203.

BEATON, G. H. 1974. Epidemiology of iron deficiency. *In* Iron in Biochemistry and Medicine. A. Jacobs and M. Worwood (Editors). Academic Press, New York.

BEISEL, W. R. 1966. Effect of infection on human protein metabolism. Fed. Proc. *25*, 1682.

BRICKER, M. L. and SMITH, J. M. 1951. A study of endogenous nitrogen output of college women, with particular reference to the use of the creatinine output in the calculation of the biological values of the protein of egg and sunflower seed flour. J. Nutr. *44*, 553.

CALLOWAY, D. H. 1975. Nitrogen balance of men with marginal intakes of protein and energy. J. Nutr. *105*, 914

CONSOLAZIO, C. F. *et al.* 1963. Excretion of sodium, potassium, magnesium and iron in human sweat and the relation of each to balance and requirements. J. Nutr. *79*, 407.

COOK, J. D., LAYRISSE, M., and FINCH, C. A. 1969. The measurement of iron absorption. Blood *33*, 421.

COOK, J. D., and MONSEN, E. R. 1975. Food iron absorption. I. Use of a semisynthetic diet to study absorption of nonheme iron. Am. J. Clin. Nutr. *28*, 1289.

FAO/WHO. 1965. Protein Requirements. WHO Technical Reprint Ser. *301*. World Health Organization, Geneva, Switzerland.

FAO/WHO. 1973. Energy and Protein Requirements. WHO Technical Reprint Ser. *522*. World Health Organization, Geneva, Switzerland.

FISHER, H., BRUSH, M. K., and GRIMINGER, P. 1969. Reassessment of amino acid requirements of young women on low nitrogen diets. I. Lysine and tryptophan. Am. J. Clin. Nutr. *22*, 1190.

FISHER, H., BRUSH, M. K., and GRIMINGER, P. 1971. Reassessment of young women on low nitrogen diets. II. Leucine, methionine and valine. Am. J. Clin. Nutr. *24*, 1216.

FAO. 1975. Handbook of Human Nutritional Requirements. FAO Nutrition Studies *28*. Food and Agriculture Organization of the United Nations, Rome, Italy.

FORBES, G. B. 1974. Stature and lean body mass. Am. J. Clin. Nutr. *27*, 595.

FORBES, G. B., and REINA, J. C. 1970. Adult lean body mass declines with age: Some longitudinal observations. Metabolism *19*, 653.

GARZA, C., SCRIMSHAW, N. S., and YOUNG, V. R. 1976. Human protein requirements: The effect of variations in energy intake within the maintenance range. Am. J. Clin. Nutr. *29*, 280.

GREEN, R. *et al.* 1968. Body iron excretion in man: A collaborative study. Am. J. Med. *45*, 336.

HALLBERG, L. *et al.* 1974. Iron absorption from Southeast Asian Diets. Am. J. Clin. Nutr. *27*, 826.

HEGSTED, D. M. 1963. Variations in requirements of nutrients - amino acids. Fed. Proc. *22*, 1424.

HEGSTED, D. M. 1972. Problems in the interpretation of the Recommended Dietary Allowances. Ecol. Food Nutr. *1*, 255.

HOLT, L. E., and SNYDERMAN, S. E. 1965. Protein and amino acid requirements of children. Nutr. Abstr. Rev. *35*, 1.

HUANG, P. C., CHONG, H. E., and RAND, W. M. 1972. Obligatory urinary and fecal nitrogen losses in young Chinese men. J. Nutr. *102*, 1605.

HUANG, P. C., YOUNG, V. R., CHOLAKOS, B. and SCRIMSHAW, N. S. 1966. Determination of the minimum dietary essential amino acid-to-total nitrogen ratio for beef protein fed to young men. J. Nutr. *90*, 416.

INOUE, G., FUJITA, Y., and NIIYAMA, Y. 1973. Studies on protein requirements of young men fed egg protein and rice protein with excess and maintenance energy intakes. J. Nutr. *103*, 1673.

IRWIN, M. J., and KIENHOLZ, E. W. 1973. A conspectus of research on calcium requirements of man. J. Nutr. *103*, 1019.

KESSNER, J., and KALK, L. 1973. A strategy for evaluating health services. Institute of Medicine, National Academy of Sciences, Washington, D. C.

KIMURA, K. 1967. A consideration of the secular trend in Japanese for height and weight by a graphic method. Am. J. Phys. Anthrop. *27*, 89.

LEVERTON, R. M. *et al.* 1956A. The quantitative amino acid requirements of young women. V. Leucine. J. Nutr. *58*, 355.

LEVERTON, R. M. *et al.* 1956B. The quantitative requirements of young women. II. Valine. J. Nutr. *58*, 83.

LEVERTON, R. M., JOHNSON, M., PAZUR, J., and ELLISON, J. 1956C. The quantitative amino acid requirements of young women. III. Tryptophan. J. Nutr. *58*, 219.

LINKSWILER, H., FOX, H. M., GESCHWENDER, D., and FRY, P. C. 1958. Availability to man of amino acids from foods. II. Valine from corn. J. Nutr. *65*, 455.

LINKSWILER, H., FOX, H. M., and FRY, P. C. 1960. Availability to man of amino acids from foods. IV. Isoleucine from corn. J. Nutr. *72*, 397.

MASEK, J. 1959. Recommended Nutrient Allowances. *In* World Review of Nutrition and Dietetics, Vol. 3. Hafner Publishing Co., New York.

MATA, L. J. 1975. Malnutrition-infection interactions in the tropics. Am. J. Trop. Med. Hyg. *24*, 564.

MUDD, S. H. *et al.* 1970. Homocystinuria due to cystothionine synthase deficiency: The effect of pyridoxine. J. Clin. Invest. *49*, 1762.

NAGESWARA RAO, C., NAIDU, N., and NARASINGA RAO, B. S. 1975. Influence of varying energy intake on nitrogen balance in men on two levels of protein intake. Am. J. Clin. Nutr. *28*, 1116.

N A S. 1975A. Population and Food. Crucial Issues. Committee on World Food, Health and Population. National Academy of Sciences, Washington, D. C.

N A S. 1975B. The Effect of Genetic Variance on Nutritional Requirements of Animals. National Academy of Sciences, Washington, D. C.

NOVAK, L. P., HAMAMOTO, K., ORVES, A. L., and BURKE, E. C. 1970. Total body potassium in infants. Am. J. Dis. Child. *119*, 325.

RAND, W. M., YOUNG, V. R., and SCRIMSHAW, N. S. 1976. Change of urinary nitrogen excretion in response to low-protein diets in adults. Am. J. Clin. Nutr. *29*, 639.

ROSE, W. C. 1957. The amino acid requirements of adult men. Nutr. Abstr. Rev. *27*, 631.

ROSE, W. C., EADES, C. H., and COON, M. J. 1955. The amino acid requirements of man. XII. The leucine and isoleucine requirement. J. Biol. Chem. *216*, 225.

ROSE, W. C., LAMBERT, G. F., and COON, M. J. 1954. The amino acid requirements of man. VII. General procedures: The tryptophan requirement. J. Biol. Chem. *211*, 815.

ROSE, W. C. WIXOM, R. L., LOCKHART, H. B., and LAMBERT, G. F. 1955. The amino acid requirements of man. XV. The valine requirement; Summary and final observations. J. Biol. Chem. *217*, 987.

SCRIMSHAW, N. S. 1963. Factors influencing protein requirements. Harvey Lecture Series *58*, 181.

SCRIMSHAW, N. S. 1968. An epidemiological approach to the causes and control of nutritional anemias. *In* Vitamins and Hormones, Vol. 26. R. S. Harris, I. G. Wool, and J. A. Loraine (Editors). Academic Press, New York.

SCRIMSHAW, N. S., and GORDON, J. E. 1968. Malnutrition, Learning and Behavior. MIT Press, Cambridge, Mass.

SCRIMSHAW, N. S. *et al.* 1972. Protein requirements of man: Variations in obligatory and fecal nitrogen losses in young men. J. Nutr. *102*, 1595.

SCRIMSHAW, N. S., PERERA, W. D. A., and YOUNG, V. R. 1976. Protein requirements of man: Obligatory urinary and fecal nitrogen losses in elderly women. J. Nutr. *106*, 665.

SCRIMSHAW, N. S., TAYLOR, C. E., and GORDON, J. E. 1968. Interactions of Nutrition and Infection. World Health Organization, Geneva, Switzerland.

SCRIMSHAW, N. S. *et al.* 1966A. Minimum dietary essential amino acid to total nitrogen ratio for whole egg protein fed to young men. J. Nutr. *89*, 9.

SCRIMSHAW, N. S. *et al.* 1966B. Protein metabolism in young men during university examinations. Am. J. Clin. Nutr. *18*, 321.

SCRIVER, C. R., and ROSENBERG, L. E. 1973. Amino Acid Metabolism and its Disorders. W. B. Saunders Co., Philadelphia, Pa.

SIEST, G. *et al.* 1975. Aspartate aminotransferase and alanine aminotransferase activities in plasma: Statistical distributions, individual variations and reference values. Clin. Chem. *21*, 1077.

STREHLER, B. L. 1962. Time, Cells and Aging. Academic Press, New York.

SWENDSEID, M. E., and DUNN, M. S. 1956. Amino acid requirements of young women based on nitrogen balance data. II. Studies on isoleucine and a minimum amount of the eight essential amino acids fed simultaneously. J. Nutr. *58*, 507.

TURNBULL, A. 1974. Iron Absorption. *In* Iron in Biochemistry and Medicine. A. Jacobs and M. Worwood (Editors). Academic Press, New York.

VENKATACHALEM, P. S. 1968. Iron metabolism and iron deficiency in India. Am. J. Clin. Nutr. *21*, 1156.

WALTON, A., and HAMMOND, J. 1938. The maternal effects on growth and conformation in Shire horse-Shetland pony crosses. Proc. Roy. Soc. (London), Series B. *125*, 311.

WHO. 1968. Nutritional Anemias. World Health Organization Tech. Reprint Series *405*. World Health Organization, Geneva, Switzerland.

WIDDOWSON, E. M., and DICKERSON, J. W. T. 1964. Chemical composition of body. *In*

Mineral Metabolism, Vol II. C. L. Comar and F. Bronner (Editors). Academic Press, New York.

WILLIAMS, R. J. 1975. Physicians' Handbook of Nutritional Science. C. C. Thomas, Springfield, Ill.

WINTERER, J. C. et al. 1976. Whole body protein turnover in aging man. Exp. Gerontol. *11*, 79.

YOUNG, V. R., HUSSEIN, M. A., MURRAY, E., and SCRIMSHAW, N. S. 1971. Plasma tryptophan response curve and its relation to tryptophan requirements in young adult men. J. Nutr. *101*, 45.

YOUNG, V. R., and SCRIMSHAW, N. S. 1977. Human protein and amino acid metabolism in relation to protein quality. *In* Evaluation of Proteins for Humans. C. E. Bodwell (Editor). AVI Publishing Co. Westport, Ct.

YOUNG, V. R., WINTERER, J. C., MUNRO, H. N., and SCRIMSHAW, N. S. 1976. Muscle and whole body protein metabolism in aging, with special reference to man. Rev. Exp. Aging. Res. *1* (In press.)

CHAPTER 12

C. Gopalan

Adaptation to Low Calorie and Low Protein Intake: Does it Exist?

The term "adaptation" can be defined and interpreted in a number of ways. In the strict physiological sense, the term may be truly applied only to a situation in which an organism responds to an altered environmental situation or environmental stress in a manner which not merely insures its survival, but helps it retain optimal functional capacity and structural integrity. However, the term "adaptation" is often used to indicate an adjustment on the part of the organism which enables it to survive, even though in this process some degree of functional competence may be sacrificed.

It would seem unlikely that true physiological adaptation of the first category is ever achieved with inputs of calories and proteins which are clearly less than what have been computed as being necessary for normal growth and function. On the other hand, "adaptation" involving varying degrees of functional impairment may be possible in such situations. Identification of the degree and the nature of functional impairment in these cases will depend upon the sensitivity of the parameters employed. In many practical situations, in spite of such functional impairment, the individual may still be able to meet his occupational and social requirements. However, individuals and communities which have undergone "adaptation" of this kind obviously cannot be considered to be in a state of optimal functional efficiency which would permit full expression of their genetic potential. Adaptation of this kind, which is no more than a temporary state of uneasy equilibrium, can only perpetuate the status quo of poor communities. It cannot lead to their development and progress, and is therefore undesirable. Unfortunately, the expression "cultural adaptation to undernutrition" is often applied to poor communities in a manner suggesting that their situation is normal and acceptable.

ADAPTATION TO LOW CALORIE INTAKE

Let us now consider the various possible ways in which adaptation to variations in calorie and protein inputs can be achieved. When calorie intake exceeds requirements, as is often the case in affluent countries, obesity is inevitable. Affluent communities tend to "adapt" themselves to excessive calorie intakes through a variety of slimming exercises. Thus various types of ingenious exercise devices have become part of the culture of the technologically advanced countries.

On the other hand, in poor communities where calorie intake is inadequate to meet normal requirements, adaptation is often achieved through voluntary reduction in physical activities. The low work output of population groups with chronic energy deficiency is attributable to this. While such a low work output may insure energy balance, this cannot be considered an acceptable form of adaptation.

In the case of children, enforced reduction in physical activity arising from low energy inputs may have deleterious effects, apart from social considerations, on physical and mental development. The fascinating work of Torun et al. (1975) has in fact shown the importance of physical activity in promoting linear growth and insuring an efficient pattern of energy utilization. Restriction of physical activity in children by reducing opportunities for stimulation and learning experiences can retard mental development. Therefore, adjustment to low energy inputs through restriction of necessary physical activity cannot be considered an acceptable form of adaptation.

It is necessary to emphasize this point because of the observations of Rutishauser and Whitehead (1972) comparing the daily energy expenditure of Ugandan children to that of European children. These have unfortunately led to certain wrong interpretations and conclusions. These authors had shown that Ugandan children subsisting on 80 kcal per kg body weight (as against 100 kcal for European children) had still managed to maintain a satisfactory growth rate through reduction in their physical activity. I interpret this observation as indicating that low energy input had resulted in restriction of physical activity, which should be considered as clearly undesirable.

On the other hand, the argument is advanced that the low physical activity of these children is perhaps a "cultural attribute" and that the low energy intake is the *result* rather than the *cause* of the decreased activity. This argument will not stand scientific scrutiny. We may safely predict that if European children were to subsist on the habitual diets of Ugandan children, their activity pattern would be no different than that of Ugandan children. Several "natural" and controlled studies have clearly demonstrated that the response of human beings to calorie undernutrition is identical irrespective of their race and nationality. The picture of calorie undernutrition was the same in Belsen and Bengal, in Madras and Minnesota. There would appear no scientific foundation for the concept of "cultural adaptation" to calorie undernutrition, which implies true physiological variations with respect to nutrient requirements between different population groups under identical environments.

ADAPTATION TO LOW PROTEIN INTAKE

The mechanisms which are brought into play when there is variation in protein intake have been well-documented by a number of workers (Waterlow 1968; Munro 1970). Protein adequacy can be considered as the minimal level of intake to maintain the individual in nitrogen equilibrium. In affluent communities where protein intake far exceeds minimal requirements, adaptation is brought about by increased excretion of nitrogen through urine and sweat and by increased catabolic rates of proteins and amino acids.

The biochemical response to low protein intake consists generally of (a) conservation of nitrogen loss from the body, and (b) changes in enzymes so as to decrease the catabolic rate of proteins and amino acids or to increase protein synthesis.

As soon as protein intake is decreased, urinary nitrogen decreases and finds a new level of equilibrium. However, if the intake falls below a minimal level, such adjustment is not possible and nitrogen output exceeds intake, resulting in negative nitrogen balance. A prolonged negative nitrogen balance results in a gradual reduction in body size and total body proteins until a new equilibrium between intake and excretion is established. The obligatory nitrogen loss in urine, expressed per unit of body weight or of basal energy, in undernourished individuals is not different from that reported for well-nourished subjects (Table 12.1). However, because of the lower body size of undernourished subjects, total daily excretion of obligatory nitrogen loss is lower in them as compared to well-nourished subjects.

Calloway and co-workers (Sirbu et al. 1967; Calloway et al. 1971) have shown decreases in dermal loss of nitrogen with a reduction in protein intake. This reduction is related to a reduction in blood urea levels which accompanies low protein intake. Nitrogen loss through sweat may also be expected to increase during hard work in hot humid climates. Although such losses have been demonstrated in unacclimatized individuals (Ashworth and Harrower 1967), in acclimatized persons they are kept to a

TABLE 12.1

OBLIGATORY NITROGEN LOSS IN HUMAN SUBJECTS

	mg/kg body wt/day	mg/basal cal/day
Well-nourished subjects		
Calloway and Margen (1971)	38.0	1.44
Scrimshaw et al. (1972)	37.2	1.77
Undernourished subjects		
Gopalan and Narasinga Rao (1966)	37.2	1.50

minimum (Consolazio *et al.* 1966). There is also evidence to indicate that under conditions of excess sweat loss there is a compensatory decrease in nitrogen loss through urine (Daly and Dill 1937).

The above data would indicate that the body attempts to conserve nitrogen in the face of an inadequate intake of protein by reducing nitrogen excretion through urine and sweat. A lowered excretion of nitrogenous products indicates a lowered level of body nitrogen metabolism due to lowered amino acid flux. Such changes are also reflected in the activity of enzymes concerned with protein metabolism in the body. Urea cycle enzymes are known to decrease in parallel with a reduction in protein intake (Schimke 1962; Stephen and Waterlow 1968). Adjustment of urea cycle enzymes to alterations in protein intake is quite rapid.

Protein catabolism in the body has been shown to be reduced following low protein intakes (Picou and Waterlow 1962; Munro 1970; Waterlow and Alleyne 1971). Low protein intake also leads to a reduced catabolism of amino acids (McFarlane and Von Holt 1969; Munro 1970) and a concomitant reduction in amino acid catabolizing enzymes like tryptophan oxygenase. Amino acid activating enzymes are shown to be elevated in livers of protein-depleted rats (Stephen and Waterlow 1968). All these changes lead to an increased efficiency of protein utilization in the face of dietary inadequacy of protein. Many of these are readily reversible with a high protein diet, indicating that they are only short-term adaptive changes and do not represent any irreversible metabolic change.

PROTEIN INTAKE AND OBLIGATORY URINARY NITROGEN LOSS

Whether obligatory nitrogen loss is the same at all levels of protein intake is an important point which has not been explored. In all computations of protein requirements, it is assumed that this is a constant factor. It is conceivable that with increasing levels of protein intake, the obligatory nitrogen loss may also increase. Although there appears to be no experimental evidence, the existence of this possibility can be deduced. At zero protein intake, the amino acid pool in the body is small and is mostly derived from catabolism of body proteins. Under these conditions, enzymes of nitrogen metabolism are also low and hence urinary nitrogen excretion will be minimal. However, when the dietary protein intake is adequate, the body pool of amino acids is derived from the dietary proteins as well as from body proteins. This pool will be much larger than when the diet contained no protein, and the levels of metabolism will be high. Consequently, a higher proportion of the amino acid pool derived both from diet and tissue protein breakdown is metabolized and excreted. Under these conditions, the so-called obligatory nitrogen loss may indeed be high as compared to that on a no-protein diet. Such differences may be one of the reasons why the protein requirement computed by nitrogen balance studies is higher than the values computed by the factoral method, which is based on the obligatory nitrogen loss observed on nitrogen-free diets. The adaptive mechanisms described above can help to preserve normality only when protein deficiency is marginal and of short duration. If inadequate protein input is maintained over a prolonged period, these mechanisms notwithstanding, there will be a loss of protein from the body which will be reflected in concomitant loss of function.

IS THERE A GENETIC BASIS FOR ADAPTATION TO LOW PROTEIN INTAKE?

It is widely held that individuals vary considerably with regard to their requirement for proteins. This biological variation is believed to have a genetic basis. In any given population, the nutrient requirements of individuals follow a normal distribution. In a population group belonging to a low socioeconomic level, wherein the dietary protein intake is expected to have been low over generations, it may be theoretically expected that individuals with high protein requirements would be eliminated through natural genetic selection, leaving behind only those individuals whose requirements were low. Waterlow (1974) has in fact suggested that those children whose protein requirements are high develop kwashiorkor. Surviving individuals with low requirements may do well with low intakes without any deleterious effects. We must ask, then, if there is any evidence that natural genetic selection may be one mechanism for adaptation to low protein diets.

The above arguments are based on the premise that there are wide interindividual variations in protein requirements. It is generally recognized that variation in a population is made up of two components: variation between individuals (interindividual variation), and within individuals (intraindividual variation) from day to day. An analysis of the published data on obligatory nitrogen loss suggests that intraindividual variation is of a greater magnitude then interindividual variation (Table 12.2). Sukhatme (1974) has in fact suggested that the so-called variation between individuals

TABLE 12.2

TOTAL VARIABILITY OF OBLIGATORY NITROGEN LOSSES
ON PROTEIN-FREE DIETS IN ADULT MALES

	DF	M.Sq.	Contribution (%)
Total variability	414	0.38	100
Interindividual variability	82	1.01	39.5
Intraindividual variability	332	0.23	60.5

Adapted from Sukhatme (1974).

in protein requirement is largely accounted for by day-to-day variations within the same individuals—that is, by intraindividual variation. Therefore, it appears that biological variation between individuals, if at all present, is very small indeed. On the basis of this consideration, we cannot distinguish between high requirers and low requirers in any population group. As a result, the possibility of high requirers being eliminated by a process of natural selection is indeed remote.

However, if the above hypothesis that high requirers in the low socioeconomic groups are eliminated by natural selection is true, the survivors must be mostly low requirers. One of the parameters employed for computing protein requirements is the estimation of obligatory urinary nitrogen loss. If the community is dominated by low requirers, obligatory nitrogen loss in such communities must be lower than that seen in well-to-do communities. Available evidence suggests that it is not so. Obligatory nitrogen loss in undernourished Indian subjects belonging to the lower socioeconomic group was found to be within the range reported for well-nourished American subjects (Gopalan and Narasinga Rao 1966). In another study, one designed to determine the minimal requirement for protein in young women, no difference was seen between the values observed in well-nourished women belonging to the privileged classes and those observed in undernourished women belonging to the low socioeconomic group (Pasricha et al. 1965). The above considerations suggest that adaptation to low protein intake through natural genetic selection does not occur among the poorer segments of a population.

GROWTH RETARDATION

When an organism is subject to chronic low inputs of protein and calories, we can expect a continuous and progressive transition from a state of normality to the stage of clinically manifest malnutrition. In all poor communities subject to chronic low calorie and protein intakes, one can expect to find individuals in various stages of this transitional process. This transition can be so insidious that it is often difficult to decide where normality has ended and demonstrable malnutrition has begun. The biochemical mechanisms which are invoked in the presence of chronic protein-calorie deficit have been well-documented. These changes are largely designed to improve efficiency and insure the utmost economy with regard to the utilization of the nutrients involved. The hormonal mechanisms which are brought into play in this process have been discussed (Jaya Rao 1974).

The major objective of these "adaptive" processes is to preserve the integrity of the more essential organs at the expense of the least essential. This process has been referred to by Garrow (1959) as a contraction of the metabolic frontiers. Jaya Rao (1974) has pointed out that, with continued malnutrition, these adaptive mechanisms may eventually break down and a stage of dysadaptation, resulting in full-fledged malnutrition like kwashiorkor, will ensue. However, it must be pointed out that even in the so-called stages of adaptation, appropriate tests may reveal functional impairment of varying kinds and degrees. Apparently we do not as yet have tests of sufficiently wide range and sensitivity to enable us to detect functional impairment at different stages of this adaptative process.

An outstanding clinical manifestation of chronic protein-calorie deficiency is growth retardation. Growth retardation has, in fact, been often referred to as an attempt at adaptation. There have been, in recent years, several attempts to classify malnutrition in terms of growth retardation (Gomez et al. 1956; Seoane and Latham 1971; McLaren and Read 1972; Waterlow 1973). These classifications are largely based on quantifying the end result of the growth retardation process. Unfortunately, they do not help us to identify the *dynamics* or the qualitative aspects of the process of growth retardation. For example, the significance of a given weight for age, or weight for height, may largely depend upon the speed and route through which that end point has been reached.

There are other dimensions as well to what may be called the qualitative aspects of growth retardation. Indeed, it would appear that we have to know much more about the precise biochemical mechanisms involved in the pathogenesis of different types of growth retardation. In several cases of malnutrition associated with growth retardation, growth hormone levels have been shown to be actually increased (Pimstone et al. 1966; Hadden 1967; Raghuramulu and Jaya Rao 1974). On the other hand, there are forms of malnutrition associated with growth retardation where growth hormone levels are not raised and the growth hormone response to the usual stimuli is greatly impaired (Beas et al. 1971; Raghuramulu and Jaya Rao 1974).

Indeed, there have been very few attempts to assess the functional significance of growth retardation. The functional significance may well depend not merely on the extent of growth retardation, but on the associated dynamic and qualitative aspects. In recent studies carried out at the Indian National Institute of Nutrition, Reddy and co-workers have estimated two functions—namely, immunocompetence and intestinal function—in children suffering from varying degrees of growth retardation. Significant alterations in intestinal function could be observed only in children whose weights were below 60% of the ICMR Standards (Reddy and Mammi 1976). Studies on immunocompetence showed that impairment of phagocytic function was observed only when the weight deficit reached 20% of the standard, while cell-mediated immune response was altered when the deficit exceeded 30% (Reddy et al. 1976). On the other hand, antibody response to typhoid antigen was observed to be impaired only in children suffering from severe protein-calorie malnutrition. These observations would suggest that not all immunological functions are equally responsive to altered nutritional status, but they do show that significant evidence of impaired immunocompetence can be demonstrated only where weight deficits exceed 20% of the standard.

In these studies, however, only two functions have been investigated. There is an imperative need to study other aspects, such as mental function and physical stamina. As pointed out earlier, suitable tests of sufficient sensitivity to investigate such a wide range of functions are presently lacking.

Apart from functions which have been shown to respond only in severe types of undernutrition, the question is often asked as to whether populations with stunted stature and low body weight are in fact at a disadvantage from the point of view of work output and physical stamina. The recent studies of Satyanarayana and Naidu (1975) appear to shed some light on this question. Studying a group of industrial workers drawn from poor socioeconomic groups, all between 20 and 35 years of age with heights and weights well below the normal standards, they showed a direct correlation between productivity and body weight (Fig. 12.1). There was a less striking relationship between height and productivity. This observation would appear to be especially significant, since the occupation investigated did not involve heavy work, such as pushing.

However, the results of studies on the relationship between growth retardation and functional performance obtained with one population group

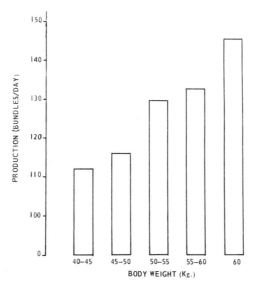

FIG. 12.1. INFLUENCE OF BODY WEIGHT ON WORK OUTPUT IN MALE INDUS-
TRIAL WORKERS DRAWN FROM POOR SOCIOECONOMIC GROUPS

may not be applicable to others. There is a clear need for studies conducted on a global basis using standard techniques to assess the true functional significance of different degrees of growth retardation in different population groups. It is only through such studies that we will be able to decide what levels of growth retardation represent true or acceptable degrees of adaptation. Such studies will also be of practical importance, as they will provide a scientific foundation to identify groups which are truly malnourished in the functional sense.

REFERENCES

ASHWORTH, A., and HARROWER, A. D. B. 1967. Protein requirements in tropical countries: Nitrogen losses in sweat and their relation to nitrogen balance. Br. J. Nutr. 21, 833–843.

BEAS, F., CONTRERAS, I., MACCIONI, A., and ARENAS, S. 1971. Growth hormone in infant malnutrition: The arginine test in marasmus and kwashiorkor. Br. J. Nutr. 26, 169–175.

CALLOWAY, D. H., and MARGEN, S. 1971. Variation in endogenous nitrogen excretion and dietary nitrogen utilization as determinants of human protein requirement. J. Nutr. 101, 205–216.

CALLOWAY, D. H., ODELL, A. C. F., and MARGEN, S. 1971. Sweat and miscellaneous nitrogen losses in human balance studies. J. Nutr. 101, 775–786.

CONSOLAZIO, C. F. et al. 1966. Comparisons of nitrogen, calcium and iodine excretion in arm and total body sweat. Am. J. Clin. Nutr. 18, 443–448.

DALY, C., and DILL, D. B. 1937. Salt economy in humid heat. Am. J. Physiol. 118, 285–289.

GARROW, J. S. 1959. The effect of protein depletion on the distribution of protein synthesis in the dog. J. Clin. Invest. 38, 1241–1250.

GOMEZ, F. et al. 1956. Mortality in second and third degree malnutrition. J. Trop. Pediat. 2, 77–83.

GOPALAN, C., and NARASINGA RAO, B. S. 1966. Effect of protein depletion on urinary nitrogen excretion in undernourished subjects. J. Nutr. 90, 213–218.

HADDEN, D. R. 1967. Glucose, free fatty acid, and insulin interrelations in kwashiorkor and marasmus. Lancet 1, 589–592.

JAYA RAO, K. S. 1974. Evolution of kwashiorkor and marasmus. Lancet 1, 709–711.

MC FARLANE, I. G., and VON HOLT, C. 1969. Metabolism of amino acids in protein-calorie deficient rats. Biochem. J. 111, 557–563.

MC LAREN, D. S., and READ, W. W. C. 1972. Classification of nutritional status in early childhood. Lancet 2, 146–148.

MUNRO, H. N. 1970. A general survey of mechanisms regulating protein metabolism in mammals. In Mammalian Protein Metabolism, Vol. IV. H. N. Munro (Editor). Academic Press, New York.

PASRICHA, S., RAO, N., MOHANRAM, K., and GOPALAN, C. 1965. Nitrogen balance studies on women in India. J. Am. Diet. Assoc. 47, 269–273.

PICOU, D., and WATERLOW, J. C. 1962. The effect of malnutrition on the metabolism of plasma albumin. Clin. Sci. 22, 459–468.

PIMSTONE, B. L., WITTMAN, W., HANSEN, J. D. L., and MURRAY, P. 1966. Growth hormone and kwashiorkor. Lancet 2, 779–780.

RAGHURAMULU, N., and JAYA RAO, K. S. 1974. Growth hormone secretion in protein-calorie malnutrition. J. Clin. Endocrinol. Metab. 38, 176–180.

REDDY, V., and MAMMI, M. V. I. 1976. Intestinal function in malnourished children. J. Trop. Pediat. 22, 3–4.

REDDY, V. et al, 1976. Functional significance of growth retardation in malnutrition. Am. J. Clin. Nutr. 29, 3–7.

RUTISHAUSER, I. H. E., and WHITEHEAD, R. G. 1972. Energy intake and expenditure in 1–3-year-old Ugandan children living in a rural environment. Br. J. Nutr. 28, 145–152.

SATYANARAYANA, K. and NAIDU, A. N. 1975. Unpublished data. National Institute of Nutrition, Hyderabad, India.

SCHIMKE, R. T. 1962. Adaptive characteristics of urea cycle enzymes in the rat. J. Biol. Chem. 237, 459–468.

SCRIMSHAW, N. S. et al. 1972. Protein requirements of man: Variations in obligatory urinary and fecal nitrogen losses in young men. J. Nutr. 102, 1595–1604.

SEOANE, N., and LATHAM, M. C. 1971. Nutritional anthropometry in the identification of malnutrition in childhood. J. Trop. Pediat. 17, 13, 98–104.

SIRBU, E. R., MARGEN, S., and CALLOWAY, D. H. 1967. Effect of reduced protein intake on nitrogen loss from the human integument. Am. J. Clin. Nutr. 20, 1158–1165.

STEPHEN, J. M. L., and WATERLOW, J. C. 1968. Effect of malnutrition on activity of two enzymes concerned with amino acid metabolism in human liver. Lancet 1, 118–122.

SUKHATME, P. V. 1974. Nutrition as the determinant of productivity and economic development: Some basic considerations. Proc. Nutr. Soc. India. 17, 32–43.

TORUN, B., SCHUTZ, Y., BRADFIELD, R., and VITERI, F. E. 1975. Effect of physical activity upon growth of children recovering from protein-calorie malnutrition. Tenth International Congress of Nutrition, Kyoto, Japan.

WATERLOW, J. C. 1968. The adaptation of protein metabolism to low protein intakes. In Calorie Deficiencies and Protein Deficiencies. R. A. McCance and E. M. Widdowson (Editors). J & A. Churchill Ltd., London.

WATERLOW, J. C. 1973. Note on the assessment and classification of protein-energy malnutrition in children. Lancet 2, 87–89.

WATERLOW, J. C. 1974. Evolution of kwashiorkor and marasmus. Lancet 2, 712.

WATERLOW, J. C., and ALLEYNE, G. A. O. 1971. Protein malnutrition in children: Advances in knowledge in the last ten years. Adv. Protein Chem. 25, 117–241.

CHAPTER 13

Reynaldo Martorell
Aarón Lechtig
Charles Yarbrough
Hernán Delgado
Robert E. Klein

Small Stature in Developing Nations: Its Causes and Implications

The dietary intakes of most populations from the developing nations are certainly low by common standards (INCAP and ICNND 1972; Joy 1973). This problem is compounded by the chronically high morbidity rates to which these populations are exposed (Marsden 1964; Banik et al. 1967) in that illnesses lead to reductions in nutritional resources through loss of appetite and through metabolic responses brought on by infectious processes (Beisel et al. 1967). Therefore, low dietary intakes and high morbidity rates combine to limit available nutrient supplies so that after satisfying the basic vital needs there is not much left for physical activity and growth. Consequently, growth retardation (Habicht et al. 1974) and perhaps limited physical activity (Rutishuaser and Whitehead 1972; Gandra and Bradfield 1971) are nearly universal characteristics of populations from the developing nations.

It is well-accepted that growth retardation is the end result of an adaptive process which permits an individual to adjust to a situation of nutrient deficiencies (Viteri and Arroyave 1974). Growth retardation, particularly in the first year of life (Frisancho et al. 1970), also results in smaller adults who have lower nutrient requirements than if they had grown to their full genetic potential.

The secular changes in adult height have by now practically stopped in the privileged classes of the industrialized developed nations (Tanner 1968). In other words, these populations are getting to be as tall as they could ever be. Because of overnutrition and a largely sedentary life, large fractions within these populations are also overweight and at high risk of early death from cardiovascular disease (Mayer 1968). It is interesting to speculate that the conditions which permit the growth potential for height to be realized also lead to changes in the growing child which predispose him to being overweight later on in life. In this regard, it is thought that the number of adipose cells may be increased by high caloric intakes during infancy (Brooks et al. 1972; Widdowson and McCance 1960). Moreover, numerous studies point out that overweight children tend to be taller (Eid 1970; Shukla et al. 1972; Forbes 1957). At any rate, the point we would like to emphasize is that it is not known whether realizing the full growth potential is necessarily "healthy" (MacKeith 1963; Forbes 1957).

Faced with these arguments, one might be of the opinion that growth retardation and subsequent small body size is something we should be thankful for in the developing nations. This general issue will be considered specifically (1) by identifying the extent and causes of growth retardation in developing nations, and (2) by discussing the implications of growth retardation in terms of future outcomes such as nutrition, morbidity, mortality, fertility and mental performance, both for the growing child and for the adult. In other words, we will be asking whether there is any risk associated with growth retardation. The last section will interpret the results presented and will ask whether, in view of its positive and negative aspects, growth retardation is something in and of itself good or bad, or whether it is merely an indicator of risk.

EXTENT AND CHANGES OF GROWTH RETARDATION

The aim of this section is to answer two questions: (1) what fraction of the growth differences between children from developed and developing countries is growth retardation, and (2) what are the causes of this growth retardation?

Some clarifications are in order. First of all, we define growth retardation as the difference between growth potential and growth actually achieved. Second, since we will be trying to disentangle the relative importance for growth of genetic and environmental differences between populations, we will for the most part be talking about stature, a body dimension for which it is easier to talk about growth potential, and one which is not influenced by overnutrition and patterns of activity in adults. Lastly, we will emphasize data on young children because malnutrition and disease are greater problems in preschool children (Jelliffe 1966) and because most of the differences seen in adult stature between populations from developed and developing nations are already evident by about five to seven years of age (Lechtig et al. 1975; Frisancho et al. 1970).

Rather than to try to answer these two questions separately, we will present evidence that we feel addresses both. Three lines of evidence will be reviewed: (1) secular changes which have taken place in about the last 100 years in the developed nations; (2) growth comparisons between high and low socioeconomic strata in developing countries; and (3) the results of studies investigating the effects of environmental factors on body size.

Secular Changes

The mean adult stature of populations from the industrialized nations has increased between 6.5 and 9.0 cm in the last 100 years or so. Children are also maturing earlier. For instance, girls begin menstruating 2.5 to 3.3 years earlier than a century ago. Boys now reach their final stature at 18 or 19 instead of at 26, as was the case at the turn of the century (Tanner 1968).

Although there is only scant data for preschool children, it points to a conclusion that the bulk of the secular change has occurred before the age of five. For instance, five-year-old British boys are now about 8–10 cm taller than boys from a century ago (Tanner 1968). This phenomenon of secular change has been demonstrated not only in populations native to these regions but in migrants as well (Damon 1965, 1968; Tanner 1968; Kimura 1967; Vlastovsky 1966; Lasker 1946; Greulich 1957). Further, these changes have been more marked in the lower socioeconomic strata; as a consequence, the initial class differences in stature have diminished considerably. In fact, there is evidence suggesting that the secular changes in body size have reached a ceiling in the more priviledged but not in the lower classes of the industrialized nations (Damon 1965, 1968; Tanner 1968; Barkwin and McLaughlin 1964).

Both environmental and genetic hypotheses have been proposed to explain the secular changes in stature (Damon 1965). The environmental hypothesis postulates that the increases in body size are due to the improvements in nutrition and health which have taken place in these nations in the last century. The genetic hypothesis attributes the changes to heterosis or hybrid vigor resulting from the breakdown of breeding isolates brought about by increased social and geographic mobility. However, the late Albert Damon (1965), after reviewing his own data and that in the literature, concluded that the effect of heterosis, if any, is bound to be minor in comparison to that of the environment. Thus, within the population, it would seem that environmental changes—and only environmental changes—can have a profound impact on average stature.

Ethic Characteristics and Socioeconomic Level

It has been shown repeatedly in developing nations that children from the high socioeconomic strata grow taller and heavier than those of poorer backgrounds. What is interesting is the fact that high socioeconomic groups of developing nations grow at rates similar to those observed in developed nations (Habicht et al. 1974; Guzmán 1975).

To exemplify this point, we present in Fig. 13.1 the heights of five-year-old boys from upper and lower socioeconomic groups in developing nations and compare these to the heights of boys from developed nations. The definition of upper and lower socioeconomic status varies greatly, but generally involves some combination of income, occupation and education of parents, or quality of home or living arrangements. These definitions, therefore, are not comparable across countries. Further, in those instances where intermediate groups were also examined, we present only data from the extreme strata in order to simplify the figure and highlight our findings. In all cases, the upper and lower SES groups belong to the same ethnic classification.

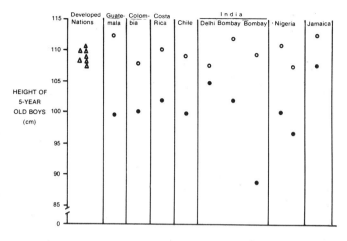

From INCAP (1975)

FIG. 13.1.   HEIGHTS OF 5-YEAR-OLD BOYS FROM DEVELOPED NATIONS (Δ) AND
FROM HIGH (o) AND LOW (•) SOCIOECONOMIC STATUS OF DEVELOPING
NATIONS

The first column shows the mean heights of five-year-old boys from developed nations and include Caucasian (Simmons 1944; Hansman 1970; Nelson 1964; Tanner *et al.* 1966; Roche and Cahn 1962), Negro (Verghese *et al.* 1969), and Japanese (Greulich 1957) samples. Clearly, the growth of these groups, in spite of ethnic and social class difference, is very similar. The top section of each subsequent column illustrates the data from upper socioeconomic groups of developing nations (Luna-Jaspe *et al.* 1970; Rea 1971; Udani 1963; Ashcroft *et al.* 1966; Barja *et al.* 1965; Johnston *et al.* 1973; Yarbrough *et al.* 1975; Banik *et al.* 1972; Currimbhoy 1963; Collis *et al.* 1962; Villarejos *et al.* 1971). It is very evident that the heights of the well-to-do from developing nations are very similar to those of children from developed nations. The wider spread in mean heights in boys from the upper socioeconomic groups of developing nations probably does not reflect differences in growth potential so much as variability due to small sample sizes in some studies, or differences in measurement techniques and in the mean ages of the children measured. For instance, the mean age of the Guatemalan high SES children presented in Fig. 13.1 is closer to 5.5 than to 5.0 years. In general, the studies from the developed nations have been carried out under more standardized conditions and at a time very close to the child's birthday. Therefore these data suggest that the genetic potential of the upper classes of these countries does not differ—at least at five years of age—from that of children from Europe or the United States.

In contrast, the heights of boys from the low socioeconomic groups of developing nations (Luna-Jaspe *et al.* 1970, Rea 1971; Udani 1963; Ashcroft

1966; Barja *et al.* 1965; Johnston *et al.* 1973; Yarbrough *et al.* 1975; Banik *et al.* 1972; Currimbhoy 1963; Collis *et al.* 1962; Villarejos *et al.* 1971) are markedly lower than those of their wealthier counterparts or than those of boys from developed nations.

The similarity of attained size in the high SES groups makes it unlikely that there are large differences in growth potential associated with social class within ethnic groups. Thus, we feel that the most likely explanation for the difference in stature associated with social class is the vast differences in health and nutrition.

Effect of Nutrition and Morbidity on Growth

To buttress this contention, we will now quickly review evidence which indicates that within the lower classes of developing nations, malnutrition and morbidity are the direct causes of the growth retardation.

Effect of Nutrition of Growth.—Although there are deficiencies of other nutrients as well, the most pervasive and serious nutritional problem in the developing countries is protein-calorie malnutrition (PCM). While severe manifestations of PCM—such as kwashiorkor and marasmus—affect less than 3% of children 1–5 years of age, mild and moderate forms of PCM probably affect nearly 75% of all such children living in developing countries (Behar 1968).

Most protein-calorie supplementation experiments conducted in the field reveal that variations in protein and calorie intake are associated with variations in growth rate. Further, the relative contribution of calories and proteins to the association seems to be dependent upon which nutrient (proteins or calories) is the most limiting in the home diet (Bancroft and Bailey 1965; Bailey 1962; Gopalan *et al.* 1973; Guzmán *et al.* 1968; Kamalanathan *et al.* 1970; King *et al.* 1963; Malcolm 1970; Rajalakshmi *et al* 1973; Subrahmanyan *et al.* 1957).

Our own ongoing study in Gautemala, where we provide a protein-calorie supplement to two villages and a caloric one to two others, reveals that caloric supplementation to the pregnant mother is causally related to birth weight. The magnitude of the association is such that the proportion of LBW babies (≤ 2.5 kg) in the group of low supplemented mothers is 19% as opposed to 9% in high supplemented mothers (Lechtig *et al.* 1975).

Our own Guatemalan data also argue that food supplementation to the child is *causally* related to physical growth (DDH/INCAP 1975). We have tentatively concluded that in this population proteins are not limiting and that this association is also due to calories. Figure 13.2 presents the differences in annual growth rates in height which we observe between children ingesting high (> 223 cal/day) and low (0–56 cal/day) amounts of calories from the supplements during the same year. It can be seen that in all

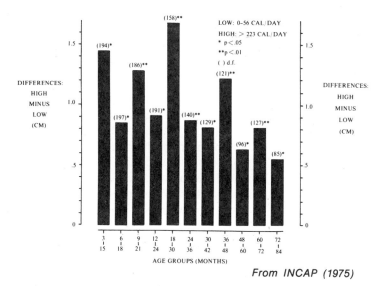

From INCAP (1975)

FIG. 13.2. DIFFERENCES IN GROWTH RATES IN HEIGHT BETWEEN HIGH AND LOW SUPPLEMENTED GROUPS (HIGH MINUS LOW)

the 11 yearly periods examined, children with high supplementation had larger height increments than children with low supplementation. The magnitude of this association is such that we expect that children with consistently high supplementation from conception to 7 years of age would be approximately 6–7 cm taller than baseline values (DDH / INCAP 1975). This is equivalent to around 50% of the difference between baseline values and USA standards

Effect of Morbidity on Growth.—One can ask why children in the high supplementation category still lag behind the standards. There are several possible reasons for this. First, the total caloric intake of the high supplemented group is still below the requirements. Second, as we shall see later, there is a generational effect. Growth retardation in the mother has an impact on her child's growth. Lastly, morbidity rates (particularly gastrointestinal problems) are highly prevalent in the study children (Martorell *et al.* 1976A).

Elsewhere we have reviewed in detail the literature on the relationship between morbidity and physical growth (Martorell *et al.* 1976A). In general, most studies from developing nations suggest that there is a negative relationship between morbidity and growth. Data from our own study in Guatemala show that diarrheal diseases are causally and negatively associated with physical growth (Martorell *et al.* 1976A). The relationship is such that children relatively free from diarrhea during the first 7 years of life would be around 4.0 cm taller than children more frequently ill with diarrhea (Martorell *et al.* 1976A). We have estimated that the current mean prevalences of diarrheal diseases in these communities account for around 10% of the differences in 7-year-old height between these communities and USA standards (Martorell *et al.* 1976B).

As is true for most human characteristics, there is wide variability between individuals in growth potential for stature (Livson *et al.* 1962; Tanner *et al.* 1970). Further, genetic differences between populations have been demonstrated for a wide range of traits (Giblett 1969). Is growth potential for stature an exception, given the data we have presented? We do not think so; we have by no means excluded the possibility that populations differ in growth potential. What we have inferred from the data, however, is that in terms of explanatory power, the overwhelming causes of the marked differences in growth between preschool children from developed and developing nations are environmental and not genetic. Therefore, we conclude that, for practical purposes, these differences in growth between groups should be interpreted as growth retardation.

It is sometimes stated that with the advent of agriculture and sedentary populations, the importance of adaptive mechanisms to malnutrition and disease became enhanced. The evidence we have presented suggests that one of the most important ways human populations have faced these problems is by achieving smaller body sizes through growth retardation—an example of what Kaplan (1954) calls plasticity, or the ability of individuals to mold the phenotype to the situation. There is no evidence, therefore, that selective pressures against individuals with greater growth potentials have produced important discernible genetic changes in growth potential of children.

IMPLICATIONS OF GROWTH RETARDATION FOR CHILDREN AND ADULTS

Having established that the differences in stature between children from developing and developed countries are mostly due to differences in the environment rather than in genetic potential, we would now like to ask a plain question: So what? In this regard we will examine the implications of growth retardation in terms of various future outcomes.

Growth Retardation in Children

The evidence we presented earlier indicated that growth retardation was principally the end result of PCM malnutrition and disease. Therefore, the magnitude of growth retardation is an indicator of the nutritional and health status of the community. But what does growth retardation mean for the individual child? Is a growth-retarded child more likely to become clinically malnourished, to be sick more often, or to die?

In terms of risk of becoming clinically malnourished, most of the evidence indicates that children who develop kwashiorkor are only slightly below or similar in stature when compared to siblings or to children from the same socioeconomic strata, either at the time of the episode or after a 5- to 10-year follow-up (Garrow and Pike 1967; Hansen *et al.* 1971; Suckling and Campbell 1957). However, as Latham (1967) points out, it must be kept in mind that the controls are also malnourished. On the other hand, children who develop marasmus tend to be smaller on admission to hospitals or later on in life (Monckeberg 1968; Viteri and Arroyave 1974). These contrasting results are probably due to the fact that kwashiorkor, unlike marasmus, is usually brought on by acute (as opposed to chronic) events. However, no studies which are prospective in nature have come to our attention, nor any which evaluate the risk of developing clinical malnutrition in children of various heights at one point in time.

A great deal has been written about the interaction between nutrition and infection (Scrimshaw *et al.* 1968). While at times the definition of nutritional status is based on nutrient intake, it is often based on weight, most commonly as categories of weight for age according to the Gómez scale. The wealth of these data suggest that not only is the risk of becoming ill increased in those with lower weight for age, but that the severity of the illness in enhanced. This has been documented for a wide variety of childhood diseases including measles, whooping cough, chickenpox and—most important—diarrhea, one of the ailments most responsible for the high child mortality rates in developing countries (Scrimshaw *et al.* 1966; Saloman *et al.* 1966; Gordon *et al.* 1965). Because growth in weight and height are so closely related, most of the information about clinically normal children given by weight for age is contained in height for age (Yarbrough *et al.* 1974). We infer from these data, therefore, that similar findings would have been obtained if height (as opposed to weight) had been employed as the measure of nutritional status.

Our own data are not in accord with the above findings (Martorell 1973). Earlier, we reviewed findings which indicated that the prevalence of diarrheal diseases was negatively related to growth rates in height. However, we found no relationship within our population between initial height at one point in time and future days ill with diarrhea in children less than seven years of age. Furthermore, the relationship between diarrhea and growth rates was similar in children above or below the local means for height. However, we did not investigate whether height was related to the frequency or the severity of diarrheal episodes. Furthermore, in contrast to most other studies, our sample did not include children with severe malnutrition, being limited to those with mild to moderate malnutrition.

It has been shown repeatedly that body weight is related to mortality. Thus, newborns weighing less than 2.5 kg have a much higher likelihood of dying during the first year of life than heavier babies (Chase 1969; Mata

1972). In children clinically defined as severely malnourished, variations in weight for age (Gómez scale) are highly related to mortality (Gómez *et al.* 1956). Similarly, numerous field studies have also found that the risk of mortality is enhanced for those with lower as opposed to those with higher percentages of weight for age (Puffer and Serrano 1973). Given these findings, we would expect that height would be related to mortality as is weight. However, weight may be markedly influenced by acute events which immediately preceed death. Thus, it may be that weight for height, rather than height or weight for age, is the variable most related to mortality. Pertinent data in this regard are those of Sommer and Loewenstein (1975), who found that the quak stick measure—or arm circumference / height ratio, which is conceptually akin to weight for height—is a good predictor of future mortality.

Studies in various parts of the world have shown that height in children is related to measures of mental development (Mora *et al.* 1974; Cravioto and Delicardie 1969; Klein *et al.* 1972; Monckeberg *et al.* 1972). Since the conditions which determine poor growth in height generally coexist with social environments not likely to stimulate optimal mental development, the question remains as to whether the relationship between height and mental development is functionally due to nutritional factors or merely reflects the results of a generally impoverished social environment or both. But whatever the reason, growth retardation in height generally correlates with suboptimal mental development.

Growth Retardation in Adults

Stature in the adult is also related to a number of outcome variables, some of which we will now discuss briefly.

First of all, it appears that greater height in women is associated with an enhanced capacity to conceive and deliver a baby more likely to survive and to have better growth and development. Many reports indicate that in poor societies, taller women tend to menstruate earlier than shorter women (Zacharias and Wurtman 1969). There is also evidence suggesting that the duration of postpartum amenorrhea—that is, the period following birth during which no menstruation occurs is greater in shorter than in taller women (Delgado 1975). Therefore, for the above two reasons, taller women may be potentially able to conceive earlier and more often than shorter women.

The incidence of abortions and stillbirths has been found to be increased in shorter women (Thompson and Billewicz 1963; Bresler 1962). By the same token, maternal height has been shown to be related to fetal growth, and thus, logically, to infant mortality as well (DDH / INCAP 1975). Figure 13.3 presents data from rural Guatemala showing the relationship between maternal height and the proportion of low birthweight babies. It

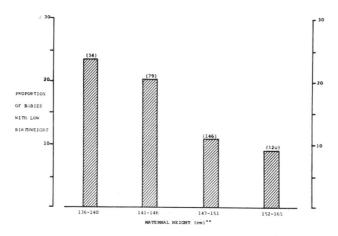

From INCAP (1975)

FIG. 13.3. RELATIONSHIP BETWEEN MATERNAL HEIGHT AND THE PROPORTION
OF LOW BIRTHWEIGHT BABIES

can be seen that in women less than 140 cm tall, the proportion of low birthweight babies is more than twice that observed in women taller than 152 cm.

Thus, the available evidence suggests that relatively taller women in developing nations have a potentially increased capacity to produce more children. Whether taller women in rural societies actually tend to have more children than shorter women is not known. If taller women tend to differ in sociocultural aspects, as is likely, then the increased biological capacity may be offset by differential practices to family planning. What seems to be clear, however, is that taller women deliver babies more likely to survive and to have better growth and development.

Earlier we referred to the fact that shorter adults have reduced nutrient needs. This is certainly advantageous in developing nations where (as is the case in rural Guatemala) caloric intake is often one of the limiting factors in productivity (Viteri 1971). There is evidence that adults from developing countries are mechanically more efficient than their taller counterparts from the developed nations; that is, that they require less oxygen per unit rate of work (Phillips 1954; Banerjee and Saha 1970; Areskog et al. 1969; Ramanamurthy and Dakshayani 1962; Wyndham 1966). Much of this difference is attributed to differences in body size. The ability of people with small body size to perform everyday tasks with less oxygen consumption (and hence, less energy) than larger ones is clearly advantageous. Put another way, in terms of common work activities there is no clear advantage to being taller.

In spite of inadequate medical care systems, poor sanitation and chronically deficient diets, the life expectancy of adults in the rural areas of developing nations is not much different from that of developed nations (UN Demographic Yearbook 1971). Although there are other intervening factors (such as stress, diet and activity), it is clear that body size and composition play a role in determining risk of cardiovascular disease or mortality. It is likely that adults who are shorter for nutritional reasons are less prone to being overweight, and therefore run less risk of hypertension and cardiovascular disease.

After evaluating the positive and negative aspects of growth retardation, one should deal with specific recommendations for action with respect to growth retardation. But the question becomes: Should one try to eradicate growth retardation or not?

The answer to this question is not an easy one. We have shown that the main causes of growth retardation are malnutrition and disease. Hence, the magnitude of growth retardation is a proportional indicator of malnutrition, morbidity, mortality and suboptimal mental performance. Growth retardation in children is likely to be associated with future risk of ill health or even death. Furthermore, growth retardation in the mother is likely to influence the health and well-being of the future generation. However, the adults themselves are probably not at a disadvantage in their daily life, for their small body size permits them to survive and carry out their work with low energy intakes. Further, the life expectancy of adults in the developing nations, while it could no doubt be higher, is at least comparable to that of the developed nations.

Thus, there are pros and cons. But should we remain passive in the face of such human misery? We think not. We do not believe that social deprivation, malnutrition, morbidity and high mortality rates during childhood should be characteristic of the greater part of mankind. Surely the quality of life must be improved. We feel, therefore, that we should try to eradicate the causes of growth retardation, not merely to increase growth, but because the causes are undesirable in and of themselves.

In seeking to bring about change in the health and well-being of the developing nations, we ought to bear in mind that fact that ill health can be produced by excess as well as by lack. As we said earlier, marked growth retardation reflects malnutrition and ill health. But is this relationship linear? Does the absence of growth retardation—that is, full growth potential—mean good health? Although this is still an open question, the evidence at hand indicates that it does not, since the achievement of full stature may also bring about the increased risk of obesity and hence, a greater tendency toward cardiovascular disease. Where the optimal point lies between these two extremes no one really knows.

What is clear, however, is that a more equitable distribution of wealth, within the developing nations themselves as well as between the rich and the poor countries of the world, will result in a healthier population than we have at present.

ACKNOWLEDGEMENTS

This research was supported by Contract N01-HD-5-0640 from the National Institute of Child Health and Human Development, National Institutes of Health, Bethesda, Maryland.

REFERENCES

ARESKOG, N.H., SELINUS, R., and VAHLQUIST, B. 1969. Physical work capacity and nutritional status in Ethiopian male children and young adults. Am. J. Clin. Nutr. 29, 471-479.

ASHCROFT, M. T., HENEAGE, P., and LOVELL, H. G. 1966. Heights and weights of Jamaican schoolchildren of various ethnic groups. Am. J. Phys. Anthrop. 24, 35-44.

BAILEY, K. V. 1962. Rural nutrition studies in Indonesia. IX. Feeding trial on schoolboys. Trop. Geogr. Med. 14, 129-139.

BANCROFT, T., and BAILEY, K. V. 1965. Supplementary feeding trial in New Guinea highland infants. J. Trop Pediat. 11, 28-34.

BANERJEE, B., and SAHA, N. 1970. Energy cost of some daily activities of tropical male and female subjects. J. Appl. Physiol. 29, 200-203.

BANIK, N. D. D., KRISHNA, R., MANE, S. I. S., and RAJ, L. 1967. Longitudinal study in morbidity and mortality pattern of children in Delhi during the first two years of life: A review of 1000 children. Indian J. Med. Res. 55, 504-512.

BANIK, N. D. D., NAYAR, S., KRISHNA, R., and RAJ, L. 1972. The effect of nutrition on growth of preschool children in different communities in Delhi. Indian Pediat. 9, 460-466.

BARJA, I. et al. 1965. Weight and height of urban preschool Chilean children of three social classes. Rev. Chilena de Pediatría. 36, 525-529. (Spanish)

BARKWIN, H., and MC LAUGHLIN, S. M. 1964. Secular increase in height. Is the end in sight? Lancet 2, 1195-1196.

BEHAR, M. 1968. Prevalence of malnutrition among preschool children in developing countries. In Malnutrition, Learning and Behavior. N.S. Scrimshaw and J.E. Gordon (Editors). MIT Press, Cambridge, Mass.

BEISEL, W. R., SAWYER, W. D., RYLL, E. D., and CROZIER, D. 1967. Metabolic effects of intracellular infections in man. Ann. Inter. Med. 67, 744-779.

BRESLER, J. B. 1962. Maternal height and the prevalence of stillbirths. Am. J. Phys. Anthrop. 20, 515-517.

BROOKS, C. G. D., LLOYD, J. K., and WOLFF, O. H. 1972. Relation between age on onset of obesity and size of number of adipose cells. Br. Med. J. 2, 25-27.

CHASE, H. C. 1969. Infant mortality and weight at birth: 1960 United States birth cohort. Am. J. Pub. Hlth. 59, 1618-1628.

COLLIS, W. R. F., DUNA, I., and LESI, F. E. A. 1962. Transverse survey of health and nutrition. Pankshari Division. Northern Nigeria. West Afr. Med. J. 11, 131-154.

CRAVIOTO, J., and DELICARDIE, S. R. 1969. Intersensory development in school age children. In Malnutrition, Learning and Behavior. N.S. Scrimshaw and J.E. Gordon (Editors). MIT Press, Cambridge, Mass.

CURRIMBHOY, Z. 1963. Growth and development of Bombay children. Indian J. Child Hlth. 12, 627-651.

DAMON, A. 1965. Stature increase among Italian-Americans: Environmental, genetic or both? Am. J. Phys. Anthrop. 23, 401-408.

DAMON, A. 1968. Secular trend in height and weight within old American families at Harvard, 1870-1965. I. Within 12 four-generation families. Am. J. Phys. Anthrop. 29, 45-50.

DDH/INCAP. 1975. Nutrition, growth and development. Bol. Of. San. Pan. *78*, 38–51. (Spanish)

DELGADO, H. *et al.* 1975. Effect of improved nutrition on the duration of postpartum amenorrhea in moderate malnourished populations. *In* Abstracts of the Xth International Congress of Nutrition. Kyoto, Japan. (In press).

EID, E. E. 1970. Follow-up study of physical growth of children who had excessive weight gain in the first six months of life. Br. Med. J. *2*, 74–76.

FORBES, G. 1957. Overnutrition for the child. Blessing or curse? Nutr. Revs. *15*, 193–196.

FRISANCHO, A. R., GARN, S. M., and ASCOLI, W. 1970. Childhood retardation resulting in reduction of adult body size due to lesser adolescent skeletal delay. Am. J. Phys. Anthrop. *33*, 325–336.

GANDRA, Y. R., and BRADFIELD, R. B. 1971. Energy expenditure and oxygen handling efficiency of anemic school children. Am. J. Clin. Nutr. *24*, 1451–1456.

GARROW, J. S., and PIKE, M. C. 1967. The long term prognosis of severe infantile malnutrition. Lancet *1*, 1–4.

GIBLETT, E. R. 1969. The Genetic Markers in Human Blood. Blackwell, London.

GÓMEZ, F. *et al.* 1956. Mortality in second and third degree malnutrition. J. Trop. Pediat. *2*, 77–83.

GOPALAN, C. *et al.* 1973. Effect of caloric supplementation on growth of undernourished children. Am. J. Clin. Nutr. *26*, 563–566.

GORDON, J. E., JANSEN, A. A. J., and ASCOLI, W. 1965. Measles in rural Guatemala. J. Trop. Pediat. *66*, 779–786.

GRUELICH, W. W. 1957. A comparison of physical growth and development of American-born and native Japanese children. Am. J. Phys. Anthrop. *15*, 489–515.

GUZMÁN, M. A. 1975. Secular trends in height and weight as indicators of the evaluation of nutritional status. *In* Proceedings of the IX Congress of Nutrition, Mexico City, 1972, *4*, 76–81.

GUZMÁN, M. A., SCRIMSHAW, N. S., BRUCH, H. A., and GORDON, J. E. 1968. Nutrition and infection field study in Guatemalan villages. 1959–1964. VII. Physical growth and development of preschool children. Arch. Environ. Hlth. *17*, 107–118.

HABICHT, J-P. *et al.* 1974. Height and weight standards for preschool children: Are there really ethnic differences in growth potential? Lancet *1*, 611–615.

HANSEN, J. D. L., FREESEMAN, C., MOODIE, A. D., and EVANS, D. E. 1971. What does nutritional growth retardation imply? Pediatrics *47*, 299–313.

HANSMAN, C. 1970. Anthropometry and related data. *In* Human Growth and Development. R. W. McCammon (Editor). C. C. Thomas, Springfield, Ill.

INCAP and ICNND. 1972. Nutritional Evaluation of the Population of Central America and Panama, 1965–67. Regional Summary 1971. Publication No. (HSM) 72–8120. U. S. Dept. of Health, Education and Welfare, Washington, D. C.

JELLIFFE, D. B. 1966. Special problems in different groups. *In* The Assessment of the Nutritional Status of the Community. WHO, Geneva.

JOHNSTON, F. E., BORDEN, M., and MAC VEAN, R. B. 1973. Height, weight and their growth velocities in Guatemalan private school children of high socioeconomic class. Hum. Biol. *45*, 627–641.

JOY, L. 1973. Food and nutrition planning. J. Agric. Econ. *24*, 165–192.

KAMALANATHAN, G., NALINAKSHI, G., and DEVADAS, R. P. 1970. Effect of a blend of protein foods on the nutritional status of preschool children in a rural Balwadi. Indian J. Nutr. Dietet. *7*, 288–292.

KAPLAN, B. 1954. Environment and human plasticity. Am. Anthrop. *56*, 780–801.

KIMURA, K. 1967. A consideration of the secular trend in Japanese for height and weight by a graphic method. Am. J. Phys. Anthrop. *27*, 89–94.

KING, K. W., SEBRELL, W. H., JR., SEVERINGHAUS, E. L., and STORVICK, W. O. 1963. Lysine fortification of wheat bread fed to Haitian school children. Am. J. Clin. Nutr. *12*, 36–48.

KLEIN, *et al.* 1972. Is big smart? The relation of growth to cognition. J. Health Soc. Behav. *13*, 219–225.

LASKER, G. W. 1946. Migration and physical differentiation. Am. J. Phys. Anthrop. *4*, 273–300.

LATHAM, M. 1967. Growth of children after malnutrition. Lancet *1*, 278–279.
LECHTIG, A. *et al.* 1975. Maternal nutrition and fetal growth in developing countries. Am. J. Dis. Child. *129*, 553–556.
LIVSON, N., MC NEILL, D., and THOMAS, K. 1962. Pooled estimates of parent-child correlations in stature from birth to maturity. Science *138*, 818–820.
LUNA-JASPE, R., *et al.* 1970. Cross-sectional study of growth, development and nutrition in 12, 138 children from Bogota, Columbia. II. Growth during the first six months of life in children of two socio-economic classes. Arch. Latinoamer. Nutr. *20*, 151–165. (Spanish)
MAC KEITH, R. C. 1963. Is a big baby healthy? Proc. Nutr. Soc. *22*, 128–134.
MALCOLM, L. A. 1970. Growth retardation in a New Guinea boarding school and its response to supplementary feeding. Br. J. Nutr. *24*, 297–305.
MARSDEN, P. D. 1964. The Sukuta project. A longitudinal study of health in Gambian children from birth to 18 months of age. Trans. Roy. Soc. Trop. Med. Hyg. *58*, 455–489.
MARTORELL, R. 1973. Illness and incremental growth in young Guatemalan children. Doctoral Dissertation, Univ. Wash., Seattle, Wash.
MARTORELL, R. *et al.* 1976A. Acute morbidity and physical growth in rural Guatemalan children. Am. J. Dis. Child. *129*, 1296–1301.
MARTORELL, R. *et al.* 1976B. Diarrheal diseases and growth retardation in preschool Guatemalan children. Am. J. Phys. Anthrop. *43*, 341–346.
MATA, L. J. *et al.* 1972. Influence of recurrent infections on nutrition and growth of children in Guatemala. Am. J. Clin. Nutr. *25*, 1267–1275.
MAYER, J. 1968. Overweight: Causes, Cost and Control. Prentice-Hall, Englewood Cliffs, N. J.
MONCKEBERG, F. 1968. Effect of early marasmic malnutrition on subsequent physical and psychological development. *In* Malnutrition, Learning and Behavior. N. S. Scrimshaw and J. E. Gordon (Editors). MIT Press, Cambridge, Mass.
MONCKEBERG, F. *et al.* 1972. Malnutrition and mental development. Am. J. Clin. Nutr. 766–772.
MORA, J. O. *et al.* 1974. Nutrition and social factors related to intellectual performance. World Rev. Nutr. Dietet. *19*, 205–236.
NELSON, W. E. 1964. Textbook of Pediatrics. Saunders, Philadelphia, Pa.
PHILLIPS, P. G. 1954. The metabolic cost of common West African agricultural activities. J. Trop. Med. Hyg. *57*, 12–20.
PUFFER, R. R., and SERRANO, C. V. 1973. Characteristics of urban mortality. Report of the Interamerican Study of Childhood Mortality. Scientific Publication No. 292. Pan American Health Organization, Washington, D. C. (Spanish)
RAJALAKSHMI, R., SAIL, S. S., SHAH, D. G., and AMBADY, S. K. 1973. The effects of supplements varying in carotene and calcium content on the physical, biochemical and skeletal status of preschool children. Br. J. Nutr. *30*, 77–86.
RAMANAMURTHY, P. S. B., and DAKSHAYANI, R. 1962. Energy intake and energy expenditure in stone cutters. Indian J. Med. Res. *50*, 804–809.
REA, J. N. 1971. Social and economic influences on the growth of preschool children in Lagos. Hum. Biol. *43*, 46–63.
ROCHE, A. F., and CAHN, A. 1962. Subcutaneous fat thickness and caloric intake in Melbourne children. Med. J. Aust. *1*, 595–597.
RUTISHAUSER, I. H. E., and WHITEHEAD, R. G. 1972. Energy intake and expenditure in 1-3-year-old Ugandan children living in a rural environment. Br. J. Nutr. *28*, 145–152.
SALOMON, J. B., GORDON, J. E., and SCRIMSHAW, N. S. 1966. Studies of diarrheal disease in Central America. X. Associated chickenpox, diarrhea and kwashiorkor in a Guatemalan village. Am. J. Trop. Med. Hyg. *15*, 997–1002.
SCRIMSHAW, N. S., SALOMON, J. B., BRUCH, H. A., and GORDON, J. E. 1966. Studies of diarrheal disease in Central America. VIII. Measles, diarrhea and nutritional deficiency in rural Guatemala. Am. J. Trop. Med. Hyg. *15*, 625–631.
SCRIMSHAW, N. S., TAYLOR, C. E., and GORDON, J. E. 1968. Interactions of Nutrition and Infection. Monograph Series *57*. WHO, Geneva.
SHULKA, A., FORSYTH, H. A., ANDERSON, C. M., and MARWAH, S. M. 1972. Infantile overnutrition in the first year of life: A field study in Dudley, Worcestershire. Br. Med. J. *4*, 507–515.

SIMMONS, K. 1944. The Brush Foundation Study of Child Growth and Development. II. Physical growth and development. Monogr. Soc. Res. Child. Develop. 9. National Research Council, Washington, D. C.

SOMMER, A., and LOEWENSTEIN, M. S. 1975. Nutritional status and mortality: A prospective validation of the Quak Stick. Am. J. Clin. Nutr. 28, 287–292.

SUBRAHMANYAN, V. et al. 1957. The effect of a supplementary multipurpose food on the growth and nutritional status of school children. Br. J. Nutr. 11, 382–388.

SUCKLING, P. V., and CAMPBELL, J. A. H. 1957. A five year follow-up of coloured children with kwashiorkor in Cape Town. J. Trop. Pediat. 2, 173–180.

TANNER, J. M., WHITEHOUSE, R. H., and TAKAISHI, M. 1966. Standards from birth to maturity for height, weight, height velocity, and weight velocity. British children, 1965. Part I. Arch. Dis. Childh. 41, 454–471.

TANNER, J. M. 1968. Earlier maturation in man. Sci. Amer. 218, 21–27.

TANNER, J. J., GOLDSTEIN, H., and WHITEHOUSE, R. H. 1970. Standards for children's height at ages 2–9 years allowing for height of parents. Arch. Dis. Childh. 45, 755–762.

THOMPSON, A. M., and BILLEWICZ, W. Z. 1963. Nutritional status, maternal physique and reproductive efficiency. Proc. Nutr. Soc. 22, 55–66.

UDANI, P. M. 1963. Physical growth of children in different socio-economic groups in Bombay. Indian J. Child Hlth. 12, 593–611.

UNITED NATIONS. 1971. Demographic Yearbook, 23rd Edition. United Nations, New York.

VERGHESE, K. P., SCOTT, R. E., TEIXEIRA, G., and FERGUSON, A. D. 1969. Studies in growth and development. XII. Physical growth of North American Negro children. Pediatrics. 44, 243–247.

VILLAREJOS, V. M., OSBORNE, J. A., PAYNE, F. J., and ARGUEDAS, G. J. A. 1971. Heights and weights of children in urban and rural Costa Rica. J. Trop. Pediat. 17, 31–43.

VITERI, F. 1971. Considerations on the effect of nutrition on body composition and physical working capacity of young Guatemalan adults. In Amino Acid Fortification of Protein Foods, N. S. Scrimshaw and A. M. Altschul (Editors). MIT Press, Cambridge, Mass.

VITERI, F. E., and ARROYAVE, G. 1974. Protein-calorie malnutrition. In Modern Nutrition in Health and Disease. R. S. Goodhart and M. E. Shils (Editors). Lea and Febiger, Philadelphia, Pa.

VLASTOVSKY, V. G. 1966. The secular trend in the growth and development of children and young persons in the Soviet Union. Hum. Biol. 38, 219–230.

WIDDOWSON, E. M., and MC CANCE, R. A. 1960. Some effects of accelerating growth. I. General somatic development. Proc. Roy. Soc. 152, 188–206.

WYNDHAM, C. H. 1966. Southern African ethnic adaptation to temperature and exercise. In The Biology of Human Adaptability. P. T. Baker and N. S. Weiner (Editors). Clarendon Press, Oxford, Eng.

YARBROUGH, C. et al. 1975. Length and weight in rural Guatemalan Ladino children, birth to seven years of age. Am. J. Phys. Anthrop. 42, 439–488.

YARBROUGH, C., HABICHT, J-P., MARTORELL, R., and KLEIN, R. E. 1974. Anthropometry as an index of nutritional status. In Nutrition and Malnutrition. A. F. Roche and F. Falkner (Editors). Plenum Press, New York.

ZACHARIAS, L., and WURTMAN, R. J. 1969. Age at menarche. Genetic and environmental influences. New Engl. Med. J. 280, 868–875.

CHAPTER 14

Doris H. Calloway

Discussion

We have been asked to consider for the first time whether or not adaptation is always beneficial. It is usually assumed that when one adapts, or when one adapts something, it is to achieve harmony with an altered situation. But what we have heard expressed is that, at least in nutritional terms, adaptation may have to be thought of more as tolerance than as genuine adaptation. Man tolerates a lot of things, much of which he probably shouldn't tolerate.

Ordinarily, we assume that variability in the biological characteristics of a population favors the survival of that population. Such variability allows us to respond to the different situations with which we are faced. But given this assumption, we must ask why some undesirable characteristics are maintained within a population. That is essentially what Dr. Palmour presents to us as a problem—why should presumably maladaptive characteristics still be prevalent? Why should such traits be carried in a population which should have adapted in a beneficial way, according to previous selection pressures?

Dr. Martorell, on the other hand, says in essence that no one has adapted at all—that no major population, for example, is any shorter than another. His thesis holds that there is a large, untapped reserve of growth throughout the world, that height is the same from one population to another, and that it is environmental factors which determine whether or not we express our genetic potential.

However, none of this really gets to the heart of the issue, nor does it provide us with any criteria against which to evaluate changes or to determine whether the shaping of individual and community behavior is beneficial or not, adaptive or not.

What man appears to have done is to use the ability to alter his environment to abridge those processes which might have led to biological selection. That is to say, if a man can't find the right things to eat, he changes his ecological niche. He accumulates goods, services and materials unequally within the population so that the dominant faction lives by exploiting the others. In the end, this allows one group to express its potential by limiting that expression in others. Man manipulates what might otherwise be natural selection forces.

So what do we say is "adaptive"? Against what criteria will we judge the

157

behavior of a culture or of an organism in attempting to deal with its environment? I don't have any answers, and I don't think any of the speakers have either. All we can do is raise questions. When conditions predispose to or provide an opportunity for changes which might be either advantageous or disadvantageous, to what extent can we alter the environment and affect the direction of changes in characteristics in a way which we could all agree was socially, culturally or biologically beneficial? How irreversible are processes once we have set them into motion? Can anything we do *now*, in nutritional terms, alter the course of what has gone before? Can nutrition in any way prevent a probable outcome which we foresee as undesirable but which arises from a change agent now in force? How do we take account of the variability, of the range of our possibilities, of our ability to take advantage of new opportunities in the environment? How do we plan, so that we can do better than we have done before? If we say that we are not simply biological creatures fitted with immutable bio-characteristics but are organisms able to respond in social and cultural ways, how can we be truly adaptive? How can we harmonize behavior so as to achieve the greatest good for the greatest number of deprived people in the population?

The specific issues which have been raised presently with respect to narrowly defined physiological nutrient requirements are, I think, almost irrelevant to what we *should* be trying to do. Dr. Scrimshaw's group, like our own, has devoted much time and effort in the attempt to precisely define man's need for protein and energy, as well as to determine the range of variability within a population. We are interested in this in a scientific and intellectual way. But in terms of the food available to a population, it is amost totally irrelevant whether the precise requirement for protein is 90 mg per kg of body weight of nitrogen or 110 or 120. This is because the food supply available to us meets our protein requirements—given almost any mix of foods accepted in the world—if we are meeting our energy requirements.

The basic issue we should be addressing is not *exactly* how much of a nutrient is minimally required, but how do we make food available? How do we distribute the food supplies that *are* available so that all people are able to meet their energy needs in order to live, to perform, to think, to grow—all the things that Dr. Gopalan would have us do better than we do now, rather than resting—as he puts it, and I think so well—uneasily on the edge of tolerance, of compensation for what can only be regarded as an unsatisfactory condition in the world.

SECTION IV

THE LIMITS OF TOLERANCE OF MAN'S
BIOLOGICAL VARIABILITY

CHAPTER 15

Tsuneo Arakawa

On the Treatment of Histidinemia

PRESENT STATUS OF TREATMENT WITH A LOW-HISTIDINE DIET

Histidinemia, an inborn error of histadine metabolism, is due to an inherited deficiency of histidase activity. In contrast to certain other inborn errors of metabolism, such as phenylketonuria or maple sugar urine disease, it is far from certain that histidinemia produces clinical disease. Although some biochemically affected children have had speech defects and mental retardation (La Du 1972), many others have been normal (Lott *et al.* 1970).

Neville *et al.* (1972) reviewed 42 cases of histidinemia, including 7 of their own. Sixteen of the 42 cases were completely normal, 12 had an intelligence quotient in the low normal range, and only 14 of the 42 were mentally retarded. They noted that there were no biochemical differences between those with or without mental retardation. And they found it difficult to decide on a dietary treatment for a neonate found (through screening) to have the biochemical features of histidinemia.

Recently (April 1974), a Lancet editorial appeared with the title "Histidinemia: To Treat or Not To Treat." The article arose from the dilemma which confronted Popkin *et al.* (1974) as to whether or not one ought to treat a child with histidinemia detected through neonatal screening. They analyzed published data to evaluate the risk of mental impairment in this condition, and found that there was a 40% chance of intellectual and/or speech impairment in histidinemic siblings of the probands. They concluded that a prospective study of dietary treatment should be undertaken. They pointed out, however, that the development of children found to have had histidinemia in the newborn period was still unknown.

Recently, Levy *et al.* (1974) reported that there was a great difference in the incidence of mental retardation and/or speech defects in histidinemic children in regard to the way in which the disorder was discovered: 85% of all histidinemic children detected through routine family screening, or as a result of medical treatment unrelated to speech or mentality, were normal. They further stated that the biochemical findings were similar in both clinically normal and clinically abnormal histidinemic children, thus raising a serious question as to whether all "biochemically histidinemic" children should be treated with a low histidine diet.

161

In regard to maternal histidinemia, both normal (Neville *et al.* 1971) and mentally retarded (Lyon *et al.* 1974) babies were observed. Thus, some investigators were in favor of prescribing a low histidine diet to children found to be biochemically histidinemic in a neonatal screening program (Komrower and Sardharwalla 1974; Lyon and Veale 1974; Ghadimi 1969; Popkin *et al.* 1974; Bulfield and Kacser 1974).

In contrast, Neville *et al.* (1972) and Levy *et al.* (1974) were inclined to point out the difficulty in deciding whether or not to treat such a child with a low histidine diet.

BRAIN DAMAGE IN HISTIDINEMIA

Since the question of the low histidine diet in treating histidinemia is somewhat confused, I think it is important to clarify the mechanism by which brain damage (if any) may result from the disorder. At least two factors may be considered: (1) a direct action of high concentrations of histidine and/or its metabolies in the serum upon the growing brain; and (2) the effect of the absence of FIGLU (formiminoglutamic acid) due to a defective histidase activity upon folic acid metabolism.

Direct Effect of High Histidine Serum Levels upon the Growing Brain

In our laboratory, Takada and Tada (1970) investigated an *in vivo* effect of an excess of a single amino acid in the serum on the incorporation of ^{14}C-leucine into the brain protein of the Wistar rats. At 17 days of age, litter mates consisting of 6 to 8 rats were divided into 2 groups (A and B). Rats in Group A were given intraperitoneal doses of 0.15 or 0.30 m-moles of a single amino acid (histidine, phenylalanine, valine or methionine) twice a day for 3 successive days. On the third day, ^{14}C-leucine (5 to 20 μCi, specific activity 7.9 mCi/mM was injected along with the amino acid. The animals were killed one hour after the ^{14}C-leucine injection. Rats in Group B served as controls, and were given an equivalent amount of saline instead of the amino acid.

The results revealed that the incorporation of ^{14}C-leucine into the brain protein was inhibited in rats when histidine (phenylalanine, valine or methionine) was loaded (Table 15.1). This suggests that the reduction of brain protein synthesis due to an imbalance of amino acid concentrations in the serum might play an important role in the development of the brain damage seen in inborn errors of amino acid metabolism.

As a result, I favor the opinion that a low histidine diet should be given to histidinemics in order to prevent an abnormal rise in serum histidine levels, even though it has been reported (Seakins and Holton 1969) that renal clearance of histidine is high as compared to that of phenylalanine, and that there is an increased efficiency in alternative pathways for the elimination of histidine in excess of that required for protein synthesis.

TABLE 15.1

RADIOACTIVITY FOUND IN THE BRAIN PROTEIN ONE HOUR AFTER AN INTRA-
PERITONEAL INJECTION OF ^{14}C-LEUCINE (5 μCi) IN RATS WITH OR
WITHOUT L-HISTIDINE LOAD (0.30 mM)

	No. of Rats	Radioactivity in the Protein (cpm/mg protein)
Group A—Control	1	213
	2	188
		Average 201
Group B—Histidine load	1	100
	2	75
	3	76
		Average 83

Note: $^B/_A \times 100 = 41\%$

The Role of Histidine in Folic Acid Metabolism

The second possible cause for the development of brain damage in histidinemia is related to the metabolic status of folic acid. It is well-known (Auerbach et al. 1962; La Du et al. 1963) that histidine-2-C is one of the major sources of carbon fragments which, when transferred to tetrahydrofolate, are used for purine and pyrimidine synthesis. La Du et al. (1963) have stated that in the case of histidinemia, a deficiency in the carbon fragments derived from histidine may develop. However, other sources of the formyl group (such as serine) apparently fulfill this need in histidinemics. Thus, there is no evidence of such a deficiency.

I would like to demonstrate here another role of histidine in folate metabolism, i.e., the mobilization of methyltetrahydrofolate from the liver into the blood stream after an oral intake of histidine, and a decreased activity of methylenetetrahydofolate reductase in the liver of rats fed on a histidine-free diet. An increase in serum folate levels after an oral histidine intake was observed in patients with various disorders, while the increase in serum folate levels was less in cases with formiminotransferase deficiency and congenital syphilis (Arakawa et al. 1972). This is shown in Fig. 15.1.

The mechanism involved with the increase in serum folate levels following an oral histidine dose may be explained on the basis of the results of Perry and Chanarin's experiment (1970), where an intravenous injection of ^{3}H-tetrahydrofolate was followed by an increase in nonlabeled methyltetrahydrofolate in the serum. Thus, it may be said that an oral intake of histidine mobilized the methyltetrahydrofolate from the liver into the bloodstream through an influx of histidine-2-C via the formiminotransferase reaction into the single carbon pool, and that the lesser increase in the serum folate after an oral histidine load in the case with formiminotransferase deficiency can be reasonably understood as being due to the deficient influx of histidine-2-C into the single carbon pool.

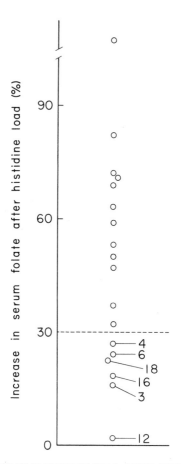

FIG. 15.1.   INCREASE (%) IN SERUM FOLATE (L. CASEI) AFTER AN ORAL LOAD
WITH HISTIDINE.

Number 18 is formiminotransferase deficiency, and number 12 is congential syphilis.

In the case of histidinemia, a lack of FIGLU develops—a condition that can also be produced in rats fed on a histidine-free diet. At 42 days of age, it was found that rats fed a histidine-free diet showed a marked decrease in $N^{5,10}$ methylenetetrahydrofolate reductase activity in the liver (Arakawa *et al.* 1972). This is illustrated in Table 15.2. Such a finding suggests that a decreased activity of $N^{5,10}$ methylenetetrahydrofolate reductase in the liver might also develop in the case of histidinemia as a result of the absence of an influx of histidine-2-C into the single carbon pool. One might assume, then, that a disturbance in folate metabolism might develop in cases marked by a defective influx of histidine-2-C into the single carbon pool, such as lack of dietary histidine and defective activity in the enzymes which

TABLE 15.2

$N^{5,10}$ METHYLENE-TETRAHYDROFOLATE REDUCTASE ACTIVITY OF
THE LIVER OF RATS (42 DAYS OLD)

Diet	No. of Rats	$N^{5,10}$ Methylene-tetrahydrofolate Reductase Activity (cpm/mg protein/hr)
Control diet	1	31,977
after weaning	2	35,550
	3	32,504
	4	36,533
	5	37,273
	6	32,027
	7	27,247
		Average 33,301
Histidine-free	8	24,819
diet after	9	30,808
weaning	10	26,079
	11	31,552
	12	27,741
	13	28,991
		Average 28,331

participate in the degradation of histidine (histidase, urocanase and formiminotransferase).

In 1963, we reported a case with an inborn error of folate metabolism characterized by mental retardation, excessive FIGLU-uria despite high serum folate levels, and a decreased activity of formiminotransferase in the liver (Arakawa et al. 1963). Since then, another four cases displaying this syndrome have been observed (Arakawa et al. 1972; Arakawa 1970). In a patient with this disorder (Arakawa et al. 1972), the incorporation of glycine-1-^{14}C into the urinary uric acid was found to be defective (Fig. 15.2). This finding may be taken as evidence that a defective purine biosynthesis in the growing brain resulted from a functional deficiency of folic acid due to the defective activity of formiminotransferase.

It was also observed (Table 15.3) that the incorporation of glycine-1-^{14}C into the RNA and DNA fraction of the brain was markedly decreased in 42-day-old rats when they were fed a diet deficient in both folate and histidine immediately after weaning (Arakawa et al. 1975). This suggests that an effective purine biosynthesis in the brain was accomplished in rats with relative folate deficiency only when there was a mobilization of folate from the liver by means of an influx of histidine-2-C into the single carbon pool.

Based on these findings, I believe that a sufficient supply of folic acid (Freeman et al. 1975) should be considered as an addition to the regimen of a low-histidine diet.

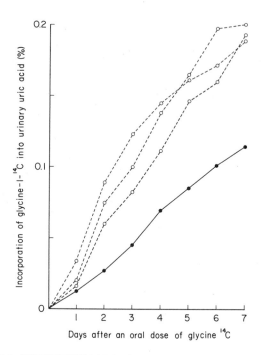

FIG. 15.2. INCORPORATION OF GLYCINE-1-¹⁴C INTO URINARY URIC ACID

(%). 0---0 = control; •-• = formiminotransferase deficiency

TABLE 15.3

INCORPORATION OF GLYCINE-1-¹⁴C INTO RNA AND DNA OF
BRAIN IN 42-DAY-OLD RATS

	No. of Rats	cpm/g of Brain (wet wt)		No. of Rats	cpm/g of Brain (wet wt)
Group A	1	180	Group B	13	660
	2	837		14	750
	3	447		15	602
	4	630		16	804
	5	569		17	662
	6	570		18	750
	7	388		19	654
	8	660		20	660
	9	659		21	1,077
	10	480		22	661
	11	542			Average 728
	12	640			
		Average 550			

Note: Group A was fed on a diet free from histidine and folic acid, Group B on a diet free from
only folic acid. Experimental feeding was carried out immediately after weaning.

A low-histidine diet and a sufficient supply of folic acid may be necessary in the treatment of histidinemia because (1) abnormally high serum histidine levels caused an impairment of the protein synthesis in the brains of growing rats, and (2) a defective influx of histidine-2-C into the single carbon pool due to the lack of histidase activity might result in functional folate deficiency which causes defective purine biosynthesis in the growing brain.

REFERENCES

ANON. 1974. Histidinemia: To treat or not to treat. Lancet *1*, 719.

ARAKAWA, TS. 1970. Congenital defects in folate utilization. Am. J. Med. *48*, 594–598.

ARAKAWA, TS. *et al.* 1963. "Hyperfolic acidemia with formiminoglutamic aciduria following histidine loading." Suggested for a case of congenital deficiency in formiminotransferase. Tohoku J. Exp. Med. *80*, 370–382.

ARAKAWA, TS., HONDA, Y., and YOSHIDA, T. 1972. Increase in serum folate following an oral histidine load. Tohoku J. Exp. Med. *108*, 239–432.

ARAKAWA, TS., and NARISAWA, K. 1975. Decrease in the $N^{5,10}$ methylenetetrahydrofolate reductase activity of the liver of rats fed on a histidine-free diet. Tohoku J. Exp. Med. (In press).

ARAKAWA, TS., NARISAWA, K., and WADA, Y. 1975. Incorporation of glycine-1-^{14}C into DNA and RNA of the brain of rats fed on a histidine-free diet. Tohoku J. Exp. Med. (In press).

ARAKAWA, TS., YOSHIDA, T., KONNO, T., and HONDA, Y. 1972. Defect of incorporation of glucine-1-^{14}C into urinary uric acid in formiminotransferase deficiency syndrome. Tohoku J. Exp. Med. *106*, 213–218.

AUERBACH, V. H. *et al.* 1962. Histidinemia. J. Pediatr. *60*, 487–497.

BULFIELD, G., and KACSER, H. 1974. Histidinaemia in mouse and man. Arch. Dis. Child. *49*, 545–552.

FREEMAN, J. M., FINKELSTEIN, J. D., and MUDD, S. H. 1975. Folate-responsive homocystinuria and "schizophrenia." New Eng. J. Med. *292*, 491–496.

GHADIMI, H. 1969. Histidinemia to date. *In* Congenital Mental Retardation. G. F. Farrell (Editor). Univ. Texas Press, Austin, Texas.

KOMROWER, G. M., and SARDHARWALLA, I. B. 1974. Histidinemia: To treat or not to treat. Lancet *1*, 1047.

LA DU, B. N. 1972. Histidinemia. *In* The Metabolic Basis of Inherited Disease. J. B. Stanbury, J. B. Wyngaarden, and D. S. Fredrickson (Editors). McGraw-Hill Book Co., New York.

LA DU, B. N. *et al.* 1963. Clinical and biochemical studies on two cases of histidinemia. Pediatrics *32*, 216–220.

LEVY, H. L., SHIH, V. E., and MADIGAN, P. M. 1974. Routine newborn screening for histidinemia. Clinical and biochemical results. New Eng. J. Med. *291*, 1214–1219.

LOTT, I. T., WHEELDEN, J. A., and LEVY, H. L. 1970. Speech and histidinemia; methodology and evaluation of four cases. Dev. Med. Child. Neurol. *12*, 596–603.

LYON, I. C. T., GARDNER, R. J. M., and VEALE, A. M. D. 1974. Maternal histidinemia. Arch. Dis. Child. *49*, 581–583.

LYON, I. C. T., and VEALE, A. M. O. 1974. Histidinemia: To treat or not to treat. Lancet *1*, 1047.

NEVILLE, B. G. R., BENTOVIM, A., CLAYTON, B. E., and SHEPHERD, J. 1972. Histidinemia. Study of relation between clinical and biological findings in seven cases. Arch. Dis. Child. *47*, 190–200.

NEVILLE, B. G. R., HARRIS, S. F., STERN, D. J., and STERN, J. 1971. Maternal histidinemia. Arch. Dis. Child. *46*, 119–121.

PERRY, J., and CHANARIN, I. 1970. Intestinal absorption of reduced folate compounds in man. Br. J. Haematol. *18*, 329–339.

POPKIN, J. S., CLOW, C. L., SCRIVER, C. R., and GROVE, J. 1974. Is hereditary histidinemia harmful? Lancet *1*, 721–722.
SEAKINS, J. W. T. and HOLTON, J. B. 1969. Histidinemia. Biochem. J. *111*, 4–6.
TAKADA, G., and TADA, K. 1970. Incorporation of ^{14}C-leucine into brain protein in rats
with hyperaminoacidemia. Tohoku J. Exp. Med. *102*, 103–111.

CHAPTER 16

Gilbert S. Omenn

Polymorphisms, Genetic Load
and the Malaria Story

The aims of the field of population genetics are to describe and to explain differing frequencies of genes. Population genetics was dominated for a long time by theoretical considerations about the fitness of genotypes for survival of the individual and survival and adaptability of the species. In the past ten years, biochemical techniques have been applied to blood samples from various human population groups around the world to identify genetically determined variation at genetic loci for many specific enzymes (Harris 1975; Giblett 1969). The extent of human variability revealed by these studies is so great that entirely new ways of thinking about genetic differences and human adaptability have emerged.

POLYMORPHISMS AND HETEROZYGOSITY
Geneticists share with poets, I think, a consuming interest in the uniqueness of the individual. With a small sampling of genetic loci, one obtains biochemical proof that all persons, except for identical twins, are indeed "unique." Combining the common polymorphisms of blood group antigens, serum proteins and blood enzymes with histocompatibility-linked leukocyte antigens (Table 16.1), the probability of identical profiles for any 2 unrelated persons is less than 1 in 3,000,000,000 (the world's present human population). The polymorphic loci listed in Table 16.1 include many which have been used extensively as genetic markers by physical and cultural anthropologists. The term *polymorphic* is applied to genetic loci at which a second allele is found in at least 1% frequency in the population, a frequency much too great to be attributed to mutation alone. Variant alleles must arise as rare mutants and achieve higher prevalence through selective advantage or through the stochastic process of random genetic drift. One source of genetic drift is the founder effect in communitites of small effective population size.

Table 16.2 indicates how incomplete is the sampling of such polymorphic loci. The number studied thus far is less than 100, or about 0.2% of the polymorphic systems expected to be found, assuming that 30% of all loci are polymorphic—a figure derived from studies in many species, including man (Lewontin and Hubby 1966; Harris and Hopkinson 1972). Harris has calculated the average heterozygosity for man to be 0.067, based on electrophoretic analysis of enzymes representing 20 polymorphic and 51 non-

169

TABLE 16.1

GENETIC MARKERS IN HUMAN BLOOD

Genetic System	Probability That Two Randomly Selected People Have the Same Phenotype	Combined Probability
MNSs	.16	.16
Rh(CC^{w}cDEe)	.20	.032
ABO(A$_1$A$_2$B)	.33	.011
Acid phosphatase	.34	.0037
Glutamic pyruvic transaminase (GPT)	.38	.0014
Kidd (Jk^{a}Jk^b)	.38	.0005
Duffy (Fy^{a}Fy^b)	.38	.0002
Dombrock blood group	.38	7.5×10^{-5}
Haptoglobin	.39	2.9×10^{-5}
G1m, G3m (Gm 1,5)	.40	1.2×10^{-5}
Glyoxalase	.45	5.2×10^{-6}
Gc	.45	2.4×10^{-6}
Cytidine deaminase (CDA)	.45	1.0×10^{-6}
Phosphoglucomutase (PGM)	.47	5.0×10^{-7}
Lewis (Le^{a}Le^b)	.57	2.9×10^{-7}
P (P$_1$P$_2$)	.67	1.9×10^{-7}
Adenosine deaminase (ADA)	.78	1.5×10^{-7}
Adenylate kinase (AK)	.82	1.2×10^{-7}
Pseudocholinesterase, E$_2$	.82	1.0×10^{-7}
Kell (Kk)	.84	8.4×10^{-8}
Uridine monophosphate kinase (UMPK)	.84	7.1×10^{-8}
Lutheran (Lu^{a}Lu^b)	.86	6.1×10^{-8}
6-Phosphogluconate dehydrogenase (6PGD)	.92	5.6×10^{-8}
Histocompatibility-linked antigens (HLA A,B)	<.003	$<0.2 \times 10^{-9}$
Xg blood group (X-linked)		
Males	.56	
Females	.81	

polymorphic loci. Average heterozygosity of 0.067 means that each person is heterozygous at one of every 16 gene loci.

Less common variant alleles also contribute to the heterozygosity of man. For example, the rare inborn errors of metabolism discussed by Professor Arakawa are due to homozygous recessive inheritance of alleles which have an appreciable frequency in the general population. Based on the random mating and the Hardy-Weinberg equation ($p^2 + 2pq + q^2 = 1$, where p^2 is the frequency of the homozygote for the normal allele p, $2pq$ is the frequency of the heterozygote, and q^2 is the frequency of the homozygote for the allele producing the disease), heterozygotes will constitute 2% of the population for diseases with frequency (q^2) of 1 in 10,000, and heterozygotes will occur in 0.2% of the population even for very rare

TABLE 16.2

ESTIMATE OF NUMBER OF PROTEIN POLYMORPHISMS IN MAN

Total nucleotide pairs in haploid human chromosome set	3 billion
Maximum number of genes (1 gene per 1000 nucleotide pairs)	3 million
Probable number of structural genes (5% of DNA)	150,000
Probable number of polymorphic genes (30% of structural genes)	45,000
Number of human polymorphisms known	~80
Percentage of polymorphic genes discovered (80/45,000)	~0.2%

diseases with frequency of 1 in 1,000,000. About 11% of the population are heterozygous carriers for one or another of the 14 metabolic disorders for which newborns are screened in this country in Massachusetts (Harris 1975).

Finally, we should note that many other types of polymorphic variation can be demonstrated with other techniques for which very few data have been collected thus far in populations. The new staining methods in cytogenetics (Hoehn 1975) show common variants in the morphological features of certain human chromosomes, especially chromosomes 9 and 16. An entirely different example is the demonstration of common variants in the features of the electroencephalogram (EEG) which are inherited as single-gene autosomal dominant traits (Vogel 1970).

GENETIC LOAD

Genetic load is defined as the relative decrease in the average fitness of a population, compared with its fitness if all individuals in the population had the genotype of maximal fitness (Crow 1958; Cavalli-Sforza and Bodmer 1971). Fitness is determined by survival of zygotes and children through adulthood, and by fertility of adults. Relative fitness can be measured as the number of surviving offspring in successive generations. Muller (1950) introduced the concept of *load* to explain the equilibrium frequency of deleterious genes maintained by a balance between new mutations and negative selection; as previously estimated by Haldane (1949), the equilibrium frequency $q^2 = \mu$, and the genetic load for this locus (L) $= \mu$, the mutation rate. The mutational load increases, of course, with inbreeding in the population, a variable that has been of particular interest in Japan (Crow and Kimura 1970).

Morton *et al.* (1956) distinguished *segregational load* from mutational load. Segregational load is of special importance to the analysis of polymorphisms and of relatively common recessive diseases, such as sickle-cell anemia and cystic fibrosis. A major problem in evaluating frequencies of alleles at a given gene locus is the possibility that the observed frequencies represent not a stable equilibrium, but a transition destined to end relatively soon in the replacement of one allele by another. It is difficult to measure changes in human gene frequencies over sufficiently long times to be significant, but some data are available for samples stratified according to age, and efforts have been made to measure ABO blood groups in Egyptian and American Indian mummies (Boyd and Boyd 1937). Most important, we must recognize that selection acts on phenotypes of the whole organism, not on specific genes. We shall return to this point later.

For a polymorphism to be stable, there must be at least two opposing forces acting upon it, and their effects must be balanced. When the heterozygote has survival advantages over both homozygotes, the selection is termed *overdominant*. By far the most instructive example known is the relationship between the sickle hemoglobin polymorphism and malaria. As you probably know, sickle-cell anemia (Hb SS disease) is a severe disease with low survival. Heterozygotes have sickle trait (Hb SA) and are essentially normal in survival in modern America; normal homozygotes (Hb AA) are relatively disadvantaged, compared with sickle-cell trait individuals in areas of hyperendemic malaria, especially due to *Plasmodium falciparum*. The relative fitness in malarious regions may be estimated as 1.0 for normal (Hb A), 1.26 for sickle-cell trait, and 0.19 for sickle-cell disease (Lerner 1968).

MALARIA AS A SELECTIVE AGENT

The prevalence of sickle-cell trait in some regions of West Africa is about 30% at birth, and rises to at least 35% in samples of adults. Throughout much of West and Central Africa, the heterozygote prevalence ($2pq$) is at least 20%, the gene frequently (q) is over 10%, and 1% of births have sickle-cell anemia (q^2). The sickle-cell allele is also found in high frequency in certain parts of Sicily and Greece in nonblack populations. It is not known whether separate identical mutations or a common mutation is involved. Four types of evidence support the argument that malaria is responsible for the sickle-cell heterozygote advantage in mortality and fertility:

(1) Geographic distribution of malaria is positively correlated with the frequency of the sickle-cell allele, even though several factors tend to decrease the correlation. These factors are fluctuations in intensity of malaria, migration of local populations, and other interacting genetic adaptations (see below).

(2) Mortality data, summarized by Motulsky (1964), showed a strikingly low number of sicklers among children dying of malaria at major metropolitan hospitals in the Congo, Ghana and Uganda. In addition, there was a significantly lower infant and childhood mortality for sickle-trait children compared with normal children. Age stratification studies are consistent with the hypothesis as well: Frequency of heterozygotes is greater in older age groups in malarial regions, but not in nonmalarial areas.

(3) Direct experimental studies of parasitization show relative resistance

of heterozygotes. *In vivo* infection led to observable parasites in blood smears of only 2/15 Luo sicklers versus 14/15 Luo nonsicklers from a hyperendemic area (Allison 1954). Less striking effects were obtained in 16 American Negro volunteers (Beutler *et al.* 1955), but treatment was required in 5/8 nonsicklers versus 0/8 sicklers. Parasite counts in children showed significant differences as well (Allison 1961):

Maximum Plasmodium Number/ml Blood

Locality	Hb Type			Author
	(SS)	(A + S)	(AA)	
Congo	11,500	250,000	1,050,000	Vandepette & Delaisse
Uganda	10,000	160,000	800,000	Raper

Luzzato *et al.* (1970) have extended these studies and demonstrated sickling of parasitized erythrocytes in sickle-cell trait as a mechanism of blocking the multiplication of the Plasmodia.

(4) Relaxation of selection is apparent in the United States, where malaria is not endemic. Relaxed selection, together with up to 20% admixture of white genes, accounts for the lower frequency (about 9%) of sickle-cell trait among American Negroes (Workman 1968).

The relationship between HbS and malaria reflects interventions made by man many generations ago, with consequences obviously not foreseen.

Origins of Malaria as Selective Agent

Malaria became hyperendemic in West Africa when large tracts of tropical rain forest were reclaimed for agriculture by slash-and-burn techniques which created ideal breeding places for mosquitoes of the *Anopheles gambiae* species complex (Livingstone 1958). Wiesenfeld (1967) has argued that not all agricultural systems have similar effects on the development of malaria, and that the Malaysian agricultural system introduced into Africa via Madagascar about 2500 years ago is intimately bound to the changes in the gene frequencies of populations using this agricultural system.

Other investigators have emphasized certain differences in the reliance on cereals versus root and tree crops. Murdock (1959) described yams and taro as the predominant root crops, and bananas and coconuts as the predominant tree crops in east and west Africa. He and Wiesenfeld attribute their cultivation to mongoloid Malagasy peoples descended from Malayo-Polynesian sailors from the coastal areas of the Sabaean Lane (a water route of antiquity connecting Indonesia, Malaya, the Phillipines, southeast China and India with Borneo).

These Ma'anyan ancestors brought from Borneo swidden agricultural techniques, dry rice, and root and tree crops. Apparently the paddy-rice cultivation technique of mainland Southeast Asia, which was established on Java and Sumatra around the beginning of the Christian era, had not yet been introduced into Borneo. The Malayan agricultural complex (or "yam belt") spread across sub-Saharan Africa from east to west, beginning about 2000 years ago, displacing the Sudanic agricultural complex of many cereal crops which were restricted to the fringes of the tropical rain forests (Murdock 1959). This development brought the expansion of the Bantu peoples through much of tropical Africa.

With the change in use of the tropical forest from hunting and gathering to slash-and-burn or swidden cultivation, there was a change in the nature of the breeding places for mosquitoes and a shift from *A. funestus* to *A. gambiae* as the major vector of malaria. *A. gambiae* are especially conducive to hyperendemic malaria, thriving in open, sunlit pools and surviving well in humid conditions. A long-lived infective mosquito with a high frequency of biting man is an essential link in the disease, since the malaria parasite needs ten days to mature in the vector. The intensity of cultivation, decrease in livestock, and higher density of people all increased the vulnerability of man to malaria.

We may note that malaria is an ancient disease of man, perhaps the greatest specific killing illness in human history (Covell 1967) and an excellent agent for selection of adaptive genes. Children, before they develop protective immunity, are most susceptible, so deaths due to malaria clearly decrease reproductive fitness. Hippocrates fully described the several types of malarial fever patterns and the signs of acute and chronic malaria. Both Greeks and Romans constructed drainage systems to mitigate the effects of stagnant water and noxious vapors. In fact, the word "malaria" is derived from the Italian "mala" and "aria," meaning "bad air" (Covell 1967).

Estimation of the Selection Coefficient

In the model of malaria selection and overdominance for sickle-cell trait, let us assume fitness of heterozygotes as 1.0, fitness for sickle-cell disease ($1-t$) as 0.15, and equilibrium frequency of the sickle gene (q_e) as 0.15. The value of the selection coefficient may be estimated as follows (based on Cavalli-Sforza and Bodmer 1971):

Genotypes:	AA	AS	SS
Fitness:	$1-s$	1.0	$1-t$

If $q_e = 0.15 = s / (s+t)$, then $s = tq_e / (1-q_e) = (.85 \times .15) / .85 = 0.15$

A selection coefficient of 0.15 or 15% represents a very great selective advantage, sufficient to increase the frequency of a new allele (HbS mutant) from 1 in 100,000 at time of occurrence to 1 in 10 within 60 generations (Cavalli-Sforza and Bodmer 1971). At a value of $s = 0.10$, approximately one hundred generations would be required to reach an allele frequency of 10%, corresponding to sickle-cell trait frequency of almost 20%.

Other Polymorphisms That May Be Adaptations to Malaria

Hemoglobinopathies (HbC).—The distribution of HbC overlaps very significantly with that of HbS in West Africa. Molecular studies, it may be noted, have identified these mutations as changes in the very same nucleotide base of the DNA codon for the sixth amino acid of the Hb beta chain. HbCC disease is quite a mild anemia, with very little selective disadvantage, so a correspondingly very small selective advantage of the AC heterozygote would suffice to generate and maintain the polymorphism. There is no direct evidence from mortality studies or parasitization counts to prove the role of HbC in adaptation to malaria.

HbC and HbS interact in the doubly heterozygous person to produce a moderate anemia called HbSC disease. For this reason, it is to be expected that in regions with substantial frequencies of HbC, such as Liberia, the frequency of HbS will not increase as greatly as in other areas with lower prevalence of HbC. Cavalli-Sforza and Bodmer analyzed Hardy and Weinberg equations for these three alleles (A,S,C) at the Hb beta chain locus. A striking negative correlation (-0.20) between HbS and HbC was found, based upon Livingstone's (1967) literature survey of 72 West African populations, with relative fitnesses of SC = 0.70, AC 0.89, and AS 1.0. It is possible that the frequency of HbC gene is still increasing, supplanting HbS.

Hemoglobinopathies (HbE).—This beta chain mutant is widely distributed in southeastern Asia from eastern India to Borneo and Sumatra, with highest frequencies in the Khmers of Thailand and Cambodia. As in the case of HbC, homozygotes with HbEE have only a mild anemia. There is striking geographic correlation with prevalence of malaria, and mortality rates from *P. falciparum* malaria among young children appear to be lower in those with HbE; no differences in parasite counts were found (Kruatrachue 1973). Again, the selection coefficient could be very small, since the selection against HbEE disease is also very small.

Hemoglobin deficiency (thalassemias).—Beta-thalassemias are disorders which produce anemia because of insufficient synthesis of beta chains of hemoglobin; similarly, alpha-thalassemias produce anemia, including anemia during fetal life, due to deficient synthesis of alpha chains (Motulsky 1975). The geographic correlation between frequency of the beta-thalassemia gene and endemicity of malaria is high in Greece and Sardinia, and alpha-thalassemia is common throughout the malarial regions of Southeast Asia. It is of interest that the first suggestion of a genetic adaptation to malaria was made by Haldane in 1949 for the case of beta-thalassemia. Direct proof is still lacking. Haldane also suggested that thalassemia protects against iron-deficiency anemia through increased absorption of dietary iron by the gastrointestinal tract. Such a phenomenon is now well recognized in anemias due to ineffective erythropoiesis of any cause.

Deficiency of the red blood cell enzyme glucose-6-phosphate dehydrogenase (G6PD).—G6PD deficiency, due to a gene on the X-chromosome, hence manifested primarily in males, is a cause of hemolytic anemia. The frequency of alleles for G6PD deficiency is highly correlated with malarial prevalences. Several different types of G6PD deficiency have reached high frequencies in different parts of the world, including the Mediterranean area, Africa, Thailand and the Philippines (Motulsky 1975). G6PD deficiency is correlated in frequency also with sickle-trait and with beta-thalassemia in areas where these traits coexist. By contrast, Hb S and beta-thalassemia in Greece and Hb E and thalassemia in Thailand are negatively correlated, just as Hb S and Hb C are negatively correlated, since such combinations generate more serious anemias in double heterozygotes (Motulsky 1975).

Luzzato et al. (1969) employed cytochemical tests on blood samples from girls heterozygous for G6PD deficiency who have both normal and G6PD-deficient red blood cells. The normal cells always contained more malarial parasites than did the G6PD-deficient cells in the same patient. In an extensive study of families in two Greek villages, Stamatoyannopoulos et al. (1973 and personal communication) found a significant decrease in the gene frequency of Hb S and suggestive declines for beta-thalassemia and G6PD-deficiency in the generation born since malaria was eradicated there in 1945-46, compared with the generation born before malaria was eliminated as a selective agent.

Of particular interest is the dietary phenomenon called favism. Among G6PD-deficient individuals in Greece and Asia Minor, some are at risk to develop acute hemolytic anemia upon ingesting or inhaling the broad bean Vicia fava. An additional gene apparently is necessary to account for favism in certain families with G6PD-deficiency. In Graves' book (1955) on the Greek myths, there is a tale about Pythagoreans who surrendered to a pursuing enemy force rather than enter a field of Vicia fava! This genetic susceptibility to favism probably represents only an early example of very many genetic predispositions to mishaps from foods, food additives, drugs and other environmental agents (Omenn & Motulsky 1975).

It is a total coincidence that modern antimalarial drugs, such as primaquine, cannot be tolerated by G6PD-deficient men. These mildly oxidizing drugs trigger the hemolytic reaction.

Histocompatibility-linked antigens (HLA).—Liability to or protection from a broad array of diseases has been associated with particular histocompatability antigens on cell surfaces (McDevitt and Bodmer 1974; Schaller and Omenn 1976). In large part, these associations may be due to immune response genes, and genes for cell-mediated immunity closely linked to the genes determining the HLA phenotypes. Immune responses could be highly important in malaria, as well as other infections. A thorough study of microgeographic variation was carried out in Sardinia (Piazza *et al.* 1972). Two lowland villages were compared with two highland villages, with very high and low prevalences of malaria respectively. The expected large differences in gene frequencies for G6PD deficiency and for beta-thalassemia were confirmed. Hb S is totally absent in Sardinia, although these people have some Negroid features. Some 22 marker enzymes and antigens (polymorphic systems listed in Table 16.1) were used to assess unrelated differences in the village populations. HLA typing showed significant heterogeneity by Wahlund's test of variance, especially for the FOUR or B locus and especially involving antigens A1, W5 and W21. Confirmation of these results would be desirable.

Duffy blood group.—All studies referred to above reflect protective mechanisms against malaria due to *Plasmodium falciparum*. It is possible that sickle trait is protective also against *P. malariae*, since this plasmodium is responsible for the nephrotic syndrome of childhood malaria, which may be less common in heterozygotes (Motulsky 1975). However, some other mechanism has been suspected (Motulsky 1964) of being responsible for the well-known resistance of most West Africans and their nonimmune descendants in the United States against infections with *P. vivax* (Bray 1958). The vivax resistance factor completely blocks infection, an entirely different mechanism of resistance from the impaired multiplication of the infecting parasite in red blood cells with hemoglobin abnormalities. Miller *et al.* (1975) have demonstrated that red blood cells lacking the Duffy antigenic determinant on the cell surface are resistant to invasion by the related *Plasmodium knowlesi*. The Duffy antigen may serve as a receptor for entry of the parasite, since treatment of Duffy-positive cells with antiserum against Duffy, or removal of the Duffy antigen by enzyme treatment, confers resistance upon the cells. Approximately 90% of West Africans are Duffy-negative, whereas this phenotype is extremely rare in other racial groups.

HOW IS THE SEGREGATIONAL LOAD TOLERATED?

Let us return now to the definition of genetic load and explanations for the very large number of polymorphisms. If each heterozygote were given a fitness of 1.0 and homozygotes (which segregate as one-half of the offspring of all matings between heterozygotes) have even a 1% disadvantage, the effect of such negative selection, multiplied over many thousands of loci, would make us all incapable of survival and reproduction. Even for n = 5000 loci, the probability of survival would be $(0.99)^{5000} = 10^{-22}$. Given the population explosion, this conclusion can hardly be true!

It is unreasonable to assign a fitness of 1.0 to that hypothetical individual who is heterozygous at all loci, consigning all others to a lower fitness. First, such a genotype, over the thousands of loci, is extremely improbable.

Second, a much smaller than maximal number of heterozygous loci may confer maximal fitness through combinations which achieve necessary thresholds for normal development and for resistance to disease-producing factors. Third, selection must be viewed as acting on the total organism, not on the specific, direct effect of every individual gene.

Several explanations have been put forth (all of which may contribute to some degree) to account for the surprisingly great amount of genetic variation within a species. These explanations will be described only briefly here:

(1) *Polymorphisms may be neutral with regard to selection.* Kimura and his associates (Kimura 1968; Kimura and Ohta 1974) have argued that the segregational load is grossly overestimated, because the vast majority of protein differences represent the occurrence and persistence of mutations with no functional consequences. Such variant proteins and their genes are described as "selectively neutral." According to this hypothesis, the high frequency of some of these alleles, including the polymorphic loci, results from random genetic drift. This hypothesis has been based upon data about the molecular evolution of a few proteins that have been sequenced in several widely separated species.

For any one protein, the rate of evolutionary change by amino acid substitution appears to be uniform over widely divergent lines of descent—not just along the same evolutionary path. For example, the average rate of amino acid substitution in hemoglobins has been about 10^{-9} per amino acid site per year in the different evolutionary lines leading to the alpha chains of the carp and of man (diverged from a common ancestor 350–400 million years ago), leading to the alpha or beta chains of such mammals as man, mouse, rabbit, horse, pig and cow (diverged some 80 million years ago), and leading to human alpha and beta chains (originated by gene duplication some 450 million years ago).

Of course, not all mutations can be neutral; the differing proportions of sites that can sustain an amino acid substitution without affecting function must be related to the structure and function of the particular protein. The rate of evolution of hemoglobins is about 2.5 times that of cytochrome c, and the rate for fibrino-peptides is about ten times that of cytochrome c. There is no good explanation for the observation that the mutation rate per gene is related to time in years, rather than time in generations.

Migration of members of a species, introducing new genes (alleles) into the recipient pool, has the same effect as new mutations. If the size of the population for reproduction is small, the new allele (whether produced by mutation or by migration) may have a very good chance of being passed on to subsequent generations. One testable hypothesis of the neutral mutation/ random drift hypothesis follows from the random nature of the probability of survival and accumulation of the variant allele. Kimura has estimated that the effective number of alleles (n_e) maintained at equilibrium in a population of effective size N_e, with mutation rate μ per locus is $n_e = 4 \, N_e \, \mu +$ 1. The probability of finding variation and heterozygosity at specific loci, then, depends upon the mutation rate and the effective population size. Different subpopulations, with similar relative values of μ and N_e, would be expected to have different complements of mutant alleles, given the randomness of genetic drift; despite a constant mean gene frequency for the sum of many subpopulations after many generations, there should, with time, be an increasing variance of the gene frequency (Crow and Kimura 1970). This effect of random drift is due primarily to fixation of one or another allele in the homozygous condition in many subpopulations. If 4 $N\mu$ exceeds a value of 1, then most populations will be able to maintain more than one allele; however, with a mutation rate of 10^{-6} and an effective subpopulation size not greater than 10^4 individuals, which are reasonable estimates, 4 $N\mu$ would be much smaller than 1 and heterozygosity should be low.

Ayala and his associates (1974) have presented extensive data on wide-spread subpopulations of several Drosophila species. These data document high values of heterozygosity and, even more significantly, persistence of electrophoretically indistiguishable (presumably identical) alleles in different subpopulations. Supportive results have been obtained with other species (Clegg et al. 1972; Selander and Kaufman 1973). Such data are not compatible with the hypothesis of selective neutrality of protein polymorphisms. To argue that the mutations are "nearly neutral" muddies the issue, by relying upon selection coefficients that are too small to demonstrate or to rule out.

(2) *Selection may no longer be acting on certain loci.* This explanation must certainly account for some polymorphic loci. The statement clearly implies that the presently observable gene frequencies are not in equilibrium. A good example, already cited, is the sickle hemoglobin allele, whose frequency is falling in the absence of the selective action of malaria in the environment. If malaria had not been recognized as a potential selective factor, the high frequency of sickle-cell trait would be just as perplexing as the high frequency of the carriers for the disease cystic fibrosis (5% of the general Caucasian population) or for Tay-Sachs disease (3% of Ashkenazi Jews).

In our electrophoretic analyses of human enzymes, the lack of polymorphisms for the entire pathway of glycolysis in either brain or erythrocytes was interpreted as a fixed pattern of alleles, presumably after a long evolutionary period of negative selection against mutants affecting these essential enzymes (Cohen et al. 1973).

One approach to learning about selection in non-Western or non-modern societies has been field study of so-called "primitive peoples" (Neel 1970). Particular attention has been paid to susceptibility to viral, bacterial and parasitic diseases, which are presumed to be potent agents of natural selection. Haldane (1949) emphasized the role of immune or inherited resistance to infections as a powerful competitive weapon. He concluded that Europeans, who were resistant against the rubeola virus (measles), used this infectious disease as a more effective weapon than firearms against primitive peoples. Nowadays we recognize that human chromosomes carry genes that determine cell receptors for virus infection and multiplication; it is likely that variation, possibly even polymorphic variation, exists at such genetic loci.

Genetic and immunological adaptation to the environment can be exemplified by the American Indians' freedom from all allergic reactions to North American plants, including poison ivy, poison oak and poison sumac (Post 1971). Post examined the gene frequencies for color blindness, myopia, anomalies of the nasal septum, and tear duct stenosis in primitive populations who are still hunters and gatherers, and in Japanese, Chinese and European populations with a long history of "civilization." In all cases, the frequencies are much lower among the hunters and gatherers, consistent with the interpretation that negative selection has diminished or disappeared. The frequency of color blindness is significantly higher among Chinese than among Japanese and Koreans, perhaps related to the earlier cultural advances in China. Post even related the much higher frequency of breast carcinoma and inadequate lactation among Caucasian women to the cultural practice over many generations of feeding infants domestic animal milk.

(3) *The selection coefficient may be too small to be demonstrated in contemporary populations.* If the homozygous condition of the variant allele is not highly deleterious, as sickle-cell anemia is, then the coefficient for positive or favorable selection of the heterozygote may be very small. Hb E, Hb C, and G6PD deficiency are examples. Another dramatic example, discussed by Dr. Kretchmer, is the phenomenon of lactose tolerance. Briefly, nearly all mammals have an intestinal enzyme called *lactase* which digests the disaccharide *lactose* in milk. Ordinarily, mammals obtain milk only from the mother's breast. However, in certain human populations, milk-producing animals were domesticated for dairying—first goats and sheep, and later cattle. An excellent anthropological / biological correlation has been demonstrated between the introduction of dairying about 10,000 years ago and the present-day frequencies of lactase activity (lactose tolerance) in the intestine of various postweaning human population groups (Simoons 1970). Persons lacking lactase activity may experience nausea, gas, bleeding and pain from the ingestion of a pint of milk. Since 80% of American Negroes, 95% of American Indians and 98% of Orientals are lactose-intolerant, milk does not provide an ideal food for programs of nutritional supplementation in many parts of the world.

What selection coefficient would be required to account for phenotype frequencies of 90% lactose-tolerance in northern European populations versus 90% intolerance among Negro populations? The corresponding gene frequencies (q) for adult lactase production would be 0.60 and 0.05, assuming that lactose-intolerance is due to an autosomal recessive gene (Lisker *et al.* 1975). A selection coefficient of 0.01 is sufficient to increase the gene frequency from 0.05 to 0.60 within 400 human generations, or about 8000 years (Gottesman and Heston 1972). Much smaller coefficients would be sufficient for smaller increases in gene frequency.

(4) *Selection coefficients may vary with the frequency of the gene.* Kojima and Yarbrough (1967) observed at the locus for the enzyme esterase-6 in *Drosophila melanogaster* the phenomenon termed gene-frequency-dependent selection. Wild-type inbred lines of flies were random-mated in a large population to presumed genic equilibrium after 30 generations. A frequency of 0.3 for the F allele was maintained for 15 subsequent generations.

However, breeding experiments indicated large differences in viability among the three genotypes when gene frequency deviated from the equilibrium value; the direction of selective advantage was opposite when F was greater than 0.3, compared to values less than 0.3. At the equilibrium gene frequency, there were no differences in viability. The interpretation was confirmed by use of population cage experiments, starting with any desired proportions of the genotypes. Similar results were obtained for the alcohol dehydrogenase locus (Kojima and Tobari 1969).

Both of these enzymes are examples of what Kojima termed group II or non-glucose-metabolizing enzymes, utilizing substrates from the external environment. Frequency-dependent models, based upon laboratory manipulations, may well reflect ecologic heterogeneity of natural environments. Thus, small differences in the chemical features of the natural environments, including nutritional factors, would serve to subdivide the population into subpopulations with differing selection coefficients for the relevant phenotypes and alleles.

This challenge to models of constant fitness seems biologically sound. The electrophoretic evidence is paralleled by studies of fitnesses of individuals with chromosomal inversions in Drosophila and grasshoppers, and by the phenomenon of the "advantage of the rare male" in mating experiments in Drosophila (Ehrman and Petit 1968).

(5) *Coadapted gene complexes as the unit of selection.* As noted above, selection acts upon the cumulative phenotypic effects of interacting gene products. The relationship between selection pressure on individuals and on loci has been calculated (Milkman 1967). Since individuals with totally heterozygous genotypes do not exist, it is appropriate to estimate relative fitness among existing individuals, rather than to estimate load as the

number of deaths in proportion to the deviation from ideal genotypes (Sved *et al.* 1967).

In one model, segregational load was recast as a component in the total variance of viability, rather than as a proportion of the population lost through selection (King 1967). Direct observations of electrophoretically detectable enzyme polymorphisms in field studies of Drosophila (Ayala *et al.* 1974) and of barley (Clegg *et all.* 1972) have shown that particular combinations or sets of alleles at different loci occur together. Clines of gene frequency across geographical ranges further suggest adaptativeness for the particular sets of loci examined and hypothesized to represent "coadapted gene pools" (Dobzhansky 1951). Often these enzymes have little in common in terms of their metabolic pathways, but most of the enzymes studied utilize substrates from the outside environment.

Coadapted gene complexes could result from selection on phenotypes determined by many physiologically related enzymes or other gene products. In addition, sets of alleles may be associated through the phenomenon of linkage disequilibrium, due to close physical coupling along a chromosome of particular alleles at successive loci, over distances too short for significant rates of recombination. Selection at one locus might carry along alleles at many additional loci. Linkage disequilibrium could reduce the segregational load quite substantially (Wills *et al.* 1970; Franklin and Lewontin 1971). Linkage disequilibrium, involving hundreds of loci, has now been deduced for the major histocompatibility region (McDevitt and Bodmer 1974; Schaller and Omenn 1976).

For all of these reasons, favorable selection may well have played a major role in the development of observable polymorphisms, which in turn provide the variability to make human and other species adaptable in diverse environments.

How will man use his capacity to modify his environment and to modify himself? The broad context of human nutrition involves major policy decisions about reclamation of large land areas, about food production, and about population control. The changes wrought by human culture bring much faster changes than do the biological processes—even with the modern agents of potential mutagenesis, including food additives and other chemicals, radiation, and other physical forces and new biological agents.

Table 16.3 presents certain contrasting features of biological and cultural evolution, while Fig. 16.1 gives some sense of the accelerating pace of cultural developments. It is possible that we are applying potent technologies to these challenges with little more ability to anticipate their consequences than did man some thousands of years ago when slash-and-burn agriculture was introduced.

Yet I conclude with an optimistic view. After all, the hallmark of our species is the capability to worry productively about the untoward con-

TABLE 16.3

COMPARISON OF BIOLOGICAL AND CULTURAL EVOLUTION

Factor	Biological Evolution	Cultural Evolution
Mediated by	Genes	Ideas
Rate of change	Slow	Rapid and exponential
Agents of change	Random variation (mutations) and selection	Usually purposeful. Directional variation and selection
Nature of new variant	Often harmful	Often beneficial
Transmission	Parents to offspring	Wide dissemination by many means
Nature of transmission	Simple	May be highly complex
Distribution in nature	All forms of life	Unique to man
Interaction	Man's biology requires cultural evolution	Human culture required biologic evolution to achieve the human brain
Complexity achieved by	Rare formation of new genes	Frequent formation of new ideas

sequences of such technologies as therapies for genetic diseases, engineering with new forms of viruses or DNA molecules, and even nuclear or geo-thermal sources of power for electricity generation.

The biological and cultural aspects of human interventions to improve nutrition in various populations and environments around the world provide many challenges. The variability, adaptiveness and creativity of man

Evolution of Man

Mean brain volume (cc)	Time scale Years ago	Generations ago	Tool use	Life style	Arts and language
400–550	1.7 million	85,000	Simplest stone & bone	Hunting & gathering	
900	600,000	30,000	More refined stone tools	Similar	
1300	50,000	2,500	Stone axes	Still hunters	Cave Painting Early languages
	30,000	1,500			
	10,000	500	Metal tools	Agriculture	Hieroglyphic, Iconic written
	8,000	400			languages
	6,000	300	More complex tools & vehicles for transportation	Cities & agriculture	Alphabetized languages
	3,500	175			
	300	15	Complex machinery	Industrialized centers	Printing
	30	1	Nuclear energy use	Atomic age	Radio, TV
	20		Computers	Post-industrial Age of "Aquarius"	

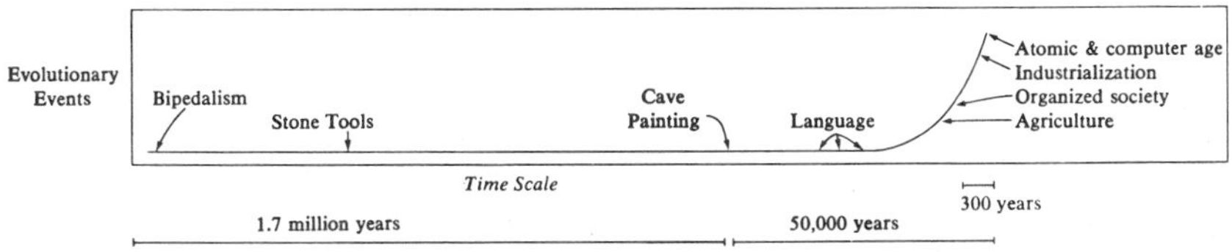

Evolutionary Events: Bipedalism / Stone Tools / Cave Painting / Language / Agriculture / Organized society / Industrialization / Atomic & computer age

Time Scale: 1.7 million years — 50,000 years — 300 years

From Omenn and Motulsky (1972)

FIG. 16.1. EVOLUTION OF MAN: A SCHEMATIC REPRESENTATION

have enabled us to prosper as a species and, hopefully, will continue to do so.

In conclusion, a truly remarkable extent of genetically determined variability exists in human populations, best demonstrated with biochemical techniques. Such variability has arisen through mutations and migration, has been enhanced by natural selection and drift, and provides the biological basis for the adaptability of our species to diverse environments. The example of the sickle hemoglobin polymorphism and its favorable selection in the face of malaria ties directly to agricultural practices of the past 2000 years in Africa. At least six other polymorphisms may be related to malaria.

The capacity of individuals to survive without "ideal genotypes" involves the selection of phenotypes of coadapted gene complexes, rather than individual genes, plus contributions of neutral mutations, frequency-dependent selection, and relaxed selection. The biological variability of man and the cultural creativity of man provide great assets for future generations.

ACKNOWLEDGEMENTS
This study was supported by Genetics Center Grant GM 15253, and by Research Career Development Award GM 43122 from the U.S. Public Health Service.

REFERENCES
ALLISON, A. C. 1954. The distribution of the sickle-cell trait in East Africa and elsewhere, and its apparent relationship to the incidence of subtertian malaria. Trans R. Soc. Trop. Med. Hyg. 48, 312–318.

ALLISON, A. C. 1961. Genetic factors in resistance to malaria. Ann. N.Y. Acad. Sci. 91, 710–729.

AYALA, F. J. et al. 1974. Genetic variation in natural populations of five Drosophila species and the hypothesis of the selective neutrality of protein polymorphisms. Genetics 77, 343–384.

BEUTLER, E., DERN, R. J., and FLANAGAN, C. L. 1955. Effect of sickle-cell trait on resistance to malaria. Brit. Med. J. 1, 1189–1191.

BOYD, W. C., and BOYD, L.G. 1937. Blood grouping tests on 300 mummies. J. Immunol. 32, 307–319.

BRAY, R. S. 1958. The susceptibility of Liberians to the Madagascar strain of Plasmodium vivax. J. Parasitol. 44, 371–373.

CAVALLI-SFORZA, L. L., and BODMER, W. F. 1971. The Genetics of Human Populations. W. H. Freeman & Co., San Francisco.

CLEGG, M. T., ALLARD, R. W., and KAHLER, A. L. 1972. Is the gene the unit of selection? Evidence from two experimental plant populations. Proc. Nat. Acad. Sci. U.S.A. 69, 2474–2478.

COHEN, P. T. W. et al. 1973. Restricted variation in the glycolytic enzymes of human brain and erythrocytes. Nature (London). New Biol. 241, 229–233.

COVELL, G. 1967. The story of malaria. J. Trop. Med. Hyg. 70, 281–285.

CROW, J. F. 1958. Some possibilities for measuring selection intensities in man. Hum. Biol. 30, 1–13.

CROW, J. F., and KIMURA, M. 1970. An Introduction to Population Genetics Theory. Harper and Row, New York.

DOBZHANSKY, T. 1951. Genetics and the Origin of Species, 3rd Edition. Columbia Univ. Press, New York.

EHRMAN, L., and PETIT, C. 1968. Genotype frequency and mating success in the *willistoni* species group of Drosophila. Evolution *22*, 649-658.

FRANKLIN, I., and LEWONTIN, R.C. 1971. Is the gene the unit of selection? Genetics *65*, 707-734.

GIBLETT, E. R. 1969. Genetic Markers in Human Blood. F. A. Davis, Philadelphia.

GOTTESMAN, I. I., and HESTON, L. L. 1972. Human behavioral adaptations: Speculations on their genesis. *In* Genetics, Environment and Behavior: Implications for Educational Policy. L. Ehrman, G. S. Omenn and E. Caspari (Editors). Academic Press, New York.

GRAVES, R. 1955. The Greek Myths, Vol. I. Penguin Books, Baltimore.

HALDANE, J. B. S. 1949. Disease and evolution. Ricerca Sci. *19* (Supp. 1), 68-76.

HARRIS, H. 1975. The Principles of Human Biochemical Genetics, 2nd Edition. North Holland Publishing Co., Amsterdam.

HARRIS, H., and HOPKINSON, D. A. 1972. Average heterozygosity per locus in man: An estimate based on the incidence of enzyme polymorphisms. Ann. Hum. Genet. *36*, 9-20.

HOEHN, H. 1975. Functional implications of differential chromosome banding. Am. J. Hum. Genet. *27*, 676-685.

KIMURA, M. 1968. Evolutionary rate at the molecular level. Nature *217*, 624-626.

KIMURA, M., and OHTA, T. 1974. On some principles governing molecular evolution. Proc. Nat. Acad. Sci. U.S.A. *71*, 2848-2852.

KING, J. L. 1967. Continuously distributed factors affecting fitness. Genetics *55*, 483-492.

KOJIMA, K., and TOBARI, Y. 1969. The pattern of viability changes associated with genotype frequency at the alcohol dehydrogenase locus in a population of *Drosophila melanogaster*. Genetics *61*, 201-209.

KOJIMA, K., and YARBROUGH, K. M. 1967. Frequency-dependent selection at the esterase 6 locus in *Drosophila melanogaster*. Proc. Nat. Acad. Sci. U.S.A. *57*, 645-649.

KRUATRACHUE, M. 1973. Genetic polymorphisms of erythrocytes and malaria in South-East Asia. *In* 9th International Congress on Tropical Medicine and Malaria, Athens. Abstracts of Invited Papers, 266-267.

LERNER, I. M. 1968. Heredity, Evolution, and Society. W. H. Freeman & Co., San Francisco.

LEWONTIN, R. C., and HUBBY, J. L. 1966. A molecular approach to the study of genetic heterozygosity in natural populations. II. Amount of variation and degree of heterozygosity in natural populations of *Drosophila pseudoobscura*. Genetics *54*, 595-609.

LISKER, R., GONZALEZ, B., and DALTABUIT, M. 1975. Recessive inheritance of the adult-type of intestinal lactase deficiency. Am. J. Hum. Genet. *27*, 662-664.

LIVINGSTONE, F. 1958. Anthropological implications of sickle-cell gene distribution. Am. Anthrop. *60*, 533-562.

LIVINGSTONE, F. 1967. Abnormal Hemoglobins in Human Populations. Aldine Publishing Co., Chicago.

LUZZATO, L., NWACHUKU-JARRETT, E. S., and REDDY, S. 1970. Increased sickling of parasitized erythrocytes as mechanism of resistance against malaria in the sickle-cell trait. Lancet. *1*, 319-321.

LUZZATO, L., USANGA, E. A., and REDDY, S. 1969. Glucose-6-phosphate dehydrogenase deficient red cells: Resistance to infection by malarial parasites. Science *164*, 839-842.

MC DEVITT, H. O., and BODMER, W. F. 1974. HL-A, immune-response genes, and disease. Lancet *1*, 1269-1275.

MILKMAN, R. D. 1967. Heterosis as a major cause of heterozygosity in nature. Genetics *55*, 493-495.

MILLER, L. H. *et al.* 1975. Erythrocyte receptors for (Plasmodium knowlesi) malaria: Duffy blood group determinants. Science *189*, 561-563.

MORTON, N. E., CROW, J. F. and MULLER, H. J. 1956. An estimate of the mutational damage in man from data on consanguineous marriages. Proc. Nat. Acad. Sci. U.S.A. *42*, 855-863.

MOTULSKY, A. G. 1964. Hereditary red cell traits and malaria. Am. J. Trop. Med. Hyg. *13*, 147-158.

MOTULSKY, A. G. 1968. Human genetics, society and medicine. J. Hered. *59*, 329–336.
MOTULSKY, A. G. 1975. Glucose-6-phosphate dehydrogenase and abnormal hemoglobin polymorphisms: Evidence regarding malarial selection. *In* The Role of Natural Selection in Human Evolution. F. M. Salzano (Editor). North Holland Publishing Co., New York.
MULLER, H. J. 1950. Our load of mutations. Am. J. Hum. Genet. *2*, 111–176.
MURDOCK, G. 1959. Africa: Its People and Their Cultural History. McGraw-Hill, New York.
NEEL, J. V. 1970. Lessons from a "primitive" people. Science *170*, 815–822.
OMENN, G. S., and MOTULSKY, A. G. 1972. Biochemical genetics and the evolution of human behavior. *In* Genetics, Environment and Behavior: Implications for Educational Policy. L. Ehrman, G. S. Omenn, and E. Caspari (Editors). Academic Press, New York.
OMENN, G. S., and MOTULSKY, A. G. 1975. Eco-genetics. *In* Genetics and Public Health, B. Cohen (Editor). Johns Hopkins Press, Baltimore.
PIAZZA, A. *et al.* 1972. HL-A variation in four Sardinian villages under differential selective pressure by malaria. *In* Histocompatibility Testing. Munksgaard, Copenhagen.
POST, R. H. 1971. Possible cases of relaxed selection in civilized populations. Humangenetik *13*, 253–284.
SCHALLER, J. G., and OMENN, G. S. 1976. The histocompatibility system and human disease. J. Pediatr. *88*, 913–925.
SELANDER, R. K., and KAUFMAN, D. W. 1973. Genic variability and strategies of adaptation in animals. Proc. Nat. Acad. Sci. U.S.A. *70*, 1875–1877.
SIMOONS, F. J. 1970. Primary adult lactose intolerance and the milking habit: A problem in biological and cultural interrelations. II. A cultural hypothesis. Am. J. Digest. Dis. *15*, 695–710.
STAMATOYANNOPOULOS, G. *et al.* 1973. Hb S. glucose-6-phosphate dehydrogenase deficiency and thalassemia in Greece before and after malarial eradication. *In* 9th International Congress on Tropical Medicine and Malaria, Athens. Abstracts of Invited Papers, 266.
SVED, J. A., REED, T. E., and BODMER, W. F. 1967. The number of balanced polymorphisms that can be maintained in a natural population. Genetics *55*, 469–481.
VOGEL, F. 1970. The genetic basis of the normal human electroencephalogram (EEG). Humangenetik *10*, 91–114.
WIESENFELD, S. L. 1967. Sickle-cell trait in human biological and cultural evolution. Science *157*, 1134–1140.
WILLS, C., CRENSHAW, J., and VITALE, J. 1970. A computer model allowing maintenance of large amounts of genetic variability in Mendelian populations. I. Assumptions and results for large populations. Genetics *64*, 107–123.
WORKMAN, P. L. 1968. Gene flow and the search for natural selection in man. Hum. Biol. *40*, 260–268.

CHAPTER 17

Robert H. Cagan
Morley R. Kare

Chemical Senses: Influence on Variability of Nutritional Adaptation

Variability among individuals in nutritional adaptation depends in part upon variability in their sensory responses. Foods to be eaten are monitored by the sensory receptors. Within the context of the present subject, it is important to consider those aspects of variability that can be introduced by the senses. Among the important properties of a food are those perceived through the chemical senses—gustation (the sense of taste) and olfaction (the sense of smell). The term "flavor" (Amerine et al. 1965) is applied to the complex of information from these senses, along with that derived from touch, temperature and mild pain—although the term "taste" is often used by the layman when "flavor" is meant.

There is ample documentation that the chemical senses are important in identifying and selecting foods (Epstein 1967; LeMagnen 1971; Mozell et al. 1969), but the sensory attributes of foods are often not considered by investigators beyond mere acceptance or rejection. In addition, there may be important physiological consequences following chemosensory stimulation. For example, the chemical stimuli in foods can affect systemic processes such as exocrine pancreatic flow (Behrman and Kare 1968; Pavlov 1902) or possibly insulin release (cf. Kipnis 1972).

Whatever the potential value of a food, it will serve no nutritional function unless it is eaten. Given a choice, individuals are less likely to eat foods that do not appeal to their flavor preferences. Appealing flavors can be used to promote good nutrition, although a current attitude among lay people and some scientists is to associate appealing flavors with poor nutrition. Not only are the sensory attributes of food important to its acceptance, but also the context of the eating situation. Dining often serves a social as well as a nutritional function, but the significance of its social aspects will not be considered here. The examples draw upon the chemical senses, especially the sense of taste.

The subjective nature of the sensory experience has undoubtedly influenced many scientists, with the exception of Kare and Maller (1967), to avoid the largely unstudied area of the chemical senses in nutrition. However, many aspects of it are susceptible to quantitative physiological and biochemical experimentation. Information from these approaches could have an important influence on the application of nutrition information to food design and development.

INFLUENCE OF CHEMICAL SENSES ON REGULATION OF NUTRIENT INTAKE

Innate Appetites

A behavioral taste response can, in principle, be entirely innate or be influenced to varying degrees by individual experience through learning, even though the ability to perceive a particular chemical is inborn. Innate behavior is defined here as the response evident the first time an individual is presented with a specific substance. There are several examples of studies showing innate taste responses; two of these are the responses to the salty taste of NaCl and to the sweet taste of sugars.

Extensive studies with animals indicate that the ability to perceive and properly respond to the presence of NaCl in a food is innate (Nachman and Cole 1971). The animal does not need to learn what is beneficial, but is able to regulate Na^+ intake to correspond with physiological requirements. The sense of taste, coupled with other physiological regulatory mechanisms, is effective in enabling a salt-deficient animal to adjust in response to the salt-deficient state by increasing its salt intake when it is available. For example, increased intake of NaCl occurs when rats are adrenalectomized. Animals without adrenal glands lose salt in the urine and rapidly show a sodium deficit. Given a two-choice preference test, adrenalectomized animals drink more of the NaCl solutions (paired with water) than do normal rats (Nachman and Cole 1971; Richter 1942). The adrenalectomized rats prefer strongly hypertonic solutions which are rejected by normal rats. Similarly, humans with adrenal cortical insufficiency (e.g., Addison's disease) show marked cravings for salt and salt-containing foods (Richter 1942). These observations point up the importance of the ability to perceive salty solutions and to distinguish their degree of saltiness in aiding regulation of salt balance. The studies reported do not, however, explain the inability of hypertensive patients, for whom restricted sodium intake is advisable, to properly regulate their sodium intake. It is reported that hypertensive patients prefer more salty solutions than do nonhypertensives (Schechter *et al.* 1974).

The response to salt has been shown to be innate in animals, because in various studies in which adrenalectomy, dietary deficiency or other techniques have been used to produce a sodium-deficient state, the selection occurs too soon in the taste-testing for learning to be important. For example, Weiner and Stellar (1951) reported that normal, but water-deprived, rats showed an immediate (within 5 min) preference for various concentrations of salt solution. They demonstrated also the familiar "preferance-aversion" behavior, with an optimum intake near isotonicity. A study by Nachman (1962) showed that the preference for sodium-containing solutions over sodium-free solutions by deficient rats occurs within

15 sec after sampling the solutions. The rats were made sodium-deficient by adrenalectomy or by dietary means.

The ability to carefully regulate NaCl intake, and the crucial role played by taste may be unique because of the pivotal role of Na^+ in the physiology of the organism. Virtually all cell types require close regulation of their internal ionic constituents. Wide variations in the ionic composition of the extracellular fluid can often have deleterious, sometimes toxic, effects.

The response to the sweet taste of sugars is another example of an innate taste preference. In an extensive and carefully controlled study by Maller and co-workers (Desor et al. 1973) newborn human infants (1–3 days old) were found to prefer the sweet taste of sugar solutions over the water control. The effective range of sugar concentrations (0.05–0.3 M) was similar to that observed in adults. In addition, the preference by the newborns for the four sugars tested (sucrose, fructose, glucose and lactose) was in the same order as the relative sweetness judged by adult humans. The fetus has also been shown to respond to taste stimuli (Mistretta and Bradley 1975). Contrary to popular misconception, the data show that newborn babies can identify a sweet taste and like it. It would be interesting to know if other naturally occurring sweet substances—such as the intensely sweet, yet carbohydrate-free protein, monellin (Cagan 1973)—are also preferred by the human newborn.

Steiner (1973) has photographically documented changes in facial expressions when newborn infants were stimulated on the tongue with various types of taste solutions. This phenomenon (the "gustofacial reflex") is suggested to be innate. Steiner interpreted the reaction as "a stimulus-dependent human nonverbal communication pattern." In particular, stimulation with sweet (sucrose), bitter (quinine) and sour (citric acid) substances elicited recognizable facial expressions. The infants studied included a group tested between birth and the first feeding to exclude previous extra-uterine experience with taste.

Role of Learning in Taste Preferences

A number of studies indicate the possible complex roles that taste can play during feeding. In a classic study, Harris and co-workers (1933) showed that rats deficient in vitamin B-1 were able to select from among several choices the food that contained the vitamin. In a series of elegant experiments, they showed that this ability to select the vitamin-containing diet was learned. The animals were able to make the correct choice by learning to associate the sensory qualities (probably the taste or odor) of the diet with the beneficial effect. For example, when the vitamin was added to the deficient diet as a concentrate, which presumably did *not* change the taste of the food, the animals were unable to distinguish the correct food. On the other hand, when the vitamin was added to a natural food source which had a taste or odor they could learn to recognize, they were able to select the vitamin-containing diet from among several choices. But once having learned the correct choice, the animals could be deceived: Even after the vitamin was removed from the now-preferred diet, they continued to select it. Therefore it was not the taste of the nutrient itself which guided the selection.

The innate ability to taste salt and properly respond to it provides another opportunity to demonstrate the effects of learning. In a two-choice preference test between NaCl solutions and water, the normal rat shows a "preference-aversion" behavior, with increasing preference for hypotonic solutions over water, and a decline as the solutions become increasingly hypertonic (Nachman and Cole 1971). The *initial* taste response to LiCl is similar to that of NaCl in being preferred to water, although the rat can discriminate between LiCl and NaCl (Harriman and Kare 1964). LiCl is highly toxic, and after a single trial the rats learn to avoid it—a "conditioned aversion" (Nachman and Cole 1971). This aversion is presumably the result of the animal associating its illness with the distinctive taste. The aversion generalizes to NaCl, apparently because of the similarity in their tastes to rats. Thus, although the ability to taste NaCl and the basic behavioral taste preference for it are innate, the behavioral taste response can be modified by learning.

Exposure to a particular flavor early in life can affect subsequent preference for that flavor. Galef and Henderson (1972) showed that the diet of a lactating female rat influences the early food preference of the young during weaning, apparently by having transmitted sensory cues in the milk. Nursing rats exposed to garlic flavor in the mother's milk showed a higher preference for garlic when later tested than did control rats (Capretta and Rawls 1974).

Learning is undoubtedly involved in many aspects of eating, and is probably responsible for considerable variability in food preferences of humans. In addition to learning, other influences could conceivably affect selection and eating of foods, although in some cases the information is anecdotal. Various types of stress might lead to alterations in eating, including stress introduced by unfamiliar situations. Experimental studies with rats indicate the important influence that the novelty of a food can exert on eating; the effect of the novel food can also depend upon prior nutritional deficiencies which developed while eating a familiar food (Rozin and Kalat 1971).

Species and Individual Variations in Taste Responses

Each species lives in its own sensory world. The range of variation in species responses to taste stimuli is well-documented (Kare 1971). Anthropomorphic interpretations about taste responses to a particular chemical are often not valid. For instance, many sugars taste sweet to humans (Cameron 1947) and to some animals, but not to all species (Kare 1971). Many other examples of species differences in taste are known.

Less well-studied than species variability are intraspecies variations. As in many areas of biological research, intraspecies variability is often viewed as a nuisance or difficulty to be circumvented by adept statistical procedures. Casual observations indicate that preferences among individuals for various foods differ widely. Relatively few studies, however, have critically examined this question of individual variability.

Some experimental evidence documents individual variability towards particular taste stimuli. In humans, for example, an extensive number of studies show that the distribution of taste sensitivity of a population to the bitter taste of one class of compounds, the phenylthiocarbamides (PTC), differs from that to other bitter compounds (Fisher 1967). Compounds of the PTC type have the chemical grouping -N-C=S. Taste sensitivity to these compounds is known to have a genetic basis, and appears to be due to an autosomal recessive inheritance. It has been widely exploited in genetic and anthropological studies in various parts of the world (Alsbirk and Alsbirk 1972; Bhalla 1972; Bonné et al. 1972). In addition to providing an explanation of one type of variability of taste sensitivity, the phenomenon of taste polymorphism also suggests that there are at least two different types of bitter taste.

Recent studies have reported differences in sweet and salt preferences between younger and adult groups and between racial groups in the United States (Desor et al. 1975), and cultural differences in taste preferences for sour and bitter between two groups in India (Moskowitz et al. 1975). Relatively few systematic studies in these areas have been carried out, however, and the possibilities for important research seem considerable.

Two examples from animal taste studies are noted which address the question of intraspecies variability. During a study of taste responses in pigs, taste preferences of the members of a single litter for saccharin solutions were studied (Kare et al. 1965). Two-choice taste preference tests were used in which a water control was paired with a saccharin solution. A litter of eight pigs contained six individuals who preferred saccharin, and two who consistently rejected the saccharin, preferring the unflavored water.

Individual variability in animal taste responses may sometimes have a genetic basis. For example, Nachman (1959) observed that in a population of rats taste-tested for saccharin preference, some preferred saccharin and others preferred water. Those with a high saccharin preference were selectively bred, as were those with a low preference. The offspring (the F_1 generation) were taste-tested, and the high saccharin preference and low preference rats were again selectively bred. The resulting two groups of offspring (the F_2 generation) were found to show quite different saccharin preference behaviors. The "saccharin-bred" had a higher overall preference for saccharin solutions compared with the preferences of the "water-bred." This occurred over a wide range of concentrations; in addition, the "saccharin-bred" animals showed less aversion to the higher saccharin concentrations. It was also noted that the saccharin preference of an animal was highly stable; those which had an extremely high preference for saccharin were consistent in their behavior, as were those at the other extreme, consuming almost no saccharin solution.

In addition to genetic components, disease states and nutritional deficiencies could also influence eating through effects on sensory receptors. For example, vitamin A-deficient rats show changes in taste preference behavior (Bernard *et al.* 1961), and there may be other deficiency states that lead to taste changes. The roles of disease and nutritional deficiencies or sensory function are important areas for further study.

Protective Functions of Taste

The possible survival value of acute senses of smell and taste is illustrated by much anecdotal material. For example, among the few indications that food has spoiled are the malodor and taste which may develop. Aside from this type of example, what is known of the role of the chemical senses in a direct interplay with nutritional status?

A recent field study made in the Andean highlands of Ecuador points up the possible importance of bitter taste sensitivity during evolution (Greene 1974). Goiter is endemic in the northeastern part of the Pichincha province of Ecuador, where the study was carried out. In general, endemic goiter stems from insufficient iodine intake. Interference with its metabolism might also be an influence, in which case naturally occurring goitrogens could be the cause (Gaitan *et al.* 1974). A goitrogen is a substance which causes hypothyroidism, with consequent enlargement of the thyroid gland (goiter).

Many compounds with goitrogenic activity occur in natural products, some of which are consumed by humans (Van Etten 1969). For example, members of the plant genus *Brassica* (family Cruciferae)—which includes such plants as cabbage and turnips—contain thioglucosides whose breakdown products include small amounts of goitrogenic compounds. It is important to note that the same compounds are also responsible for the flavor characteristics which have led to the food and condiment uses of these plants. Among the goitrogenic products formed from the thioglucosides are isothiocyanates $(R-N=C=S)$(Van Etten 1969). The related bitter-tasting synthetic compound, phenylthiocarbamide (PTC), mentioned above, has been used extensively in studies of genetic taste polymorphism (Alsbirk and Alsbirk 1972; Bhalla 1972; Bonné *et al.* 1972; Fischer 1967).

Those members of a population who are relatively sensitive to the taste of compounds of this type are called "tasters." "Nontasters" are those individuals who are relatively insensitive to the taste of such compounds, although they are generally able to detect them at a sufficiently high concentration.

A portion of the study by Greene (1974) in Ecuador included taste sensitivity measurements using PTC as a bitter taste-testing compound. The populations studied were two communities where goiter and cretinism are endemic. Earlier, in 1966, the children in one community had received iodine while those in the other community had not (Fierro-Benitez *et al.* 1969). This earlier program attempted to reduce the prevalence of goiter and cretinism, and the iodine was therefore administered by a route (intramuscular injection of iodized oil) which would insure a long-lasting effect. In the noniodized population, PTC taste sensitivity and visual-motor maturation were positively correlated, although to a small degree (Greene 1974). Children sensitive to the taste of PTC had somewhat higher visual-motor maturation scores than those who were insensitive tasters of PTC.

In the iodized population, this correlation was not found. The hypothesis proposed to explain this difference was that sensitive tasters of PTC have an adaptive advantage in being better able to limit ingestion of naturally occurring goitrogens through the sense of taste. By limiting their intake of goitrogens, they therefore put less stress on the thyroid and are consequently less likely to be retarded in visual-motor development. In the iodized population, however, no such thyroid stress occurs and there is no relationship between taste sensitivity and neurological development. This study therefore provides an example of the influence that taste sensitivity can have on nutritional status and neurological maturation.

INFLUENCE OF CHEMICAL SENSES ON REGULATION OF SYSTEMIC PROCESSES

Digestive Consequences

Less widely appreciated than the role of the chemical senses in selecting foods is their possible role in systemic physiological processes. The classic studies of Pavlov (1902) showed that stimuli associated with food can increase salivary flow. It is perhaps less well known that Pavlov's studies also demonstrated changes in gastric and exocrine pancreatic flows. In more recent work, Behrman and Kare (1968) documented an increase in exocrine pancreatic flow rate and protein content in dogs when the animals were stimulated orally with food that contained different flavoring agents. Presumably the protein content reflected an increase in pancreatic digestive enzymes.

Responses of Blood Glucose and Insulin

A number of investigators have reported conflicting results of the effects on blood glucose levels due to oral stimulation with sweet substances. In studies in which blood glucose levels of rats were continuously monitored *in vivo*, Nicolaïdis (1969) showed that stimulation in the oral cavity with sucrose or saccharin led to a hyperglycemic effect. The effect occurred within the first few minutes following stimulation and appeared to depend in part upon the time interval between the most recent meal and stimulation, an observation which might explain some of the discrepancies among earlier reports.

In studies on human patients, Kipnis and co-workers (1972) observed that a glucose load administered orally has a different effect on plasma insulin than a load given by intravenous infusion. Oral administration leads to a larger release of insulin into the bloodstream, pointing to the possibility of oral or gastrointestinal receptors.

These examples suggest important influences of the chemical senses on systemic physiology which extend far beyond the question of the acceptance of food. The influence of sensory stimulation in the oral cavity could thereby affect nutritional adaptation through influences on digestive and metabolic processes.

CONCLUSION

Variability in sensory responses among individuals to the chemical stimuli in foods could result in variability in nutritional adaptation. In some cases individual responses to the taste of foods can be demonstrated at birth. With other foods, the response may be influenced to varying degrees by learning. Two examples of an innate ability to taste a substance and respond behaviorally to it are the salty taste of sodium chloride (in a number of animal studies) and the sweet taste of sugars (in human studies).

The responses to stimuli can be influenced to varying degrees by learning. For example, a classic study showed that vitamin B-1-deficient rats are able to select a vitamin-containing diet from among several choices. In this case, the selection is based upon learned responses to sensory cues in the diet, rather than on the taste of the vitamin itself.

Anthropomorphic interpretation of the particular sensory responses in animals may not be valid. A number of studies involving the taste responses of various species show that each lives in its own sensory world. On the other hand, intraspecies variations in taste responses have been studied relatively little, even though they could account for part of the variability in nutrition. The chemical senses also serve a protective function. For example, evidence suggests that an acute sense of taste for certain bitter compounds might play a protective role in iodine-deficient individuals who are also exposed to naturally occurring goitrogens.

Influences of chemosensory stimulation on systemic processes have been demonstrated. Particularly important could be the effects of oral stimulation on digestion in the intestine, and on carbohydrate metabolism systemically. These are areas that require further consideration in relation to the nutritional consequences of gustatory stimulation.

The complexities introduced by varied individual responses to sensory stimuli in foods must be seriously considered in nutritional programs. Taste and olfaction are important to humans, as seen from their influence on selecting foods to eat and the pleasure derived from this sensory stimulation. This fact should be more carefully considered in using sensory aspects to aid in providing good nutrition.

ACKNOWLEDGEMENTS
Dr. Gary Beauchamp of the Monell Chemical Senses Center provided scholarly critiques at important stages during the development of this manuscript, for which we are most appreciative.

REFERENCES
ALSBIRK, K. E., and ALSBIRK, P. H. 1972. PTC taste sensitivity in Greenland Eskimos from Umanaq. Distribution and correlation to anterior chamber depth. Hum. Hered. 22, 445–452.

AMERINE, M. A., PANGBORN, R. M., and ROESSLER, E. 1965. Principles of Sensory Evaluation of Food. Academic Press, New York.

BEHRMAN, H. R., and KARE, M. R. 1968. Canine pancreatic secretion in response to acceptable and aversive taste stimuli. Proc. Soc. Exp. Biol. Med. 129, 343–346.

BERNARD, R. A., HALPERN, B. P., and KARE, M. R. 1961. Effect of vitamin A deficiency on taste. Proc. Soc. Exp. Biol. Med. 108, 784–786.

BHALLA, V. 1972. Variations in taste threshold for PTC in populations of Tibet and Ladakh. Hum. Hered. 22, 453–458.

BONNÉ, B., ASHBEL, S., BERLIN, G., and SELA, B. 1972. The Habbanite isolate. III. Anthropometrics, taste sensitivity and color vision. Hum. Hered. 22, 430–444.

CAGAN, R. H. 1973. Chemostimulatory protein: A new type of taste stimulus. Science 181, 32–35.

CAMERON, A. T. 1947. The taste sense and the relative sweetness of sugars and other sweet substances. Sci. Rept. Ser. 9, Sugar Research Foundation, New York.

CAPRETTA, P. J., and RAWLS, L. H., III. 1974. Establishment of a flavor preference in rats: Importance of nursing and weaning experience. J. Comp. Physiol. Psychol. 86, 670–673.

DESOR, J. A., GREENE, L. S., and MALLER, O. 1975. Preferences for sweet and salty in 9- to 15-year-old and adult humans. Science 190, 686–687.

DESOR, J. A., MALLER, O., and TURNER, R. E. 1973. Taste in acceptance of sugars by human infants. J. Comp. Physiol. Psychol. 84, 496–501.

EPSTEIN, A. N. 1967. Oropharyngeal factors in feeding and drinking. In Handbook of Physiology, Vol. I. C. F. Code (Editor). Am. Physiol. Soc., Washington, D. C.

FIERRO-BENITEZ, R. et al. 1969. Iodized oil in the prevention of endemic goiter and associated defects in the Andean region of Ecuador. I. Program design, effects on goiter prevalence, thyroid function, and iodine excretion. In Endemic Goiter. J. B. Stanbury (Editor). Sci. Pub.193, Pan Am. Health Org., WHO, Washington, D. C.

FISCHER, R. 1967. Genetics and gustatory chemoreception in man and other primates. In The Chemical Senses and Nutrition. M. R. Kare and O. Maller (Editors). Johns Hopkins Press, Baltimore.

GAITAN, E., MEYER, J. D., and MERINO, H. 1974. Environmental goitrogens in Colombia. *In* Endemic Goiter and Cretinism: Continuing Threats to World Health. J. T. Dunn and G. A. Medeiros-Neto (Editors). Sci. Pub. *292*, Pan Am. Health Org., WHO, Washington, D. C.

GALEF, B. G., JR., and HENDERSON, P. W. 1972. Mother's milk: A determinant of the feeding preferences of weaning rat pups. J. Comp. Physiol. Psychol. *78*, 213–219.

GREENE, L. S. 1974. Physical growth and development, neurological maturation, and behavioral functioning in two Ecuadorian Andean communities in which goiter is endemic. II. PTC taste sensitivity and neurological maturation. Am. J. Phys. Anthrop. *41*, 139–151.

HARRIMAN, A. E., and KARE, M. R. 1964. Preference of sodium chloride over lithium chloride by adrenalectomized rats. Am. J. Physiol. *207*, 941–943.

HARRIS, L. J., CLAY, J., HARGREAVES, F. J., and WARD, A. 1933. Appetite and choice of diet. The ability of the vitamin B deficient rat to discriminate between diets containing and lacking the vitamin. Proc. Roy. Soc. (Biol.) *113*, 161–190.

KARE, M. 1971. Comparative study of taste. *In* Handbook of Sensory Physiology, Vol. IV. L. M. Beidler (Editor). Springer-Verlag, New York.

KARE, M. R., and MALLER, O. 1967. The Chemical Senses and Nutrition. Johns Hopkins Press, Baltimore.

KARE, M. R., POND, W. C., and CAMPBELL, J. 1965. Observations on the taste reactions in pigs. Anim. Behav. *13*, 265–269.

KIPNIS, D. M. 1972. Nutrient regulation of insulin secretion in human subjects. Diabetes *21*, Suppl. 2, 606–616.

LE MAGNEN, J. 1971. Olfaction and nutrition. *In* Handbook of Sensory Physiology, Vol. IV. L. M. Beidler (Editor). Springer-Verlag, New York.

MISTRETTA, C. M., and BRADLEY, R. M. 1975. Taste and swallowing in utero. A discussion of fetal sensory function. Br. Med. Bull. *31*, 80–84.

MOSKOWITZ, H. W. *et al.* 1975. Cross-cultural differences in simple taste preferences. Science *190*, 1217–1218.

MOZELL, M. M. *et al.* 1969. Nasal chemoreception in flavor identification. Arch. Otolaryng. *90*, 367–373.

NACHMAN, M. 1959. The inheritance of saccharin preference. J. Comp. Physiol. Psychol. *52*, 451–457.

NACHMAN, M. 1962. Taste preferences for sodium salts by adrenalectomized rats. J. Comp. Physiol. Psychol. *55*, 1124–1129.

NACHMAN, M., and COLE, L. P. 1971. Role of taste in specific hungers. *In* Handbook of Sensory Physiology, Vol. IV. L. M. Beidler (Editor) Springer-Verlag, New York.

NICOLAIDIS, S. 1969. Early systemic responses to orogastric stimulation in the regulation of food and water balance: Functional and electrophysiological data. Ann. N. Y. Acad. Sci. *157*, 1176–1200.

PAVLOV, J. P. 1902. The Work of the Digestive Glands. Charles Griffin and Co., Ltd., London.

RICHTER, C. P. 1942. Total self-regulatory functions in animals and human beings. Harvey Lect. *38*, 63–103.

ROZIN, P., and KALAT, J. W. 1971. Specific hungers and poison avoidance as adaptive specializations of learning. Psychol. Rev. *78*, 459–486.

SCHECHTER, P. J., HORWITZ, D., and HENKIN, R. I. 1974. Salt preference in patients with untreated and treated essential hypertension. Am. J. Med. Sci. *267*, 320–326.

STEINER, J. E. 1973. The gustofacial response: Observation on normal and anencephalic newborn infants. *In* 4th Symposium on Oral Sensation and Perception. J. F. Bosma (Editor). U. S. Dept. of Health, Education, and Welfare, N.I.H., Bethesda, Md.

VAN ETTEN, C. H. 1969. Goitrogens. *In* Toxic Constituents of Plant Foodstuffs. I. E. Liener (Editor). Academic Press, New York.

WEINER, I. H. and STELLAR, E. 1951. Salt preference of the rat determined by a single-stimulus method. J. Comp. Physiol. Psychol. *44*, 394–401.

CHAPTER 18

Norman Kretchmer

Genetic Variability and Lactose Tolerance

Throughout eons of evolutionary history, milk has been the chief food of young mammals, and the milk sugar lactose has been their prime source of carbohydrate. Yet it is only among certain subgroups of one species (*Homo sapiens*), and only in the last 6 to 10 thousand years, that milk and lactose have played a role in adult nutrition. The Neolithic discovery of domestication of plants and animals, followed by the adoption of dairying, allowed certain human groups to extend the consumption of milk into a phase of the life span in which there had previously been no need for the enzymatic capacity to digest lactose. This paper will describe the response of individuals and populations to the nutritional challenge of adult lactose consumption, insofar as we have been able to discern it from our own studies and a review of the world literature (Johnson *et al.* 1974).

The individual response of greatest concern to the clinician, of course, is lactose intolerance; or, to use a more generally applicable term, lactose malabsorption. There are three basic forms of lactose malabsorption, each associated with low activity of the intestinal enzyme lactase, which is specific for the substrate lactose. The three forms of lactose malabsorption are distinguishable from one another by etiology and time of onset.

CONGENITAL MALABSORPTION

This condition is rarely observed in humans. A few cases of infantile diarrhea resulting from congenital lactose malabsorption have been reported in the medical literature, including several by Holzel in England (1967) and two by Durand in Italy (1958). Congenital malabsorption of lactose is universal at all ages among the seals, sea lions and walruses (*Pinnipedia*) of the Pacific Basin. These sea mammals have no lactase in their intestines at any age, and no lactose in their milk. This does not hold true, however, for the pinnipeds of the Atlantic Basin, which follow the typical mammalian pattern with respect to synthesis of lactase and lactose. It has been suggested that the two groups of seal mammals may have evolved from different ancestors—the Pacific *Pinnipedia* from a bear-like progenitor, and their Atlantic counterparts from some sort of ancient land otter (Kretchmer and Sunshine 1967).

SECONDARY LACTOSE MALABSORPTION

This phenomenon occurs rather frequently among infants or adults who have been subjected to gastrointestinal stress. It may be observed in association with specific or nonspecific diarrhea, postoperative reactions, the use of various drugs, etc. In each case, the inciting agent has caused the enzyme lactase to be obliterated from the intestine. Activity of lactase generally reappears within one to two months, as the cells of the villi regenerate. Secondary lactose malabsorption often appears in infants suffering from diarrhea (Sunshine and Kretchmer 1964), and has been familiar to pediatricians since it was first described by Abraham Jacobi in 1898.

HEREDITARY (POST-WEANING) MALABSORPTION

This form of lactose malabsorption is common among persons older than 3 to 5 years of age, and represents the typical mammalian pattern with respect to lactase activity.

In the vast majority of mammalian species, lactase activity is at its highest during the perinatal period; thereafter it decreases to very low values. Figure 18.1 shows the developmental profile of lactase activity in the intestine of the rat, with the characteristic elevation at about the time of birth, and a gradual decline with increasing maturity of the animal (Doell and Kretchmer 1962). In most species, there are about 10 units of lactase activity per g of intestinal mucosa in the perinatal period for every 1 unit per g of material in the adult animal. For example, the newborn kitten exhibits 4 units of enzymic activity per g of intestinal material, as com-

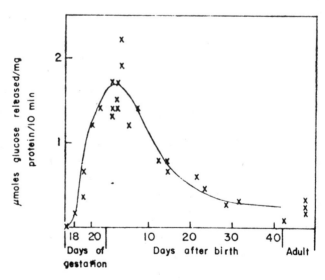

FIG. 18.1. LACTOSE ACTIVITY IN THE INTESTINE OF THE RAT

pared with 0.5 units per g in the adult cat. In the dog, there are 6 units per g of intestinal material at birth, and 0.7 units in adulthood.

One exception to the general rule is the guinea pig, which is known for its early maturation; in this case, lactase activity remains almost constant from birth to maturity. The Pacific pinnipeds are also atypical, as mentioned earlier. But the most remarkable exception to the typical mammalian pattern of lactase activity is found in the human species, some of whose adult members exhibit little or none. Although the enzyme is present in high activity (29 ± 6 units per g of intestinal mucosa) in all healthy infants, the value decreases to 2.7 ± 2 units for the adult malabsorber, as compared with 17 ± 7 units for the adult absorber.

In recent years there has been a steady accumulation of evidence, which demonstrates that lactose malabsorption in otherwise healthy adults is not only hereditary, but closely correlated with ethnic origin. Johnson *et al.* (1974) have surveyed the world literature on lactose malabsorption in adults and have divided the populations for which data is available into three major groups:

(1) Populations in which lactose absorbers predominate. This group includes the Danes, the Finns, the Dutch and the French, together with Poles, Czechs, Northern Italians and those Greeks living in the vicinity of Athens. In general, Northern European populations show a malabsorption rate of about 10 to 15%. A recent study of Hungarians indicates that their rate of malabsorption is about the same as that of the Finns, to whom they are linguistically related. Also included among the ethnic groups composed predominantly of absorbers are three African tribes—the Fulani of the Western sub-Saharan region, the Tussi of Uganda and Rwanda, and the Masai of Kenya and Tanzania.

(2) Populations in which the majority of adults are lactose malabsorbers. This category may well include most of the peoples of the earth. Known examples are populations of the Mediterranean Basin, Southeastern Europe, the Orient, Polynesia and Micronesia, together with a number of African tribes, Eskimos, and the Pima and Apache Indians of Arizona. Among the Yoruba of Western Nigeria, Ransome-Kuti *et al.* (1975) found a malabsorption rate of 99%, while the Ibo of Eastern Nigeria attained a perfect 100%. Although few populations exhibit a 100% malabsorption rate (among the rare examples are the New Guineans, the Fijians, and those Italians in the area of Naples), the world literature indicates that major regions of the globe are inhabited by peoples who cannot digest lactose (Fig. 18.2).

(3) Populations formed by recent admixture between lactose-absorbing and nonabsorbing ethnic groups. These mixed populations exhibit frequencies of malabsorption intermediate between those of the parent groups. Among the mixed populations, the author has had the most experience

DIFFERENCES IN LACTOSE MALABSORPTION AMONG THE WORLD'S PEOPLES (ADULTS)

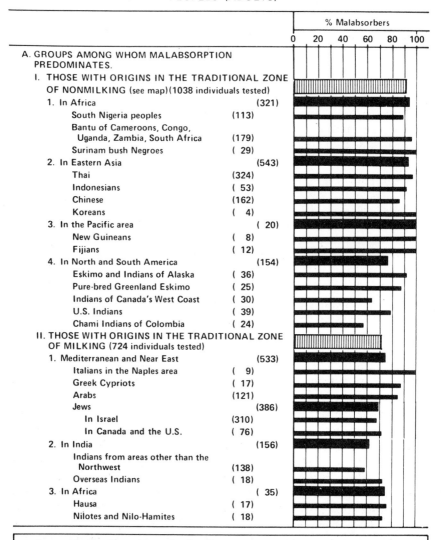

	% Malabsorbers 0 20 40 60 80 100
A. GROUPS AMONG WHOM MALABSORPTION PREDOMINATES.	
I. THOSE WITH ORIGINS IN THE TRADITIONAL ZONE OF NONMILKING (see map)(1038 individuals tested)	
1. In Africa (321)	
South Nigeria peoples (113)	
Bantu of Cameroons, Congo, Uganda, Zambia, South Africa (179)	
Surinam bush Negroes (29)	
2. In Eastern Asia (543)	
Thai (324)	
Indonesians (53)	
Chinese (162)	
Koreans (4)	
3. In the Pacific area (20)	
New Guineans (8)	
Fijians (12)	
4. In North and South America (154)	
Eskimo and Indians of Alaska (36)	
Pure-bred Greenland Eskimo (25)	
Indians of Canada's West Coast (30)	
U.S. Indians (39)	
Chami Indians of Colombia (24)	
II. THOSE WITH ORIGINS IN THE TRADITIONAL ZONE OF MILKING (724 individuals tested)	
1. Mediterranean and Near East (533)	
Italians in the Naples area (9)	
Greek Cypriots (17)	
Arabs (121)	
Jews (386)	
In Israel (310)	
In Canada and the U.S. (76)	
2. In India (156)	
Indians from areas other than the Northwest (138)	
Overseas Indians (18)	
3. In Africa (35)	
Hausa (17)	
Nilotes and Nilo-Hamites (18)	

In preparing the above table results of studies were used only if they involved one of the two most reliable, widely used tests of malabsorption: (1) lactose loading test, which measures the rise of blood glucose, and (2) assay of lactase activity following intestinal biopsy. Excluded from consideration were all studies using testing procedures of questionable reliability or studies focusing on symptoms rather than on absorption per se.

Excluded were all studies of children. Also eliminated, insofar as possible, were individuals among whom malabsorption may have been secondary, in cases where the incidence of malabsorption in the study group may have been significantly influenced. Also not taken into our account were those studies in which data presented did not permit the determination of percentage of malabsorption in the group in question.

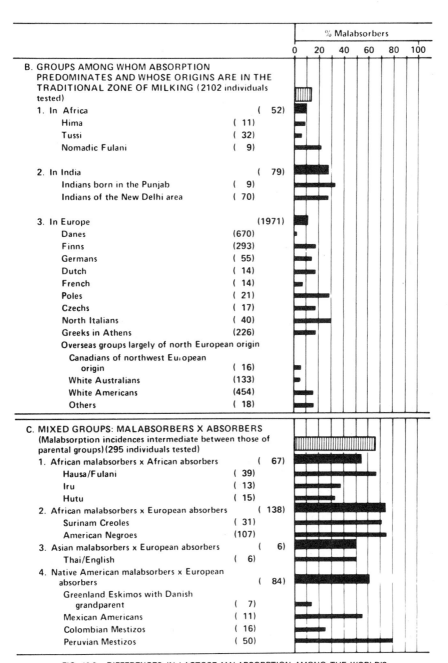

FIG. 18.2. DIFFERENCES IN LACTOSE MALABSORPTION AMONG THE WORLD'S
PEOPLES (ADULTS)
A. Groups among whom malabsorption predominates; B. Groups among whom absorption predominates and whose origins are in the traditional zone of milking; C. Mixed groups: Malabsorbers x absorbers.

with the Fulani-Hausa of Northern Nigeria. The Fulani, who are thought to be descendants of ancient Saharan cattle herders, are predominantly lactose absorbers. The Hausa, who are descended from ancient Berbers, are malabsorbers. In the population formed by intermarriage between the two groups, 60–70% of the adults are malabsorbers. American Negroes exhibit a malabsorption rate of approximately 80%, but the average for mixed populations is about 70%.

The data summarized above indicate that the capacity for adult lactose absorption is not randomly distributed among the peoples of the world. Populations in which absorbers predominate seem to be derived exclusively from those portions of the Old World in which dairying has been practiced for centuries. Figure 18.3 illustrates the extent of dairying as of 1500 A.D. At that time, there was a single large region of milk-using peoples extending from Tibet and Mongolia in the East to the Iberian Peninsula in the West, and southward into the Indian subcontinent and sub-Saharan Africa. There were also several large zones where milking was not practiced: in the Far East, Equatorial Africa, Oceania and the Americas. Populations which contain a significant minority of absorbers will generally have some history of admixture with a population from the traditional dairying zone.

This correlation between the ethnic and geographical distribution of lactose malabsorption and the traditional geographical distribution of dairying has led Simoons (1970) to formulate the so-called *cultural-historical hypothesis* which, simply stated, suggests that those peoples whose origins lie in the traditionally milk-drinking regions of the world are likely to have become, by genetic selection, lactose absorbers, while peoples whose origins lie elsewhere would never have acquired the enzymatic capacity for lactose digestion in adulthood.

Obviously, it is not possible to devise a direct test of the cultural-historical hypothesis. However, we can identify certain questions whose answers will have a strong bearing on the ultimate acceptance or rejection of the hypothesis. First, what is the pattern of inheritance of lactose malabsorption? Second, which was the original "wild type"—the absorber or the malabsorber? Third, has adequate time elapsed since the advent of dairying to account for the present-day frequency of lactose absorption in the peoples of the so-called "milking zone"?

Investigations aimed at delineating the pattern of inheritance of lactose malabsorption have recently been carried out by Ransome-Kuti *et al.* (1975) in Nigeria and by Simoons *et al.* (unpub.) among the Pima and related American Indian tribes of the Phoenix, Arizona, area. In both instances, the investigators have taken advantage of a situation in which the recent admixture of absorbing and nonabsorbing ethnic stocks guarantees a large number of marriages between individuals who differ in their capacity for lactose absorption.

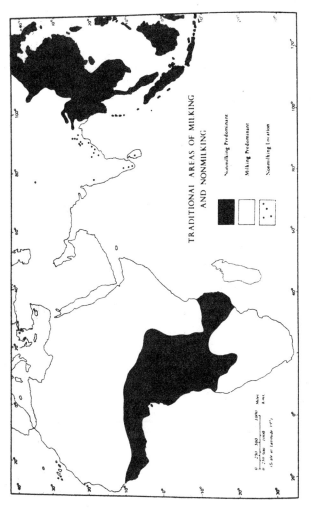

FIG. 18.3. TRADITIONAL AREAS OF MILKING AND NON-MILKING

The results of these and other family studies, summarized in Table 18.1, suggest that the ability to absorb lactose by an adult human is inherited as a dominant trait. Thus, when a heterozygous lactose digestor (Dd) marries either a homozygous lactose nondigestor (dd) or another heterozygous lactose digestor (Dd), statistically the progeny could be expected to be a mixture of both types, i.e., digestors (50–75%) and nondigestors (25–50%). However, in the case of a cross between two lactose nondigestors (dd), none of the progeny should be capable of digesting lactose. There is one report in the literature (Welsh *et al.* 1968) of a digestor arising out of a cross between two nondigestors, but this case is exceptional and may indicate nonpaternity.

TABLE 18.1

SUMMARY OF FAMILIES IN THIS STUDY AND FROM THE LITERATURE

Predicted Genetic Notation	No. of Families	Digestors (D–)	Nondigestors (dd)
		Progeny[1]	
A. Families taken from the literature			
dd × dd	12	1	34
D– × dd	15	24	23
D– × D–	3	8	4
B. Nigerian families (Ransome-Kuti *et al.* 1975)			
dd × dd	9	0	21
D– × dd	10	18	11

[1]The progeny are listed as lactose digestors and nondigestors. The marriages are given a predicted genetic notation.

Continuous intermarriage between a small population of lactose absorbers and a larger population of nonabsorbers should eventually lead to dilution of the gene for adult lactase in the population. This has been the case in Northern Nigeria, where descendants of the nomadic, lactose-absorbing Fulani began to intermarry 200 years ago with the Hausa, a sedentary group of nonabsorbers. The progeny from the Hausa-Fulani crosses have continued to marry into the larger population of Hausa town dwellers, giving rise to a population which is relatively incapable of digesting lactose, but retains many of the cultural traits of the Fulani.

Although the American Negro population is derived primarily from West African peoples who are nondigestors of lactose, it has a surprising frequency of 20–30% adult lactose digestors. This observation could be explained on the basis of unions with Northern European groups composed predominantly (about 90%) of lactose digestors, and fits with information derived from studies of the Gm genotype among American Caucasians and Negroes (Ransome-Kuti *et al.* 1975).

It is probable that the human ability to digest lactose in adulthood is the result of a mutation in a gene affecting the level of intestinal lactase activity, such that a value of 17 ± 7 units is attained in place of the 2.7 ± 2 units typically present in the nondigestor. Since the usual characteristic of mammals is elevated activity of the enzyme during infancy and markedly diminished activity in the adult, it seems reasonable to suppose that the nondigestor represents the original "wild type" and the digestor the mutant type. If this is the case, then it seems reasonable to hypothesize that selective pressure may have increased the frequency of lactose digestors in those ethic groups which practiced milk-drinking.

Cavalli-Sforza (1973) has calculated that a coefficient of selection of 3% operating over a span of 10,000 years would be sufficient to give rise to the high frequency of adult lactose absorption observed among Northern Europeans and certain African tribes today. Direct evidence for the antiquity of dairying can be found in certain rock drawings from the Sahara which depict the milking of cattle, and are dated at ca. 4000 to 3000 B.C. However, the earliest known domestication of a herd animal, that of the sheep, dates to about 9000 B.C. in the Near East. Presumably the initiation of dairying must have occurred sometime between these two events. Further investigations by archaeologists and palaeoanthropologists are needed to determine whether dairying has in fact existed long enough to produce the postulated changes in gene frequency.

If the cultural-historical hypothesis does indeed withstand the test of further investigation, the implications for future nutritional research—and even more significantly, for future nutritional planning—will be enormous. For milk-drinking is only one of dozens of food consumption patterns which have arisen and spread across the world in the last ten thousand years. If differences in milk consumption have in fact led to genetic divergence among human populations, it may well be that other differences have arisen in response to other foodstuffs. There is a definite need for research to determine the true extent of individual and ethnic idiosyncrasies with respect to the most common elements of our diet.

REFERENCES

CAVALLI-SFORZA, L. L. 1973. Analytic review: Some current problems of human genetics. Am. J. Hum. Gen. *25*, 82–104.

DOELL, R. G., and KRETCHMER, N. 1962. Studies of small intestine during development. I. Distribution and activity of β-galactosidase. Biochem. Biophys. Acta *62*, 353.

DURAND, P. 1958. Idiopathic lactosuria in a patient with chronic acidic diarrhea. Minerva Pediatr. *10*, 706. (Italian)

HOLZEL, A. 1967. Sugar malabsorption due to deficiences of disaccharidase activities and of monosaccharide transport. Arch. Dis. Child. *42*, 341.

JOHNSON, J. D., KRETCHMER, N., and SIMOONS, F. J. 1974. Lactose malabsorption: Its biology and history. Adv. in Pediatr. *21*, 197–238.

KRETCHMER, N., and SUNSHINE, P. 1967. Intestinal disaccharidase deficiency in the sea lion, Gastroenterology *53*, 123.

RANSOME-KUTI, O., KRETCHMER, N., JOHNSON, J., and GRIBBLE, J. T. 1975. A genetic study of lactose digestion in Nigerian families. Gastroenterology *68*, 431–436.

SIMOONS, F. J. 1970. Primary adult lactose intolerance and the milking habit: A problem in biological and cultural interrelations. II. A cultural-historical hypothesis. Am. J. Dig. Dis. *15*, 695.

SIMOONS, F. J. *et al.* Lactose malabsorption among the Indians of the American Southwest. (Two unpublished papers)

SUNSHINE, P., and KRETCHMER, N. 1964. Studies of the small intestine during development. III. Infantile diarrhea associated with intolerance to disaccharides. Pediatrics *34*, 38–50.

WELSH, J. D. *et al.* 1968. Studies of lactose intolerance in families. Arch. Intern. Med. *122*, 315–316.

CHAPTER 19

Toshio Oiso

Anthropometric and Disease Pattern Changes in the Japanese Population: Nutritional or Other?

During the past half century (1925-1975), Japan has undergone drastic changes in all areas. Following the close of World War II, we entered an age of democracy. Because the food situation was very grave at that time, the government attempted to rebuild Japan's economic capability through industrial growth. After a period of endurance, diligence and hard work, living conditions became gradually improved. Because the food problem was so urgent, the Japanese people felt that elevating their economy was of great importance. They strongly wished to promote industrial production and to participate in the free economy of the world. Within 10 or 15 years (1955-1960), Japan's latent economic power came to bear fruit (Fig. 19.1), and rose rapidly from that point on.

The abrupt changes, especially between 1940 and the present day, have influenced the Japanese both materially and spiritually. During the past 50 years, the older generation died out, a new generation continued on. But while this younger generation had grown up with far greater material benefits, they still did not possess physical well-being. It is difficult to find a clear explanation for the changes in the patterns of disease which occured during this period of biological stress, but it seems obvious that a number of environmental and nutritional factors were involved. These changes in previous life patterns produced certain alterations in the metabolism of the human body which have led to different disease states and causes of death. This point will become more clear in relation to the data presented here.

One of the most important factors to be considered is the nearly two-fold increase in the Japanese population over the past 50 years. In 1925, the population numbered 60 million, creating a population density of 146 persons per square km. The population is now 110 million, with a population density of nearly 300 persons per square km. The natural increase in population is rather high, owing to recent decreases in both birth and mortality rates (Table 19.1). Of special interest is the decrease in infant mortality, and the reduced rate of death from tuberculosis among younger people.

The increase in population naturally brings the question of food supply into the forefront. From 1930 to 1945, Japan underwent a serious food shortage, and much of the population suffered hunger. In the years following World War II, the urban population consumed a very small number

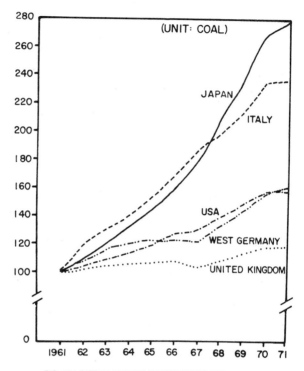

FIG. 19.1 RISE IN JAPAN'S ECONOMIC POWER, 1961-67

of calories—about 1700 calories per day per capita. In the rural areas, the situation was somewhat better (Tables 19.2 – 19.4) As social conditions gradually improved and the level of industry rose, the economic status of the cities took an upward turn. The rural farming and fishing populations were then urbanized.

TABLE 19.1

POPULATION STATISTICS

Year	Total Population (1000)	No. of Families (1000)	No. of Persons per Family	Rate of Birth (%)	Rate of Death (%)	Life Expectancy (years) Male	Life Expectancy (years) Female
1935	68,662	13,378	5.13	31.6	16.8	46.9	49.6
1945	71,998	15,871	4.92	–	–	23.9	37.5
1950	83,200	16,580	5.02	28.1	10.9	58.0	61.5
1955	89,276	17,960	4.97	19.4	7.8	63.9	68.4
1960	93,419	20,639	4.53	17.2	7.6	65.4	70.3
1965	98,275	24,104	4.08	18.5	7.1	67.7	72.9
1970	103,720	29,146	3.72	18.8	6.9	69.3	74.7

TABLE 19.2
NATIONAL ANNUAL CHANGES IN NUTRIENT INTAKE

		1949	1953	1958	1963	1968	1968/1949
				(per capita per day)			(ratio)
Calories		2087	2041	2108	2090	2214	1.1
Total protein	(g)	68	69	71	71	77	1.1
Animal protein	(g)	16	22	24	29	32	2.0
Fat	(g)	18	20	23	29	45	2.6
Vitamin A	(I.U.)	–	–	1240	1423	1421	1.2
Vitamin B-1	(mg)	1.51	1.11	1.05	1.03	1.10	0.7
Vitamin B-2	(mg)	0.65	0.72	0.83	0.81	0.96	1.5
Vitamin C	(mg)	95	75	72	66	96	1.0
Calcium	(mg)	258	373	394	415	529	2.1

Although lacking industrial resources, Japan was able to import the techniques of more advanced countries during the years following the war; the result was a remarkable recovery of the Japanese economy, an extremely high level of industrialization and participation in world trade. In 1920, about half of the population was engaged in primary industry—agriculture, forestry and fishing. At the present time, only about 16% of the people are involved with primary industry, the rest having moved into secondary (such as iron or textile mills) or tertiary (such as trade and service work) fields (Table 19.5).

TABLE 19.3
ANNUAL CHANGES IN URBAN FOOD CONSUMPTION

	1946	1951	1956	1961	1966	1968
			(g per capita per day)			
Rice	190	329	340	341	316	293
Wheat	141	109	80	74	76	73
Other cereals	–	52	37	11	5	4
Potatoes	250	78	57	54	67	46
Sugars	1	14	17	13	14	20
Fats and oils	3	4	6	7	12	14
Pulses	27	67	77	70	78	72
Fruits	24	62	78	81	136	–
Green vegetables	158	64	44	35	46	46
Other vegetables	200	133	172	159	188	201
Seasonings	24	41	45	84	95	119
Fish and shellfish	–	85	77	79	86	84
Meat and poultry	67	12	23	29	42	44
Eggs	9	11	17	28	39	41
Milk	3	11	26	45	66	71
Animal food	80	120	143	181	234	240

TABLE 19.4

ANNUAL CHANGES IN RURAL NUTRIENT INTAKE

		1946	1951	1956	1961	1966	1968
				(per capita per day)			
Calories		2084	2171	2152	2210	2243	2225
Total protein	(g)	59	67	68	69	74	75
Animal protein	(g)	6	17	20	21	27	29
Fat	(g)	13	16	19	23	36	39
Vitamin A	(I.U.)	–	–	–	1071	1407	1325
Vitamin B-1	(mg)	1.98	1.58	1.07	1.00	1.02	1.00
Vitamin B-2	(mg)	0.71	0.74	0.69	0.74	0.82	0.93
Vitamin C	(mg)	186	105	78	79	113	–
Calcium	(mg)	253	270	377	387	486	519

Industrialization led to urbanization; at present, approximately 72% of the population lives in urban areas (Table 19.6). Urbanization brought about an imbalance in the rural and urban income levels, leading many of the young rural inhabitants into city life. Since the distribution of everyday commodities (especially foodstuffs) was unsatisfactory, there was an accompanying imbalance in food consumption.

An awareness of this imbalance brought about the National Nutrition Survey which has been conducted every year since 1946. Early surveys showed that those people who lived in rural areas had a higher caloric intake than did city dwellers, but fell noticeably behind in total protein intake, especially in regard to animal protein, fats and oils (Figs. 19.1–19.5). In recent years, the protein gap between rural and urban populations has begun to narrow, partly because the economy has improved, and partly as the result of the development of frozen and processed foods.

Industrialization required steady sources of energy, and the demand for low cost, high yield petroleum rose year after year (Table 19.7). This increase in the consumption of petroleum and petroleum-based products

TABLE 19.5

ANNUAL CHANGE IN THE NUMBER OF WORKERS
(15-19 YEARS OLD) BY INDUSTRIAL STRUCTURE

Year	Primary Industry	Secondary Industry	Tertiary Industry	All Industry
1920	52.1	28.6	19.4	100.0
1930	41.4	28.4	30.2	100.0
1940	32.3	37.2	30.5	100.0
1950	47.6	28.1	24.3	100.0
1955	33.0	34.0	33.0	100.0
1960	16.8	46.5	36.7	100.0

Source: Census Report Data

TABLE 19.6

AN INDEX OF URBANIZATION

Year	No. of Cities	Total (10,000)	Population Urban (10,000)	Ratio (%)	Area Urban (km²)	Ratio (%)
1935	125	6,866	2,258	32.9	5,087	1.3
1940	125	7,254	2,749	37.9	8,844	2.3
1945	205	7,200	2,002	27.8	14,520	3.9
1950	248	8,320	3,120	37.5	19,815	5.4
1955	490	8,928	5,029	56.3	67,761	18.3
1960	555	9,342	5,933	63.5	82,559	22.3
1965	560	9,827	6,693	68.1	88,068	23.8
1970	579	10,372	7,485	72.2	94,685	25.1

produced serious pollution problems, as did the increasing use of other mineral resources. Among the harmful effects to the human body caused by this pollution is an abnormally high incidence of bronchial asthma. Wastes generated by industrial plants polluted rivers and harbors, leading to chronic cadmium or mercury poisoning among those people who were used to eating fish and shellfish from these regions.

Pollution stemming from industrial waste created political disputes between local citizens and area businessmen, leading to a number of suits for damages. This sort of public unrest has extended into such areas as food additives, agricultural fertilizers, pharmaceuticals and animal feeds.

As more and more agricultural land was put to industrial use, the rural populations were also exposed to the effects of air and water pollution. And the increase in economic prosperity, coupled with the move toward secondary and tertiary industry, led to increased use of the automobile, thus creating traffic congestion and added pollutants in the air. The loss in farmland meant a decrease in domestic food production, so that more and more food items had to be imported.

As a result, food patterns were drastically altered. The original Japanese diet was centered around rice, with the addition of fish, shellfish and vegetables. With the introduction of a Westernized, industrial culture, people began to turn away from simple and economic meals to more extravagant foodstuffs. The appearance of "labor-saving" devices reduced the amount of work done in the home, and food preparation time was decreased by means of "pre-cooked," "instant" and "convenience" foods. In addition, the industrial work week has been shortened. Thus, energy requirements have dropped at the same time that the intake of animal proteins, fats and oils has increased per capita per day. The result is increased obesity in the cities, especially among middle-aged men and women (Fig. 19.6).

Medical care and public health services remained in the background of such overwhelming social and cultural changes. In the periods of food

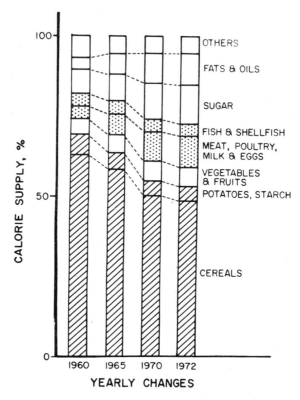

FIG. 19.2. YEARLY CHANGES IN CALORIE SUPPLY (%)

scarcity, nutritional improvement played an important role in the daily life of the people. As a result, physical status improved in the years following the war, as did the labor capacity in industry; morbidity, on the other hand, decreased. But while the Japanese people are much better off economically, the resulting problems of pollution have become serious impairments to national health.

Viewed in this perspective, one can detect many changes in the health and disease patterns of the population. As an example, around 1925, the death rate from tuberculosis, infant mortality and beriberi was at its highest (Fig. 19.7). The diet at that time centered around white rice, soy bean soup (*miso*) and salted, pickled vegetables. Children complained of colds, chilblains and sniffles in the winter, and of diarrhea and enteritis in the summer. Thirty years later (1955), these ailments had completely disappeared; people had begun eating more high quality protein, along with greater quantities of fat, oil, milk, eggs and raw vegetables.

These improvements in the traditional diet elevated the physical status of children and led to early maturation. Infant mortality rates dropped as a

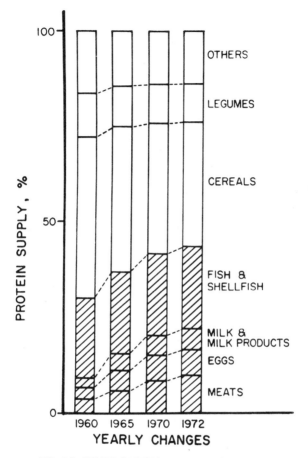

FIG. 19.3. YEARLY CHANGES IN PROTEIN SUPPLY (%)

result of the increased consumption of milk and dairy products. This added dietary protein and calcium (lacking in the traditional diet) brought about remarkable increases in the heights of children (Fig. 19.8). Another factor in this height increase might be the shift from Japanese to Western living conditions (sitting down on chairs, sleeping in beds, etc., leading to an elongation of the legs).

Diseases frequently seen in children, such as trachoma, tuberculosis, parasites and infectious illnesses, tended to decrease while short-sightedness, tooth decay, kidney trouble and asthma increased. While children born after 1955 reach conspicuously greater heights, they are not always physically fit. In fact, physical fitness among city dwellers is much less than that of rural populations. This is partly due to the fact that there is little space in the cities for physical exercise.

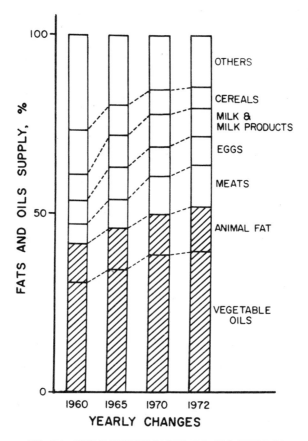

FIG. 19.4.   YEARLY CHANGES IN FATS AND OILS SUPPLY (%)

Infectious diseases, such as tuberculosis, have sharply decreased since 1945 (Table 19.8). Longevity in Japan is approaching that found in the Scandinavian countries. On the other hand, there has been a marked increase in such adult diseases as cerebral hemorrhage, malignant tumors and heart/circulation disorders (Fig. 19.9). (It might be noted that cerebral hemorrhage and heart diseases occupy a reversed position when compared with Western nations.) This causes for disease pattern may lie in the changed diet and living conditions; this question calls for further investigation.

It is expected that pollution problems will continue to rise, with concomitant physiological and psychological effects on the human body. On the other hand, efforts are being made to remove many of these new stresses. In the near future, we will either see an improvement in the disease patterns and physical status of the Japanese people, or new disease patterns resulting from environmental hazards will present new problems.

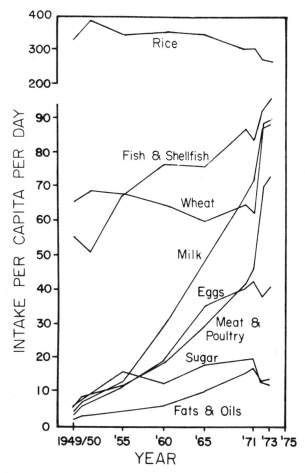

FIG. 19.5. YEARLY INTAKE PER CAPITA PER DAY

TABLE 19.7

CONSUMPTION TREND OF PETROLEUM PRODUCTS IN JAPAN (1000 KL)

Year	Gasoline	Naptha	Jet Fuel	Kerosene	Light Oil	Crude Petroleum	Total
1935	1,025	–	–	137	134	2,381	3,677
1950	413	–	–	77	208	1,111	1,809
1965	10,577	7,316	529	5,064	5,396	47,504	76,386
1969	18,051	20,532	911	11,975	10,155	87,870	149,494
1970	20,440	26,483	1,119	15,311	11,703	105,387	180,442
1971	22,380	29,068	1,225	16,052	12,647	114,402	195,773
1972	24,282	32,022	1,459	17,075	14,028	115,623	204,489

Source: Ministry of International Trade and Industry (1972)

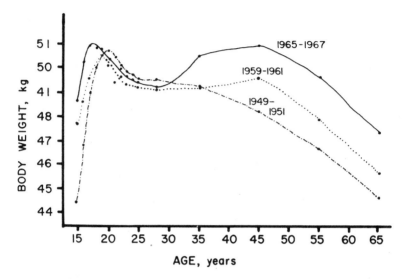

FIG. 19.6. RESULTS OF INCREASE IN ANIMAL PROTEIN REFLECTING INCREASED
OBESITY AMONG MIDDLE-AGED MEN AND WOMEN

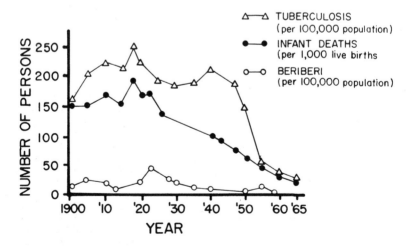

FIG. 19.7. DEATH RATE CHANGES DUE TO HEALTH AND DISEASE PATTERN
CHANGES

TABLE 19.8

LEADING CAUSES OF DEATH IN JAPAN (PER 100,000 POPULATION)

Year	Cerebro- vascular Diseases B30	Malignant Neoplasmas B19	Heart Diseases B26 B29 B28 B29	Accidents BE47 BE48	Senility Without Psychosis B45a	Pneumonia Bronchitis B32 B33a B46d	Tuber- culosis (All forms) B5 B6	Suicide BE49
1900	159	46	48	45	131	226	164	13
1910	132	67	65	44	120	262	230	19
1920	158	73	64	47	131	408	224	19
1935	165	72	58	42	114	187	191	21
1940	178	72	63	40	125	186	213	14
1945	–	–	–	–	–	–	–	–
1950	127	77	64	40	70	93	146	20
1955	136	87	61	37	67	48	52	25
1960	161	100	73	42	58	49	34	22
1965	176	108	77	41	50	37	23	15
1970	175	116	86	42	38	34	15	15
1972	167	120	81	40	31	28	12	17

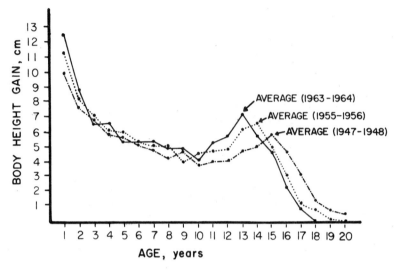

FIG. 19.8. INCREASED HEIGHT CHANGE DUE TO PROTEIN AND CALCIUM INTAKE

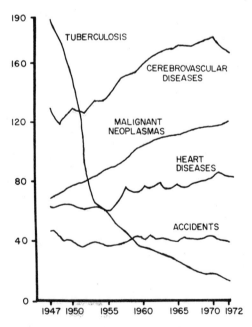

FIG. 19.9. YEARLY CHANGES IN INCREASED ADULT DISEASES AND DISORDERS

CHAPTER 20

S. Onaka
S. Hori
N. Saito
K. Shiraki
Panata Migasena
Hisato Yoshimura

The Role of Food Habits in Physiological Adaptation of Inhabitants of Southeast Asia to the Habitat of Tropical Countries

About 20 years ago, our colleague Dr. S. Osiba began studies on the seasonal variations in basal metabolism (B.M.) with Japanese subjects. At that time, Japanese investigators unanimously claimed that B.M. changed seasonally—that it was higher in the winter and lower in the summer. The maximal change amounted to about 18% of the annual mean. On the other hand, most American authors believed that B.M. is nearly constant throughout the year, and noted that the experimental conditions in the Japanese studies were not constant throughout the time involved in the studies. For example, a rise in metabolism as the result of shivering in winter might have been included in their data.

In an attempt to confirm this issue, Osiba (1957) measured the B.M. of subjects who had spent the previous night in an air-conditioned room at 25°C. All of the subjects clearly showed an individual seasonal variation (Fig. 20.1). The broken lines indicate the seasonal variation of the same subject as measured the previous year at the standardized condition, but in a natural environment where the subject was still in bed. The results in both cases were the same, indicating that the Japanese do manifest a seasonal variation in B.M. As measured by Baker's method, protein-bound iodine (P.B.I.) also showed a seasonal variation parallel to that found in the B.M.

Osiba assumed that the findings in regard to American subjects differed from those of the Japanese because the latter have poor home heating facilities and must therefore adapt to the cold of winter by raising their own B.M. Americans, on the other hand, live in moderate temperatures even in the winter. In an attempt to confirm his assumption, he constructed an experiment in B.M. acclimation using two volunteers. To get the control values for winter, the basal metabolism and P.B.I. of the volunteers was measured after they had become acclimated to a room temperature of 10°–14°C. The subjects then entered a hot room (dry temperature [D. T.] 30°C and wet temperature [W. T.] 24°C) and remained there for about 10 days, leaving for only about 8 hours to go to school. The B.M. was measured daily and the P.B.I. once a week.

As seen in Fig. 20.2, the B.M. at the beginning of winter was reasonably high, but gradually fell each day in the hot room and attained its minimum value for about ten days. Similar experiments were conducted with five

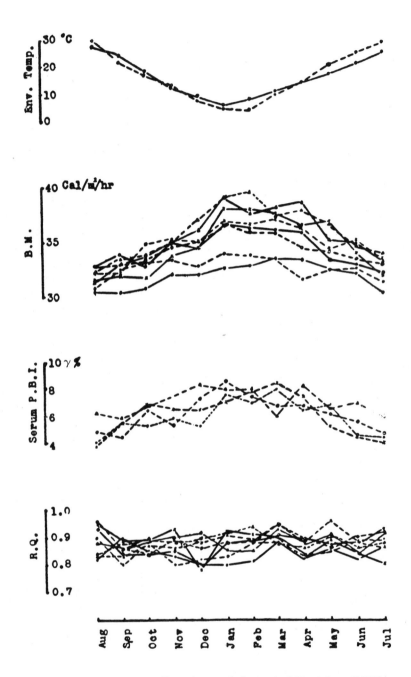

From Japanese Journal of Physiology (1957)

FIG. 20.1. SEASONAL VARIATION OF BM AND SERUM PBI (FOUR SUBJECTS)

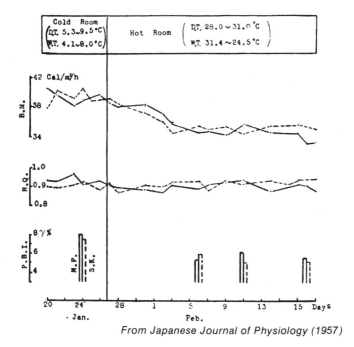

From Japanese Journal of Physiology (1957)

FIG. 20.2. HEAT ADAPTATION OF BASAL METABOLISM (TWO SUBJECTS)

subjects and the changes in B.M. were confirmed. The mean reduction of B.M.R. from the initial control value was about 10.5%. By plotting the B.M.R. against the P.B.I. observed in these acclimation experiments, it can be seen that these seasonal changes in B.M. are closely related to P.B.I., presumably due to the activity of the thyroid gland (Fig. 20.3).

In the next step, Yoshimura *et al.* (1966) attempted to determine why the Caucasians did not show this seasonal variation in B.M. They found a group of Canadian missionaries living in Kyoto in a Japanese-style house that was not equipped with temperature controls, and compared them with Japanese living under similar conditions. The results of the monthly B.M. measurements taken from the Canadians are shown in Fig. 20.4. They demonstrate that the basal metabolism of the Canadian missionaries is maintained at respective constant levels for each subject; some inconsistent variation can be found in some subjects. In Fig. 20.5, we see that the Japanese control subjects, measured at the same time, show a consistent seasonal variation of B.M., with some individual differences among the group.

Differences in living conditions and racial characteristics were each considered as possible causal factors. In regard to living conditions, the most striking difference between the two groups was that the Canadians con-

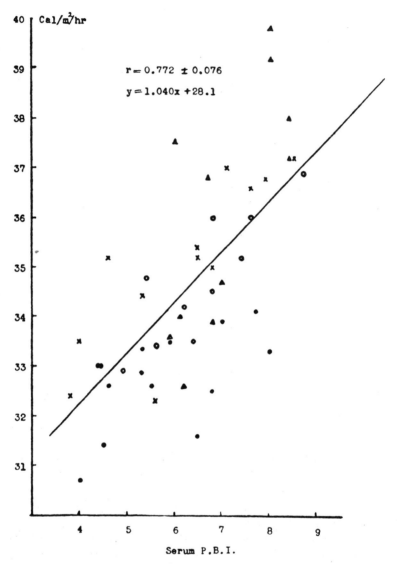

From Japanese Journal of Physiology (1957)

FIG. 20.3. CORRELATION BETWEEN BM AND SERUM PBI

sumed twice as much fat as the Japanese (Fig. 20.6). However, several facts tend to dispute any racial hypothesis in regard to seasonal variation. The first piece of contrary evidence is that M. Yoshimura (1970), one of the control subjects in the Canadian experiments, later spent two years in

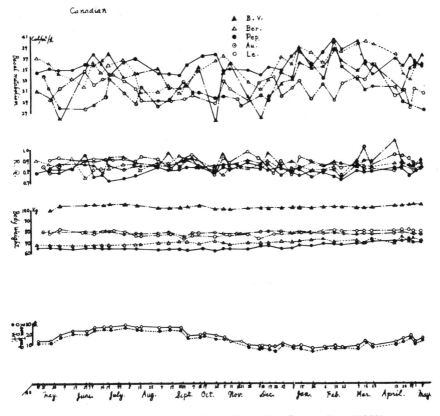

From Federation Proceedings (1966)

FIG. 20.4.   BASAL METABOLISM OF CANADIAN MISSIONARIES DURING MAY 1964
TO MAY 1965. BASAL METABOLISM WAS MEASURED THREE TIMES EACH MONTH

Santa Barbara, California. While there, his basal metabolism and thyroid activity were measured monthly, and seasonal variations recorded; his thyroid activity was found to be higher than it had been in Japan (Fig. 20.7). The two most striking differences in his living conditions involved the composition of his diet in the United States, and the climate in Santa Barbara. He took in over twice as much fat while in the U. S. than he had in Japan, and his intake of carbohydrates decreased. And unlike Japan, the local ambient temperature was nearly constant throughout the year. It seems likely, then, that the seasonal changes in B.M. were caused by differences in living conditions (Yoshimura and Yoshimura 1970).

On the other hand, Dr. Sasaki went to Lexington, Kentucky, where the ambient temperature was similar to that of his native city, Kumamoto. As shown in Fig. 20.8, the seasonal variation in B.M. was greater in Kuma-

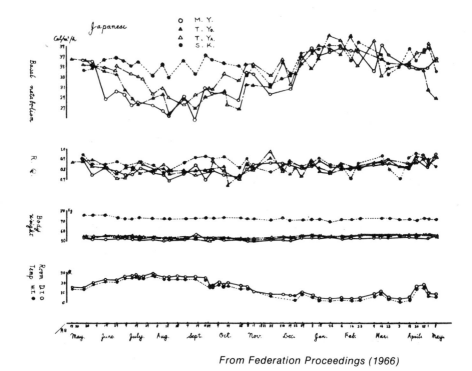

From Federation Proceedings (1966)

FIG. 20.5. BASAL METABOLISM OF JAPANESE DURING MAY 1964 TO MAY 1965.
SUBJECT SK (CLOSED CIRCLE) SHOWS THE DIFFERENT VALUE FROM OTHER
SUBJECTS

moto than it was in Lexington (Ogata *et al.* 1966). Further evidence against
the racial hypothesis was reported by M. Nakamura (1975), who measured
the monthly variation in ten Japanese and ten Caucasian subjects living in
Nagasaki. The Caucasians exhibited clear seasonal changes in B.M. remarkably similar to those of the Japanese (Fig. 20.9). The subjects' dietary
composition was not analyzed in these two experiments, but judging from
the respiratory quotient (R.Q.) graph in Fig. 20.9, the Caucasians' diet
seems to have been close to that of the Japanese; that is, their fat intake
was not as great as that of the Canadians shown in Fig. 20.6. Thus, racial
differences can be completely excluded from any explanation of the causes
for seasonal variation in B.M.

On the positive side, the role of living conditions as a cause for such
variations can be verified by a number of facts. To those experimental data
derived from the study involving Japanese and Canadians, and to the
studies conducted by Dr. Yoshimura and Dr. Sasaki, we can add an annual
trend toward a reduction in the annual range of seasonal variation in B.M.
(Table 20.1), accompanied by an annual increase in fat intake as demon-

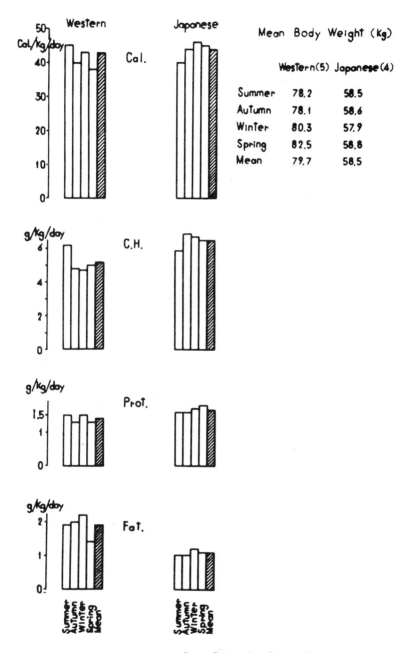

Mean Body Weight (kg)

Western(5) Japanese(4)

	Western(5)	Japanese(4)
Summer	78.2	58.5
Autumn	78.1	58.6
Winter	80.3	57.9
Spring	82.5	58.8
Mean	79.7	58.5

From Federation Proceedings (1966)

FIG. 20.6. COMPARISON OF DIETARY COMPOSITION BETWEEN CANADIAN AND
JAPANESE, AND SEASONAL CHANGES OF BODY WEIGHT

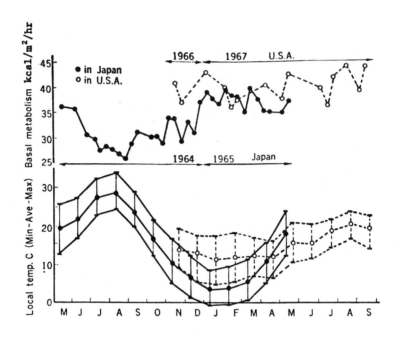

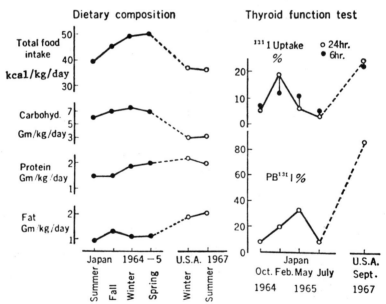

From Itoh, Ogata and Yoshimura (1972)

FIG. 20.7. DIETARY COMPOSITION DURING FOUR SEASONS IN KYOTO COM-
PARED WITH THAT IN THE U.S.A.

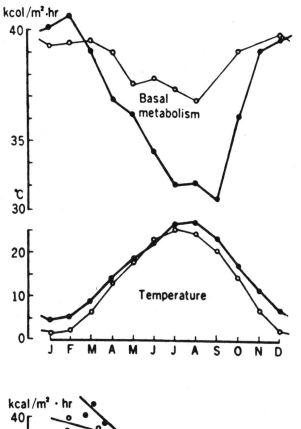

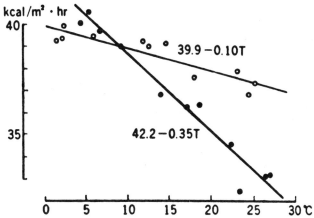

From Itoh, Ogata and Yoshimura (1972)

FIG. 20.8. ANNUAL PERIODICITY OF BM IN THE SAME SUBJECT AT DIFFERENT
LOCATIONS; KUMAMOTO, JAPAN (SOLID CIRCLE) AND LEXINGTON, KY., U.S.A.
(OPEN CIRCLE)

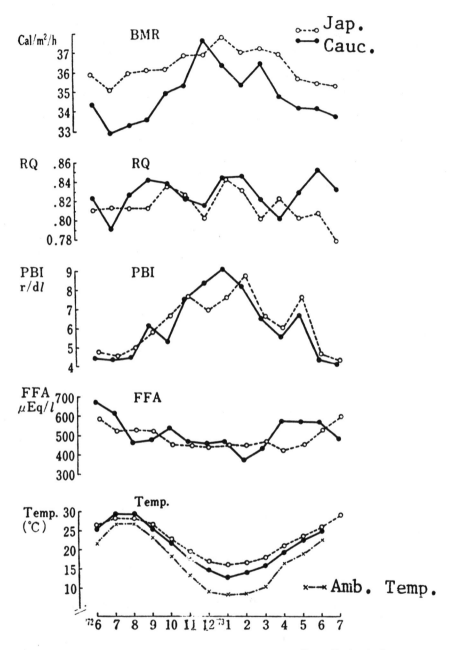

From Koshueisei

FIG. 20.9. SEASONAL VARIATION OF BMR OF JAPANESE AND CAUCASIANS
LIVING IN NAGASAKI (NAKAMURA *ET AL.*)

TABLE 20.1
PROGRESSIVE CHANGE IN ANNUAL RATE OF BM AND DIETARY COMPOSITION IN THE JAPANESE

Series	Year	No. of Subject	Sex	Annual Range (%)	Total Caloric Intake (kcal)	Protein (%)	Fat (%)	Carbohydrate (%)	F/C Ratio	Author
A	1949–50	9	M	17.3	2204	13.4	8.7	77.9	0.112	Sasaki (1954)
		6	F	21.2	2425	12.5	10.6	76.9	0.138	
B	1950	8	M	19.8						Sasaki (1954)
C	1951	4	F	15.2						Sakamoto (1953)
D	1952–53	9	M	12.2						Fukuda (1953)
		3	F	12.4						Masuko (1958)
E	1953–55	9	M	17.6						Osiba (1957)
F	1956–57	29	M	16.1						Koga (1959)
G	1957–58	4	M	9.9						Tashiro (1961)
H	1958–59	total	M	15.9	2858	15.0	12.4	72.7	0.171	Miyazaki (1970)
I	1961–62	201	M	11.3	2860	14.0	12.4	73.6	0.168	Masuda (1967)
		5			2743	14.9	14.8	70.2	0.211	
					2735	16.5	16.2	67.3	0.241	
J	1966–67	5	M	9.6						Sasaki et al. (1969)
K	1967	7	M	7.7	3255	14.6	18.3	67.1	0.277	Yurugi et al. (1968)

strated in the national survey of food consumption (Table 20.2). Thus, the annual range in seasonal variation was about 8% of the mean in 1967, as compared to about 20% in 1950. In sum, the above analytical investigation indicates that the seasonal variation in B.M. is due to adaptation to climatic changes, and seems to be reduced by an increased fat intake; and no racial differences can be found.

TABLE 20.2
ANNUAL SURVEY OF NUTRITION IN JAPAN (MALE ADULTS)

Year	Total Caloric Intake (kcal)	Protein (g)	Fat (g)	Carbo-hydrate (g)	Protein (%)	Fat (%)	Carbo-hydrate (%)	F / C Ratio
1946	1963	59.0	14.0	400.0	12.0	6.4	81.6	0.078
1948	2047	63.0	13.0	419.0	12.3	5.7	81.9	0.070
1952	2109	69.9	20.1	412.0	13.3	8.6	78.1	0.110
1956	2092	69.1	21.8	405.0	13.2	9.4	77.4	0.121
1960	2096	69.7	24.7	398.8	13.3	10.6	76.1	0.139
1964	2223	74.4	34.3	398.0	13.4	14.0	72.5	0.194
(1970)	2300	75.0	38.0	(414.5)	13.0	14.9	72.1	0.207
(1975)	2500	75.0	56.0	(407.7)	12.3	20.8	66.9	0.311

Note: Figures for 1970 and 1975 are target figures for a dietary improvement program under way.

In an effort to determine whether or not B.M. can be affected by the climate of various countries, group means for B.M. in Japanese, Koreans (Kim 1965), Thais (Berry 1962) and Indians (Malhotra et al. 1960) were plotted against the monthly mean temperatures of the various locales involved in the B.M. data. These results are summarized in Fig. 20.10, which shows that the B.M. is well correlated with the monthly mean ambient temperatures. The regression line is represented by the equation y = -0.22x + 42, which indicates that B.M. decreases by 2 cal/m²/h by decreasing the ambient temperature 10°C.

On the other hand, the B.M. plots for the Canadians (Yoshimura et al. (1966) stick out of the 95% confidence line of the correlation. The reason for this seems to lie in the differences in the Canadian living conditions, and especially in their dietary habits. As seen in Fig. 20.6, the Canadian missionaries usually took in 2g/kg/day of fat, which corresponds to 42% of their total caloric intake. In comparison, the Japanese took in less than 1g/kg/day of fat, or about 20% of their total caloric intake. Fat intake among Thai soldiers (Berry 1962) was 16.6%, and that of Indian soldiers 23.6% (Malhotra et al. 1960). At any rate, the B.M.R. of Asian people (including Caucasians living on an Eastern diet) presents a seasonal variation in response to climate.

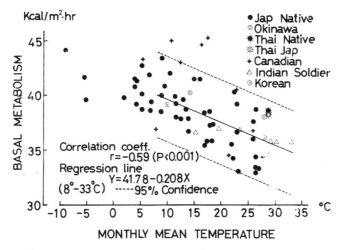

FIG. 20.10 CLIMATIC EFFECT ON GROUP MEANS OF BM IN ASIA

The underlying mechanism in these seasonal variations in B.M. involves a change in thyroid activity which accompanies the ambient temperature; fat intake seems also to be related to this change in thyroid activity. But how does a high fat intake disturb this climatic change in B.M.R.? To answer this question, Yoshimura *et al.* (1972) devised an experiment using 50 rats. Thirty of the rats were divided into groups of 15; one group was fed on a high carbohydrate diet, the other on a high fat diet, for a period of 5 weeks in a chamber at 30°C. These rats were the acclimated group. The remaining 20 rats were divided into control groups of 10, and fed either high fat or high carbohydrate diets for 5 weeks in a chamber at 20°C. After 5 weeks, the resting metabolism of each rat was measured at the ambient temperature of 20°C., and again at 30°C. Afterwards, 1 μc of ^{131}I was injected intraperitoneally, and the rats sacrificed 15 hours later. Blood samples and the thyroid gland from each animal were collected, and the thyroid activity was measured. A portion of the results is presented in Table 20.3.

From these data, it can be seen that the thyroid weight per body weight and the iodine uptake per unit g of thyroid gland were significantly higher in the high fat group, while thyroid weight in the heat-acclimated group was lower than the control group on either diet. Thus, high-fat feeding tends to accelerate thyroid activity.

In another experiment (Yoshimura *et al.* 1972), the effect of high fat and high carbohydrate intake on thyroid activity was examined in 55 rats. Half were fed a high fat diet, the rest a high carbohydrate food for 5 weeks at 20°C. (The composition of the foods was similar to that of the previous experiment). The T / S ratio was measured by the Vanderlan and Greer

TABLE 20.3

DIETARY COMPOSITION AND THYROID FUNCTION (MEAN VALUE)

		Heat Acclimate	Control
Fat Diet	B.W. (g)	233 ± 23	179 ± 35
	Thyroid weight (g)	16.03 ± 3.15	17.8 ± 2.5
	″/B.W. (mg/g)	0.074 ± 0.012*	0.108 ± 0.028
	C.R. % (8)	23.8 ± 2.4	23.1 ± 9.4
	I uptake %	19.0 ± 5.4	21.3 ± 6.1
	″/Thyroid (g)	1.34 ± 0.18*	1.26 ± 0.46
CHO diet	B.W. (g)	277 ± 18	222 ± 33
	Thyroid weight (g)	15.4 ± 4.6	20.1 ± 3.3
	″/B.W. (mg/g)	0.055 ± 0.015*	0.083 ± 0.012
	C.R. % (8)	21.0 ± 4.4	21.9 ± 6.0
	I uptake %	19.2 ± 4.0	16.8 ± 7.1
	″/Thyroid (g)	1.08 ± 0.20*	0.79 ± 0.33

	Fat diet	Carbohydrate (CHO) diet
Casein	25 g%	25 g%
Starch	6	66
Lard	60	–
Cottonseed oil	2	2
Liver oil	1	1
Salt	4	4
Vitamin mixt.	2	2

(1950) procedure, and the PB[131]I conversion ratio was measured in blood samples collected successively in time following subcutaneous injections of $15\,\mu$c of [131]I. Chemical PBI in this experiment was determined by Grossman's procedure (1955). As seen in Table 20.4, T/S and PB[131]I of the high fat group was significantly higher than that of the high carbohydrate group; other values were not statistically significant. Thus, while a high fat intake cannot be said to definitely elevate thyroid activity, these data show that there is a tendency toward such acceleration.

However, as seen in Fig. 20.11 (Yoshimura et al. 1972), the high fat group always shows a higher resting metabolism than does the high carbohydrate group. This high metabolism (or oxygen consumption) of the high fat group was the same in the heat-acclimated group as in the controls when the measurements were made at 20°C. On the other hand, the high carbohydrate group showed a reduction in resting metabolism in the heat acclimated group; the reduction was even more remarkable when the measurement was made at 30°C.

From these experiments, it may be presumed that a high fat intake tends to inhibit the reduction in resting metabolism due to heat acclimatization, and that this inhibition may be initiated by high thyroid activity which seems to be accelerated by a high fat diet. This means that the high intake of carbohydrates seems to accelerate the acclimatization of the thyroid

TABLE 20.4

EFFECT OF DIETARY COMPOSITION ON THYROID ACTIVITY

Subjects			Carbohydrate	Fat
Diet group A	Number		17	25
	Body weight (g)		273 ± 31	281 ± 27
	T/S		48.6 ± 14.3[1]	64.1 ± 22.9[1]
Diet group B	Number		22	21
	Body weight (g)		274 ± 29	284 ± 28
	Conversion ratio (%)	24 hr	47.6 ± 9.9	55.7 ± 9.0
		48 hr	80.3 ± 5.5	79.6 ± 6.9
	PB^{131}I	24 hr	50.5 ± 18.2[2]	60.2 ± 27.0[2]
		48 hr	47.0 ± 9.1	57.2 ± 14.2
	PB^{127}I (γ/dl)		3.6 ± 0.5	4.0 ± 0.9
	^{131}I Urinary output (%) (first 24 hr)		33.0 ± 4.5	31.0 ± 12.2
	^{131}I Fecal output (%) (first 24 hr)		1.1 ± 0.5	1.6 ± 0.7

Note: Values are mean ±SE. PB^{131}I: (cpm of PB^{131}I per ml plasma) × 10^5/total cpm of ^{131}I solution injected.
[1]Difference of T/S was statistically significant between these two figures (P<0.0025).
[2]Difference of PB^{131}I (24 hr) was statistically significant (P<0.004).

gland to heat, causing a reduction of the B.M. in heat among Asian people on a high carbohydrate diet.

It is well-known that the climate of Southeast Asia is hot and humid, that damp or wet agriculture is well-developed, and that the rice crop is large. People living in this area use rice as a staple food, making it their main source of both protein and calories. This increases the carbohydrate intake, allowing rice eaters to acclimate themselves to hot weather by reducing the heat production in their own bodies. Thus, their lives are well-adapted to both climate and mode of agriculture.

Of course, neither Japan nor Korea has such a hot climate. But the rice-based diet seems to originate in more tropical countries—which is not to suggest that all people living in tropical areas should eat rice. The point is simply that in such cases the acclimatization of the human body is well-coordinated with rice production, thus forming a well-developed ecosystem.

ACKNOWLEDGEMENTS

The authors wish to offer their deep appreciation to Dr. Mayurie Balankura, Col. Paja Sirivorasarn, who cooperated with us in making measurements and surveys in Bangkok, and Ms. Laddavan and other technicians in the Department of Tropical Nutrition and Food Sciences, Faculty of Tropical Medicine, Mahidol University, Bangkok. Thanks are also owed to Rev. K. Wakugami, Chairman of the Foundation of Sekai Kyuseikyo, Taikyokai, and his friends; to Dr. Y. Kaida, Liaison Officer of

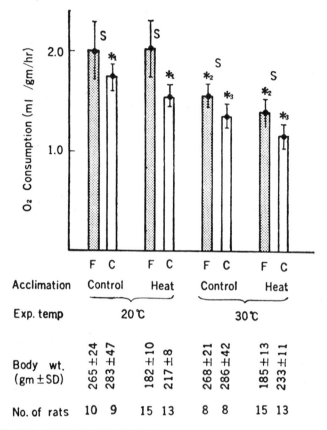

FIG. 20.11. EFFECT OF DIET ON THERMAL ACCLIMATION OF O^2 CONSUMPTION
IN HIGH FAT (F) AND HIGH CARBOHYDRATE (C) DIET GROUPS

Bangkok, Center for Southeast Asian Studies, Kyoto University; and to Dr. Asai, President of Ajinomoto Co., Ltd., in Thailand who offered us valuable information on the Japanese in Bangkok and also helped in taking various measurements among them. The authors' studies in Bangkok were supported by a research grant from the Center for Southeast Asian Studies, Kyoto University, and by the Malnutrition Panel of the U.S.-Japan Cooperative Medical Sciences Program.

REFERENCES

BERRY, F.B. 1962. A Report of the Interdepartmental Committee on Nutrition for National Defense. Office of the Assist. Sec. Def., Washington, D.C.

ITOH, S., OGATA, K., and YOSHIMURA, M. 1972. Advances in Climatic Physiology, Springer-Verlag New York, Inc., New York.

KIM, K.J. 1965. Studies on basal metabolism, caloric expenditure and daily energy expenditure of Korean students in middle school, high school and college. J. Kor. Mod. Med. *3*, 291-294.

MALHOTRA, M.S., RAMASWAMY, S.S., and RAY, S.N. 1960. Effect of environmental temperature on work and resting metabolism. J. Appl. Physiol. *15*, 769-770.

NAKAMURA, M. 1975. Racial difference in acclimatization. Koshu Eisei *39*, 548-555. (Japanese)

OGATA, K. SASAKI, T., and MURAKAMI, N. 1966. Central nervous and metabolic aspects of body temperature. Bull. Inst. Constit. Med.. Kumamoto Univ. *16* (Suppl.), 36-42.

OSIBA, S. 1957. The seasonal variation of basal metabolism and activity of thyroid gland in man. Jap. J. Physiol. *7*, 355-365.

YOSHIMURA, M., HORI, S., and YOSHIMURA, H. 1972. Effect of high fat diet on thermal acclimation with special reference to thyroid activity. Jap. J. Physiol. *22*, 517-531.

YOSHIMURA, M., and YOSHIMURA, H. 1970. Dietary composition and acclimatization. Nippon Rinsho *28*, 166-171. (Japanese)

YOSHIMURA, M., YUKIYOSHI, K., YOSHIOKA, T., and TAKEDA, H. 1966. Climatic adaptation of basal metabolism. Fed. Proc. *25*, 1169-1176.

SECTION V

MAN'S COMPLEX CULTURE OF TODAY AND TOMORROW: CAN MAN'S BIOLOGICAL ADAPTATION COPE WITH CULTURAL CHANGE, ESPECIALLY AS REGARDS NUTRITION?

CHAPTER 21

J. Leonard Joy

As Seen from the Perspective of International Organizations

This presentation is designed to address four major questions:
(1) Can we expect malnutrition to increase?
(2) Can international organizations do anything to prevent this?
(3) What is likely to happen?
(4) What should we be doing?
I shall need to lead up to these questions indirectly. To begin, I wish to discuss the homeostatic nature of social systems in an attempt to link the anthropological considerations with our present effort to deal with the international social system.

We have heard that social systems tend to be homeostatic, that is, to be regulated in ways that insure community survival. What is not clear is the possibility that these survival mechanisms might well depend on or result in selective malnutrition. For example, productive adults may be fed before infants, who may in fact be allowed to die. Several of these social mechanisms which insure community survival have already been mentioned, but I would like to refer to other specific examples in order to introduce the concept of breakdown in regard to these mechanisms, and then discuss what happens when several cultures exist within national and international communities under the stress of change.

The operation of community survival may be seen, perhaps, in the Sahel, which has already been discussed. Here we find communities trying to secure their survival in the most hostile of natural ecologies, where the assurance of survival (at least in the short run) depends upon population regulation. Thus, a high rate of infant mortality could be seen as a regulating mechanism necessary for the survival of the community. If this were so, any attempt to reduce this high infant mortality rate would interfere with the solution of what might be regarded as a more fundamental problem. I am not trying to present a teleological argument that a high infant mortality rate is good because it serves a purpose. I *am* saying, however, that we must be careful in defining objectives and we must examine fully the consequences of actions proposed as improvements.

I might also cite the *jajmani* system in India as a mechanism which insures minimum allocations of food to allow a labor force to survive even in bad times. One can find similar equilibrating mechanisms in a good many communities, such as the Acholi of northern Uganda, where the

239

people band together for crop cultivation, moving from one family plot to another, thus insuring that all of the crops are not planted on the same day. This sequential crop planting spreads out the risk of crop failure, much the way a banker's portfolio is a protection against any one bad investment. The process can also be linked to those systems in which food is distributed by a "chief," thus permitting those people who may have planted their crops at the wrong time to have some claim on the community's overall resources.

The point I want to make in regard to these regulatory mechanisms is, first, that they do not necessarily insure adequate nutrition for everyone all the time; and second, that they are related to values, to expected patterns of behavior, to social institutions, and to leadership backed by authority and custom. Further, these patterns and their regulatory effects break down under stress, and alternative social mechanisms achieving similar results do not necessarily emerge. In other words, the culture does not necessarily adapt in this sense.

Often other aims and values become dominant. Among the Acholi, for example, the introduction of the tractor and the concept of cash crops led to the cash employment of labor, thus breaking down the reciprocal labor pattern which in turn brought about the collapse of the "portfolio diversification" mechanism. I think a similar situation exists in India, where the *jajmani* system is breaking down under various pressures (all aggravated by population growth), leading to the emergence of a great band of people who have little value to the land owners who might formerly have retained them as laborers on their holdings. These land owners now find it cheaper to simply hire labor when they need it, rather than retain a labor force for which they feel responsible. (It is even cheaper now since the cost of grain necessary to feed a stable labor force has been much increased by inflation.)

If on the one hand we see the breakdown of some of these traditional social mechanisms, on the other we find the emergence of new mechanisms associated with the development of the nation states in which many of these cultures are subsumed. In particular, we find that the basis of power is often derived from loose coalitions of interest that may not be specifically tribal, or even based on a common culture. The goals of national governments are most likely to be involved with political survival; other aims, such as the reduction of malnutrition, are apt to be secondary.

To recapitulate, I maintain that the elimination of malnutrition is not a necessary goal for traditional communities or national governments, and we must examine the implications of including it as an object of social goalseeking. We have to ask what it is we have to do in order to really eliminate malnutrition in a community. What would this require? Is it feasible? What might the consequences be?

Before proceeding to these questions, however, we must be explicit about

the forces which lead to the breakdown of the traditional social mechanisms. I wish to draw attention to three of them:
(1) The development of markets;
(2) The development or introduction of new technologies; and
(3) Population growth itself, perhaps the consequence of improved public health and markets.

All of these pressures lead to disequilibrium within traditional societies in part because they allow or encourage people to contract out of their traditional obligations. Feasts have often been cited as an important regulating mechanism in some traditional communities because they help to inhibit the accumulation of resources or capital. Moreover, it has been pointed out, such feasts are commonly ritualized in ways which insure social cohesion and reaffirm common identity. One of their major implications is stability, since they prevent individuals from becoming self-sufficient and thereby withdrawing from the social contract. However, with the advent of markets, people *can* contract out; they can flout social mores and obligations and still survive economically. And they are tempted by other values, most of them material. (Of course, they may also be tempted to use the market in order to increase their power or status within the traditional community.)

In one way or another, these forces create disequilibrium and change within the community. Among the key changes are those affecting patterns of production and distribution, and those affecting the nature of decision-making and the control of resources (both in terms of production and consumption). We find changes in interpersonal relationships, which are now governed by market exchange and legal contracts, rather than by interpersonal status. There is also an accumulation (including accumulation through inheritance) of resources which increases the disparities among people of the community in terms of social, political and economic status. The new regulators are the market and the government which—by constructing irrigation systems, roads, stores, bridges and so on create new opportunities and generate new patterns of behavior.

What are the consequences of this for nutrition? Many have already been discussed—changes in the availability and cost of foodstuffs, new technologies for storage and processing leading to changes in dietary habits, etc.—but the most important consequence is this: the change in the number of people who simply cannot afford to eat.

I would like to explicitly and directly challenge the conventional view of the world food problem; that is, that we have a serious malnutrition problem because the rate of population growth is outstripping the rate of growth in world food supplies. I would argue that this view is wrong because it leads to the conclusion that what we must do is reduce the rate of population growth and increase the food supply until the two are once again in equilibrium. Unfortunately, we are now learning that voluntary family planning programs show little success in situations where the standard of living is very low; that is, in those very situations characterized by high rates of malnutrition and infant mortality.

Therefore, it would seem that the conventional view has the cart before the horse, and that in fact the reduction of malnutrition is a precondition for effective population control. Even though the *immediate* response to a reduction of malnutrition might be an *increase* in the rate of population growth, the available evidence suggests that we could expect the population to stabilize by means of a reduction in the birth rate.

The complementary proposition—that we must increase the food supply—is equally fallacious, not because there is no need for such an increase, but because it would be a consequence of and not a means toward any real solution. What, after all, can you do to increase the food supply to people who cannot afford to pay for the food they need? American farmers would be delighted with the opportunity to grow more food. But, they ask, "Who will pay for it?" Thus, the problem is not that more food cannot be produced (at some cost), but that there is an increasing number of people who cannot afford to pay for it.

Paradoxically, then, the best way to increase the food supply to the malnourished is to reduce malnutrition; that is, to increase the productivity and income of those who are malnourished to a level at which they can support themselves. The core of the problem we shall be facing in the coming decades is that *displacement* (the growth in the number of people without land) is going to exceed *absorption* (the number of people for whom adequate wage employment can be found).

Let me explain what I mean by that. At the present time, the pressures of development and change are forcing people from the land. More and more people are born without any claim to the land resources required for their own subsistence needs. Nor do most of these people have any supplementary or alternative opportunities for productive employment. It is the growth in the number of these people who have been displaced (productively, and often socially as well) but not absorbed which constitutes our problem at the present and in the future. And the question we must ask is, "How can we make these people productive and self-reliant?" Clearly, unregulated development will aggravate this problem rather than reduce it.

To return to the concern of goal-seeking governments in regard to reducing malnutrition, I must emphasize that government leadership will have to work *explicitly* with the problem of malnutrition; to merely press for greater development will not be enough. To effectively implement such a goal, the government will have to mobilize political support. However, this generally means that it is precisely those people who are without social, economic or political power who would be *required* to benefit from development measures. As a result, I would conclude that we might reasonably expect an increase in malnutrition in many poor countries. Thus, my conditional answer to the first question I posed is, yes, we can expect malnutrition to increase unless specific and effective steps are taken to decrease it.

My second question was, "Can international organizations do anything to prevent this?" First, I think it is clear that the necessary actions must be undertaken by national governments themselves. The relevant question then becomes, "Is there anything that international organizations (especially the multinational groups) can do to induce the right actions, or to support and promote those actions?" We might also ask whether it is likely that what *should* be done *will* be done.

Let me first raise the question of international regulation of market forces, since this issue is often stressed in relation to the problems of malnutrition in poor countries. Is there anything that the rich countries can do in this area? Up to now, success in the regulation of international trade for the benefit of poor countries has been conspicuously limited, which suggests that there are problems in this field. And it is not my task, at the present time, to assess the prospects for the future. But I would like to point out that, even if they succeeded, such attempts to improve trade benefits for poor countries would only make it easier for such nations to reduce their malnutrition. In practice, these efforts might even backfire and increase malnutrition. Stimulating markets for agricultural produce would reduce malnutrition if the added production were undertaken by those who would otherwise be hungry. But if in fact this added production led to increases in estate farming, mechanization, displacement of labor and rural disparities, it would merely aggravate the problem. So while rich countries might help in the fight against malnutrition by altering their trade policies, the actual key to success would remain with the poor countries.

The same holds true for aid programs. Foreign aid can help poor countries increase their productive potential, but it can easily be provided in ways that aggravate the problem. To be effective, it must be geared toward solving the specific problem of malnutrition, and not merely toward increasing the country's overall productive capacity.

I would like now to look at two significant events in the international field as they relate to malnutrition. The first was Mr. Robert McNamara's 1974 speech in which he paid particular attention to the question of malnutrition in the world, and the effort he was making to mobilize support for a World Bank program aimed at reducing the problem. The importance of the speech owes less to the possibility that the World Bank might have a significant effect on malnutrition than to the impact of such ideas being promoted with such authority in that quarter. The second event is the World Food Conference of November 1974 which resolved to eliminate hunger and malnutrition within a decade. While that was a fine resolve, more significance can be attached to the series of resolutions which called upon the countries concerned (and upon international agencies as well) to pursue particular lines of action. But what are the chances of any effective action coming about as a result of those resolutions?

Let me first note that the initial philosophy of the World Food Conference was precisely the one I have attacked; that is, it first perceived the problem in terms of food supply and the means of increasing it. Consequently, there was a strong emphasis in its resolutions upon measures designed to increase the world food supply and to improve world food security. (The World Food Conference took place immediately after a steep rise in food prices throughout the world as the result of an unusual conjunction of poor harvests and massive demands on the international market by some large countries; this depleted world stocks and pushed up the price of internationally traded grains.) At the time, the conference showed a proper concern for world food security, and devoted much attention to the problem that would face poor countries if such a situation should recur. Efforts were made to insure that food stocks could be held in store for disbursement to poor countries in the event of a future food scarcity.

The provision of food stocks (particularly within nations, but perhaps internationally as well) for this explicit type of relief could be important, but in my view, it does not get to the heart of the problem. Instead, it deals with the acute and transient manifestations of that problem, making few (if any) substantial contributions to the fundamental, chronic difficulties. Moreover, such measures would be extremely difficult to implement. Rich countries might well believe that it was more advantageous to express their willingness to come to the aid of poor countries directly, rather than making costly, long-term commitments to the maintenance of grain stores. In that way, they would maintain their power over the dispersal of such grains.

There are difficulties, too, in deciding how these stocks should be released. Whom *do* we help? How do we determine when a nation is facing an acute situation and is in need of help? Should we help a country which does not help itself? What criteria would be used to exclude a country from such aid? What evidence would be required for the release of stocks? How could procedures be routinized so as to maintain an equity among nations, and avoid manifestations of power trying to influence events? All of these are formidable problems, and most of them have not been explicitly addressed thus far.

I would like to turn now to the question of technical assistance and the role of the United Nations. Following the resolutions of the World Food Conference, various UN agencies have met to consider what kind of support they might give to countries seeking effective solutions in the field of nutrition. Particular attention has been given to the idea of "integrated food and nutrition planning," and the concerned agencies are developing methods and approaches to such problems. The chief value of this approach is its recognition of the fact that the problem is not simply one of increased food output, but is a broad issue which will involve areas other than those covered by the ministers of health, education and agriculture. National nutritional policies will of necessity embrace a wide range of decisions and strategy issues that will affect the way in which people are absorbed into productive employment. Methods and approaches to integrated food and nutrition planning must be developed to assist those countries which wish to apply them. (Assistance in administrative decision-making is especially important.) Program assistance of many kinds is being developed, including emergency food aid related to "global nutrition surveillance," the correction of specific nutrient deficiencies (vitamin A, iron, iodine, etc.), and the more familiar child feeding and applied nutrition programs.

But can the UN provide this type of support? Let us look at what is envisaged. The first step is viewed as an informal approach to the government in question to discuss the nature of the problem (as it sees it), the steps which need to be taken to correct the problem, and the government's willingness to contract with the UN for technical support. If such willingness exists, support would be supplied under four broad headings:

(1) The construction of data systems to identify and define the nutritional problem, diagnose its causes and prescribe measures for its solution (this would include setting goals for nutritional improvement, target intakes, etc.);

(2) Policy analysis (for example, the analysis of the effects of agricultural price policy on malnutrition);

(3) Rural development planning, relating nutritional objectives to other rural needs rather than focus on food and malnutrition alone; and

(4) Program and project identification, design and implementation. In all cases, efforts to increase government capability would be linked to more material assistance.

What does such an effort really involve? In the first place, it requires a body of knowledge which would allow for coherence and consistency in all aspects of the approach, and that the people who might possess this knowledge work consistently and harmoniously together. This does not seem to be the case at the moment. Moreover, it requires that such expertise be employed in an ongoing and evolving series of programs throughout the world. I do not believe that the UN is capable of managing this at present and would face a monumental problem of development. While there are at least the beginnings of a body of knowledge, it has never been articulated, has yet to be worked out in practice, and seems likely to require important changes from previous programs.

UN personnel skilled in these fields is limited and largely preoccupied with ongoing commitments. To reorient existing programs would require recruitment and training of new personnel. Those people presently at the UN are dispersed through numberless agencies, divisions and departments, and do not come under any single management focus. Certainly there are no teams of people who have worked successfully together, sharing their views and experience.

I would argue, therefore, that UN capability in this field is very small indeed, and that it could not possibly mobilize this type of assistance in any direct fashion, whether by contract or consultancy. The required expertise does not exist in any developed or significant form, and the UN is not geared to develop it. Moreover, the UN has problems in asserting its priorities in regard to such programs. It even has difficulty in maintaining its focus on problems of malnutrition, and the idea that it ought to work with those governments which have given the reduction of malnutrition a high priority and hold compatible views as to how it might be accomplished. In fact, the UN is not very strong at all, and is especially weak in its ability to generate research and development or to provide the training required for these new approaches, whatever they might be.

Can the UN even respond to the idea that such a capability ought to be developed? Can it appreciate what is lacking? Can it understand what needs to be done to develop this capability, and in fact achieve it? My own judgement is that it cannot.

But even if it could, its effectiveness would depend on the governments in the poor countries themselves, which must first appreciate the nature of the problem and then express a willingness to implement the measures required for progress. We might well ask if there is as yet any such understanding on the part of any poor country government.

In answer to the question, "What is likely to happen?," the most probable scenario for the coming years is an increasing number of "scares," a greater manifestation of conspicuous hunger, and more frequent calls for assistance in various ways from the nations thus affected. I think that the frequency and magnitude of these problems will be so great that the developed countries will be forced to ask themselves how they should respond and under what circumstances. They are likely to become very selective about such assistance and require (as they have done in the past) that the recipients follow the policies which the donors feel will most effectively reduce the demands.

I think new approaches to the problem will be developed, not merely in terms of stimulating economic growth or even generating employment, but in terms of increasing the productivity of those who would otherwise be without a means of subsistence. What is most important is a growth of understanding, especially among the public. So long as we believe that the problem is one of food supply, that it can be cured by technology, and that the problem is one of convincing governments to implement these technologies, then we have mistaken the nature of the situation. As we begin to understand the true nature of the problem and realize that the means to a solution is largely with us already, I believe that we will see a change in attitude which will affect action and policy on all sides.

Let me now try to pull these themes together. Traditional societies often utilize social devices for the control of food production and distribution in order to insure the survival of the community, even at the expense of some of its members. As these communities fall under the influence of a cash economy, these mechanisms break down. Production and distribution are increasingly governed by the market, by law and by government. One consequence of this breakdown is increased malnutrition, since it leads to the displacement of people from the land without providing them with alternative employment in order to subsist. Those governments which act to reduce malnutrition will have to favor those with the least social and economic status. Since this group generally has the least political power, the government must curb the natural consequences of the economic and political systems which constitute their own base of support.

This does not mean that it is inherently unfeasible to reduce malnutrition. But it does suggest that the unqualified promotion of economic development will not ease the problem, and that new criteria for investment and development strategies are required. In principle, the international agencies could help countries develop and apply such criteria, and they are attempting to do so. What is implied here, however, is substantial change in the approach of both individual governments and international agencies, and in the relations between them. This sort of innovation will not come easily to the UN system.

Nonetheless, I believe that in the long run the international community will generate and disseminate an understanding of what is needed to effectively tackle the problem of malnutrition and strengthen its commitment to eliminating it. In this sense, mankind will adapt at an international level in response to the growing incidence of malnutrition, and thus promote its reduction. What we should be doing, then, is to aid in this process of understanding.

CHAPTER 22

Sol Chafkin

As Seen From National Levels: Developed World

In exploring "Man's Complex Culture of Today and Tomorrow," I am going to discuss money, which I think has a respectable position in human society and does bear a bit on nutrition. In addition, I will examine the decision-making process and the ways in which decision-making institutions operate.

To provide the proper tone of cultural anthropology to the first part of this presentation, the subject should probably be titled "Nutrition is good, but money is better." Utilizing some amateur linguistics, I might cite the slang expression "bread," as in "Lay some bread on me." "Bread," in this instance, means "money," and it would seem that there are rich opportunities—if they haven't already been seized—for an anthropological study, perhaps to be published in the *Journal of Obscure Studies*, on the equivalence of bread and money in contemporary American society. So much for the qualification in terms of culture.

In dealing with the issue of social justice, I shall examine the question of nutritional intervention and the setting in which such decisions are made. By and large, it has something to do with government. The model goes something like this: Either on his own initiative or as the result of prodding by political opponents or in response to nutritional complaints made by private groups in his own country or as a result of outside intervention (perhaps from one of the UN organizations), someone in a government position proposes that something be done to alleviate the nutritional problems in his country. And almost invariably, what he proposes will cost money.

If it's a small amount of money, the chances that his proposal will be acted upon are good. This is why so many programs in nutritional intervention are called "demonstrations," "pilots," "experiments," "action-oriented research" and so on. Low-cost projects allow a government to show its concern without goring any other agency's budgetary ox. As a result, "demonstrations" tend to go on for years without ever being scaled upward, since large scale interventions usually require funds which can only be obtained by reducing some other program. This latter course naturally leads to conflict.

Similarly, if what this government official proposes costs a lot of money, the chances that it will be implemented are considerably reduced. To propose an increase in food imports, for example, when the government is already having trouble with foreign exchange is almost always a lost cause.

When a government finds itself in a tight financial situation, whether internal or external, an obvious solution is to redeploy the existing monies—to spend less for X in order to spend more for Y. But this is asking a great deal from a government, since it will almost invariably be faced with protests from various established constituencies.

Unfortunately, those countries with the most serious nutritional problems are also those with the most serious financial difficulties. A classic example of the effects of external financial pressures can be found in the recent hike in oil prices engineered by the oil-exporting countries, the reverberations of which are still being felt both in developed and developing nations. As others have pointed out, the effect of that action on the price of foodstuffs in low-income countries and among low-income populations has killed people as surely (if less dramatically) as warfare or natural calamity.

We might say, then, that nations are subject to what I call the Iron Law of International Financial Survival—that is, governments will almost always subordinate internal social objectives in order to protect their international financial viability. When international financial stringencies are combined with internal fiscal problems (for example, budget cutting in an attempt to reduce inflation), it becomes extraordinarily difficult for the advocate of social or nutritional justice to suggest that money be spent on food-related problems.

Here we find the Iron Law of Budget Cuts. Certain areas of expenditure, such as a defense budget, are nearly immune to budget cuts. Generally speaking, the "soft" areas are in welfare costs—in money spent for health, education, nutrition and the like. Given this sort of financial setting, it is somewhat arrogant to insist that a government do something about improving nutrition because that is a good thing to do. It is up to the interventionist to prove that what he proposes is a better way to spend money already within the total budget. And he must also take care that the design of his proposal will minimize the potentially adverse effects on the country's internal and external financial position.

I want to make it clear that I am not arguing against advocacy. I *am* saying, however, that advocates of social justice must be sensitive to the constraints which may prevent a government from acting on even the most noble proposals.

It seems to me that as we examine the process of decision-making within a country, we find yet another Iron Law at work; that is, as governments begin to increase in size, power and sophistication, they often bring about the atrophy of the local organizations which traditionally looked after problems in the community. This phenomenon deserves our attention because it is quite possible that the most effective nutritional intervention programs will require the aid of vigorous community organizations. In fact, such organizations might be called upon to provide not only energy and initiative in problem-solving, but also a basis for continuing commitment and perhaps even an assumption of financial responsibility.

Speaking from the perspective of the developed nations (which actually means the perspective of someone living in the United States), I would have to say that the growth of the planning industry and the export of planning skills to the developing nations may well be counter-productive. That is, as governments become more sophisticated in their planning, their reach is extended down to the local level; and as they enter into problem-solving at the local level, they may well exacerbate this atrophy of local organizations.

This sort of argument has even been brought up in regard to New York City. As the problems of that city increase, people have begun to wonder aloud if perhaps that old, disreputable political organization known as Tammany Hall was really such a bad thing. In retrospect, it seems that the political machine was fairly skilled at handling the problems of the local people. The ward bosses found jobs for those who needed them; somehow a food package was assembled and delivered to the family that had fallen on hard times, and so on. As a result, I tend to become quite nervous about proposals which tend to produce very centralized economic planning.

Now let me turn my attention to the model of nutritional intervention which seems to be emerging: that is, government-financed and government-operated meal lines. These meal lines (of which there are several varieties) frequently tend to miss the people who need the food most, and they usually amount to little more than bandaids on a far more serious problem. For this and other reasons, we must ask ourselves if there are alternatives to the meal line. One such alternative is to try to solve the economic issues which underlie the problem, instead of simply to plaster it over with food stamps.

We must also ask if it is really so difficult for governments to give things away free. It seems to me that it is not. Given the resources, the problem is merely logistical and administrative. The difficult thing is to influence the decision-making of the recipient so that any additional increments of income will be used to buy things which improve the nutritional status of the family.

In this respect, I was interested to learn that the government of Columbia has begun to experiment with alternatives to the meal line. Recognizing the fact that 50% of the nation's food is produced on small, economically troubled farms, the Colombian government has placed its emphasis on providing the assistance necessary to increase the efficiency of such farms. This will not only reduce the displacement (discussed by Leonard Joy), but will also tend to stabilize the supply and the price of food in urban areas. At the same time, the farmers will have greater income to alleviate their own money-related nutritional problems.

At the present time, there seem to be three models for nutritional intervention:

(1) The China model, which flows from the philosophy of governance. This model may become more important than any programmatic notions in regard to intervention. And it should be pointed out that, while policy in China is developed centrally, there is a good deal of discretionary power within the local organizations which actually carry out the central policies.

(2) The income redistribution model, which holds that the problems of poverty and malnutrition can be solved by a redistribution of political and economic power. While it is an attractive model, it is very difficult (if not impossible) for an outsider to recommend that a government give up its own power in the name of redistribution.

(3) The incremental model, which holds that you work around the edges of a given system in the hope that over time you can produce some consequential changes. It is in this area that you find yourself making choices as to what sort of interventional program you prefer, and these choices center around techniques and delivery systems.

I would now like to propound my fourth Iron Law (and these iron laws of mine seem to be more universal than basal metabolism), which is the Iron Law of We and They. In this sense, of course, "we" applies to the developed nations, and "they" to the developing countries. According to this mode of thinking, "we" say that malnutrition is a problem which "they" have, and which "we" shall try to alleviate for them. "They" need nutritional intervention programs; "we" provide the food and technical advice.

This all sounds fine until you realize that the largest government-run nutritional intervention program in the world belongs to a "we" country— the United States. "We" spend something in excess of 7 billion dollars each year to affect the food consumption of perhaps 30 million people. This "we/they" thinking produces some strange results: "We" have made no real effort to assess the results of this enormous food program, yet we insist that "they" evaluate their programs with great rigor. "We" send experts abroad to formulate national food programs for "them," but haven't even begun such a process at home.

More of the artificial nature of this "we/they" distinction between developed and developing nations can be seen in the following quote from a recently published article:

Because the majority of individuals handicapped by malnutrition may still fall within "normal bounds," it may be questioned whether any loss has been suffered. If one focuses on the individual, only the most severe instances of retardation may be provable. But if one enlarges the scope of investigation to compare the children of undernourished mothers with the children of those who have been soundly nourished, the loss becomes obvious. It is a gratuitous retardation, and it is a retardation that imposes immense costs upon society. If [the child] is educable, he will be more expensive and difficult to educate than if he were not retarded. If his retardation is sufficiently obvious to be recognized, he will require special education. If not, he will proceed through conventional schools posing an insoluble problem, possibly all the way to college. Even if educated, he is unlikely to make any substantial contribution to the advancement of society. At best, he will be a welfare client all his life. If his retardation is mild enough not to be diagnosed, he will go through life failing at the simplest tasks, at best marginally employable and perhaps even driven into a life of crime.

This article uses the sort of language we hear in discussions of the problems of developing countries. But it happens to be from an article written by the President of Boston University, published in the *New York Times* on Sunday, November 16, 1975, and the subject is children in the United States.

Given the fact that malnutrition is a panhuman phenomenon and not a question of "we" and "they," I would like to bring to your attention some issues which the Ford Foundation is exploring. Many of us have felt that our current reliance in the United States on psychological explanations for problems like school failure and delinquency leaves much to be desired, both in terms of theoretical explanation and practical results. The rate of school failure and juvenile crime suggests that it is time to ask if deficiencies in health and nutrition might not play a significant role in social pathology in this country.

So far as I can tell, the gate-keeper for the American problem child is the school psychologist. Down the line a bit is the psychiatric social worker. And somewhere amid the lofty establishment is the psychiatrist for the school system. It seems to me that this creates a peculiar monopoly. It thus becomes rather important to examine the possible significance of health and nutritional status to provide some balance in the analysis of socially troublesome behavior.

We discovered several things. First, that many psychiatrists were unhappy that we had even mentioned health and nutrition in regard to problems of behavior, but that other psychiatrists were eager to investigate this question. We also learned that teachers who work in low-income neighborhoods frequently bring food into the classroom. When asked why, they said that they had to "calm" the children down before they could even begin to teach them.

Oddly enough, when we asked psychiatric social workers about their methods, they laid out a panoply of interventional tools—psychiatric counselling, group therapy, rap sessions, a mini-school and so on—but never a word about the children's diets. When we asked if they fed the children in the mini-school, they said that they did, and that if they didn't, the kids would tear the place apart. Clearly, then, food seems important in regard to behavior, but it is not considered to be worth mentioning.

In 1874, T. H. Huxley said that "the roots of psychology lie in the physiology of the nervous system," so that what we call operations of the mind are actually functions of the brain. In this sense, while the effects of malnutrition in a population may not be evident, they nevertheless may pose serious problems for an industrialized society. Indeed, their very subtlety constitutes a challenge to develop more specific and sensitive techniques for diagnosis and for the assessment of our therapeutic measures.

What I hope has emerged from this presentation is the panhuman character of malnutrition. During the next generation or two, we will see nutritional problems arising in developed and developing nations alike. When we export the technology of our food processing industry, when we export the practices of our own unevaluated nutritional programs, we may also be exporting the problems which these things create in the United States. There is an international interdependence which we cannot escape. We must realize that a poor wheat crop in Russia can mean higher wheat prices in the United States, which will in turn affect not only our own low-income populations but the populations of those nations which buy wheat from us.

All nations, whether developed or underdeveloped, must deal with the same three conflicting objectives:

(1) To meet balance of payment requirements, which means increasing exports. In the United States, food has become one of the most significant exports;

(2) To meet the domestic pressure for lower food prices;

(3) To provide incentives for farmers by keeping food prices high in order to maximize production.

On national levels, we must try to harmonize these conflicts. In regard to the community, we must find the best way to utilize local energy and local initiative so that nutritional intervention can really make a difference. And that holds true whether you are dealing with a village in India or a schoolroom in the United States.

CHAPTER 23

Leonardo J. Mata
Edgar Mohs

As Seen From National Levels:
Developing World

The grim realities involved with the solution of such world problems as food, energy and pollution make it difficult to address such issues with optimism (Meadows *et al.* 1972; Mesarovic and Pestel 1974). On the other hand, these challenges to man's survival stimulate the search for explanations, causes and corrective strategies.

The evolution of nutritional concepts over the past twenty years demonstates that well-established principles have broken down while unorthodox ideas have been embraced with almost religious fervor. Until recently, malnutrition was thought to be caused solely by a lack of food; to cure it, one merely provided additional foodstuffs. In the past, the emphasis was on protein, with little regard for calories. It was also believed that some kind of development was needed to improve the quality of life; more often than not, this meant industrialization.

We now know that culture plays a decisive role in the appearance of malnutrition, whatever the society. We shall attempt to describe the cultural and biological changes which have affected health and nutrition, using concepts and examples which can be applied to the inhabitants of the Americas (particularly those living in tropical and subtropical regions). Our emphasis will be on the evolution of our own country, Costa Rica.

EVOLUTIONARY CHANGES AND THE ORIGINS OF MALNUTRITION

The more we work in the field, the more we come to realize that malnutrition is a disease caused by man himself, and more specifically, by human society. Apparently primates (like other animals living in the wild) do not suffer from malnutrition unless handicapped by a birth defect or postnatal injury, or exposed to natural or man-made disasters. Such events generally eliminate the individual (Morris 1967; van Lawick-Goodall 1971), or result in increased mortality, thus exerting control over population growth and the accumulation of defective biological attributes. While the reasons for this general absence of malnutrition in wild animals are not entirely clear, one may presume that their highly diversified diet is a determining factor. Moreover, primates constantly move away from defecation sites; when coupled with relatively low population density, this behavior makes it difficult for pathogens to persist within the community.

During man's early history in the Americas, he lived in small hunting and gathering groups. Breast-feeding was widely practiced (as it still is today among the Indians of the American Highlands). It seems likely that malnutrition was not very prevalent among such groups because their diet was diversified and infectious agents which entered the colony were eventually eliminated.

However, man was so successful in terms of reproduction that large, dense populations came into being. Such a demographic accomplishment presented logistical problems in terms of feeding the larger community. Villagers and city dwellers began to rely more heavily on maize and other domesticated plants. There were other complications as well, such as depletion of wild life, the destruction of forests and the deterioration of the land (Recinos 1950; Struever 1971).

Two important changes occurred during this process:

(1) Man shifted from a diversified diet to one consisting of a cereal and a complementary food (maize and beans, for example); and

(2) Human society evolved from tribal groups composed of a few families to communities embracing a large number of individuals.

The first shift involved a deterioration of the diet; the second increased the probability that diseases would spread, and more important, that pathogens would persist in the community and be enhanced. These social and biological changes probably marked the appearance of malnutrition as an endemic disease; before that time, the diet of early Americans seems to have been adequate (Coe 1966; Von Hagen 1960).

European involvement in the Americas, beginning at the turn of the 15th century, introduced differing food habits into aboriginal cultures. At the same time, many hitherto unknown viruses and bacteria were also introduced, causing much suffering, malnutrition and death among these susceptible populations (Dubos 1959).

There is good reason to believe that malnutrition was not very prevalent in Spain itself during this period. Writings from the 17th century describe well-balanced diets, and often manifest an innate knowledge of good nutrition (de Cervantes-Saavedra 1605). Strangely enough, the emphasis on a rich and diversified diet persisted among the Spanish descendants. For example, inhabitants of rural Costa Rica characteristically eat *olla de carne* (meat pot), a steaming casserole of vegetables, cereals and meat. When recorded some 25 years ago, the descendants of the Spaniards and the Chorotega Indians had a good diet (Wagner 1958). On the other hand, the Spanish often had to adopt such unknown foods as maize, and at times experienced hardships and famine.

The Spanish presence in the Americas seriously disrupted Indian culture. The aborigines were robbed, exploited and killed; their civilization was undermined in nearly every respect. The results of such a collision of cultures can be seen today among the Indians of the American Highlands and among the Plains Indians of the United States (Mata 1976; McLuhan 1971). It seems likely that the spread of malnutrition among Indian populations was largely the result of the social disruption brought about under European domination.

Spanish and mestizo populations were somewhat better off than the Indians, but malnutrition nonetheless occurred as the result of poor diet and infectious disease. From colonial times up to the present, malnutrition has appeared as a consequence of seasonal changes, war, or natural disasters affecting food availability.

WORLDWIDE GAINS IN NUTRITION AND HEALTH

In 19th century Europe, improvement in the way of life reduced the mortality rates in respect to many important infectious diseases (Kass 1971). It is important to note that European nations at that time were as underdeveloped as the Central American countries are today. These improvements in health were recorded before either the etiology or measures for the control and prevention of such diseases were known, thus pointing up the role of social determinants as a causal factor.

A recent analysis of the nutritional situation reveals improvement in nearly every part of the world, except where natural or man-made disasters have occurred (Mesarovic and Pestel 1974; Turnbull 1972). While such a trend points toward bettered socioeconomic conditions throughout the world, the level of improvement seems too modest to cope with current and expected projections of food availability and energetics.

Observations in a typical Guatemalan village showed that many Mayan traditions and beliefs have been preserved (Coe 1966), and that these relate principally to childbirth, infant feeding and family or communal organization. However, other features, such as ruralism and traditional agriculture, have deteriorated. In the past few decades, there has been a consistent decrease in the mean gross domestic product throughout most of rural Guatemala. In many nations, the lack of satisfactory land reform and social justice programs has caused a progressive saturation of the land, without alternative employment for the young (Mata 1976). Demographic pressure, poverty and slums have been the result. It is difficult to predict the future for nations displaying this pattern, but it is safe to say that disaster seems inevitable unless significant social transformations are effected and considerable international cooperation employed to alter present conditions (Mata 1975).

(Countries like Cuba, Jamaica and Costa Rica seem to be better off, but it is not certain whether present trends will continue, or even if the observed changes are wholly desirable).

Costa Rica is an agricultural nation of some 2 million inhabitants located 10° north of the equator. Its economy is based on the export of coffee, cattle, bananas, sugar and cacao. At the end of the 19th century, its capital city, with some 25,000 people, was described as one of the filthiest cities in the world, with a death rate (Table 23.1) of 41 per 1000 (Jiménez and Jiménez 1901). Since then, there has been a progressive decline in mortality due to diarrhea and other communicable diseases. As seen in

TABLE 23.1

DEATHS PER 1000 IN CITIES AROUND 1894

Berlin	16.3
Stockholm	16.9
London	20.0
Rome	27.6
Venice	30.1
San Jose, C.R.[1]	40.7
Alexandria	52.9

[1]Crude death rate for Costa Rica in 1974 = 5.3.

Table 23.2, the rates of mortality from diarrhea and dysentery were 82 and 157 per 100,000 respectively. The rate of death from diarrheal disease was reduced by half within 70 years; a further 50% reduction was effected in only 4 years (Moya 1975). A similar situation can be noted in regard to communicable childhood diseases and malnutrition (Table 23.3). An infant mortality rate of 250 per 1000 live births in 1920 had dropped to 84 per 1000 by 1953, and then remained stable for a decade. In 1974, the rate had declined to 38 per 1000. Even more significant is a reduction in the second year death rate from 12 per 1000 in 1953 to a mere 2 per 1000 in 1974.

These improvements in mortality statistics are particularly significant, since they were accompanied by a decline in the birth rate to 30 per 1000 in

82

TABLE 23.2

DEATHS PER 100,000 DUE TO DIARRHEA, GASTROENTERITIS AND COLITIS, SAN JOSE (1900) AND COSTA RICA (1970–1974)

Year	Diarrhea (0091)	Gastroenteritis and Colitis (0092)	All
1900	82.0	157.0[1,2]	
1970	18.4	51.5	70.7
1971	18.7	36.5	56.4
1972	24.1	29.9	55.4
1973	18.7	25.6	45.2
1974	12.1	14.2	27.4

[1]The figure 157 likely included codes 0049, 0060, 0069, 0083, 0090, 0091, and 0092.
[2]Dysentery

TABLE 23.3

HEALTH INDICATORS IN COSTA RICA

	1953	1964	1973	1974
Births per 1000	48	44	29	30
Infant[1] deaths per 1000	84	82	43	38
Deaths 1–4 years per 1000	12	7	3	2
Total infant[1] deaths				
Malnutrition	346	290	52	57
Diarrhea	937	1500	600	402
Lower respiratory disease	276	609	191	161
Immaturity	172	782[2]	556	626

[1]Deaths under one year.
[2]A change in definition of certain causes of death affected this category.

1974. In that year, there was enough room for all children entering school, and some rural schools registered fewer first grade pupils.

Until 1971, the reduction in infant mortality was primarily due to decreased mortality in the postneonatal period (Table 23.4). In recent years, however, both neonatal and postneonatal mortalities have declined, indicating improvements not only in the environment of the child, but also in that of the mother and neonate.

The gains shown in these health indicators parallel several national interventions. For example, in 1968 Costa Rica reached the 1970 goals for water supplies which had been set at the Conference of Punta del Este; the 1980 goals of the Santiago Conference were achieved by 1974. At the present time, piped water is available to nearly all city dwellers, and to a large number of rural citizens as well. The eradication of malaria has demonstrated similar success: in 1974, there were fewer than 150 reported cases of the disease, and half of those had been imported from neighboring countries. Moreover, in 1975 we had raised our per capita income to about

TABLE 23.4

NEONATAL AND POSTNEONATAL INFANT
MORTALITY RATES[1], COSTA RICA 1965–1974

Year	Neonatal (0–28 days)	Postneonatal (29 days–11 months)	Infant (0–11 months)
1965	27.2	48.9	76.0
1967	24.3	38.0	62.3
1969	25.4	41.7	67.1
1971	28.7	27.8	56.4
1973	20.8	24.0	44.8
1974	17.7	19.8	37.6

[1]Per 1000 live births.

$800. Food production has increased, with a record bean crop in 1974 and a record rice crop in 1975. We now produce an excess of both calories and proteins, a good part of which are exported. GAFICA projections suggest a favorable food situation in Costa Rica.

The interrelationship between malnutrition and mortality in Latin America has been well-documented (Mata 1975; Mata 1976; Puffer and Serrano 1973). Thus, it is no surprise that better nutrition and growth in children has run parallel to the control of infectious diseases and improvements in the quality of life. We have already mentioned the significant drop in deaths due to malnutrition, and in the communicable diseases often associated with malnutrition. Surveys conducted by INCAP (1966) and the Ministry of Health (Diaz 1975; Moya 1975; Villegas 1975) have provided a good deal of nutritional information. A representative sample of children under 5 years was examined in 30 rural communities. The comparative results (similar methods of data collection were used in each survey) showed marked changes in child nutrition over the nine-year period. Using the weight for age relationship and the Iowa standard, 41% of the children under one year in 1966 had weight for age deficits of 10% or more (Mata *et al.* 1976), as compared to only 28% in 1975 (Table 23.5). Moreover, the

TABLE 23.5

PREVALANCE (%) OF OVERWEIGHT[1] AND UNDERWEIGHT[2] CHILDREN
IN 2 SURVEYS OF 30 COSTA RICAN RURAL COMMUNITIES

Age (years)	1966 Survey (n = 791)		1975 Survey (n = 1910)	
	Over	Under	Over	Under
<1	10.6	40.9	19.7	28.3
1	2.8	56.7	6.5	47.1
2	1.7	58.1	8.4	53.4
3	2.4	54.5	5.4	50.4
4	2.8	63.9	4.1	63.8
Total	3.8	57.1	8.3	49.6

[1]Overweight = >110% for age.
[2]Underweight = <91% for age.

number of children displaying excess weight for age more than doubled during that time (3.8% in 1966, 8.3% in 1975).

Even more significant changes have occurred among infants. In this case, height is a better indicator of nutritional status. As seen in Table 23.6, 17% of the children under 5 examined in 1966 were stunted (i.e., showed a deficit in height of 10% or more) when compared to the Iowa standard (Mata *et al.* 1976); in 1975, only 7% were stunted. Again, the most dramatic changes occurred in the first year of life.

TABLE 23.6

PREVALENCE (%) OF STUNTING[1] IN CHILDREN
IN 2 SURVEYS OF 30 COSTA RICAN RURAL COMMUNITIES

Age (years)	1966 Survey (n = 791)	1975 Survey (n = 1910)
<1	4.6	1.3
1	14.8	5.8
2	20.4	9.2
3	20.6	9.1
4	21.1	9.5
Total	16.9	7.2

[1]Stunting = <91% height for age.

But while these data unquestionably demonstrate an improved nutritional status over the past nine years, they also reveal that a good many children still fail to reach their optimal growth potential. Current inflationary trends could cause this situation to worsen, and might well interfere with the consolidation of present gains. Inflation seriously affected wages and food prices in the Guatemalan village (Mata 1975), and a similar phenomenon is taking place in Costa Rica.

How can we explain this progress in Costa Rica, an agricultural society which was originally one of the poorest nations in Central America? This is, of course, an area of much speculation, but three factors seem to have played a decisive role:

(1) A relative homogeneity in the population which prevented the marked class distinctions so prevalent in other Latin American nations;

(2) Governmental emphasis on education over the past century, leading to a present illiteracy rate of only 14%; and

(3) Peaceful social reform which began in 1940 with the passage of labor legislation, the creation of a social security system, the development of housing, and the initiation of an income tax and other forms of income redistribution. In 1975, the government distributed $40 million obtained from sales taxes levied on high income groups among the rural population under the terms of the *Asignaciones Familiares* (Family Allowances).

The most important fact is that the improvements in health and nutrition were based on social reforms, better environmental sanitation and a rise in the standard of living. There is no apparent relationship to scientific developments in nutrition; in fact, few papers on nutrition have been written by Costa Ricans. Little nutritional research is being conducted, and the nation's twenty nutritionists are engaged either in applied governmental activities or collective alimentation programs. Nor does it appear that the improved health and nutrition is related to any of these applied nutrition programs. Thus, it would appear that social determinants and poor health are the most important components of malnutrition.

RELATION OF CULTURAL CHANGES TO HEALTH AND NUTRITION
No matter how strong a society's traditions and beliefs might be, Western culture is very successful at neutralizing or altering them. We do not know if cultural changes occur at different rates in capitalist or socialist industrial societies; in view of our geographical location and historical background, we prefer to refer to the former.

Cultural influences on developing nations have modified food habits, hygienic practices, family and social organization, productivity, mental and moral attitudes and health and welfare. While the results have been positive in many respects, there has also been considerable damage, much of it irreversible. A greater variety of foods in greater quantities has become available to certain sectors of the population, but the diet of the poor remains deficient. The breast-feeding period has been shortened primarily in urban populations, but the villages have not been spared. Adoption by the young of such foods as potato chips and carbonated beverages represents an economic waste which contributes to malnutrition. (Any increase in protein or calorie intake beyond that required by adults favors obesity and certain degenerative diseases.)

Consumerism is not confined to food habits, but affects every aspect of life. An emphasis on the acquisition of material goods fosters waste. This trend toward an exaggerated utilization of resources and greater environmental contamination has become increasingly evident in underdeveloped countries. To assess our responsibilities in regard to cultural evolution is beyond the scope of this paper. Nonetheless, it is evident that it is both unrealistic and dangerous to follow the model of the developed industrial nations.

ON MODELS OF DEVELOPMENT
The leaders of developing countries tend to favor models based on the United States and Western European nations. As a result, we came to believe that schools and universities would solve the problems of education, that hospitals and physicians would eliminate health deficits, and that machinery, chemical fertilizers and highways would take care of the food situation. The failure of these utopian schemes led to despair and frustration among scientists, planners and politicians.

While these concepts are still being reviewed (Wade 1975), we realize that there must be alternatives to that orthodox approach. For example, some distinguished contemporary philosophers have pointed out that the apparent health in some modern societies is a mirage (Dubos 1959; Illich

1975). And one wonders about the connections between industrial development and recent increases in prematurity, mental disorders, urban violence and drug abuse.

Referring again to Costa Rica, we are concerned that certain undesirable cultural, economic and biological changes are occurring along with the improvements in health indices, but at a faster rate. There is, for example, a marked tendency toward less physical activity. We find increases in stress and anxiety, alcoholism and drug dependence, obesity, diabetes and degenerative diseases. There is a greater dependence on imported foods such as wheat, and an increase in the export of both calories and high quality proteins (sugar, rice and meat) in order to satisfy the society's material demands.

We can see that development is not entirely relevant to health by comparing mortality statistics from Shanghai and New York (Sidel 1975). Social measures in Shanghai have cut infant mortality to 9 per 1000 live births, half of that found among Caucasians in New York. Moreover, the mortality rates of Switzerland and Sweden are lower than those of the United States and Germany. It seems clear that industrialization and increases in material wealth cannot always be equated with improved health and welfare for all sectors of the society. Unlimited growth is neither logical nor desirable.

We can learn an important lesson in community organization from the example of the Rural Health Program in Costa Rica. As malaria progressively disappeared, the infrastructure of the National Service for the Eradication of Malaria was shifted over time to the Rural Health Program (Villegas and Vargas 1975). Targeted toward 600,000 people (31% of the national population) found, for the most part, in communities numbering less than 500, the Rural Health Program began to revolutionize health delivery in 1971. At present, 60% of this population group is handled by 210 "health workers with shoes" operating out of 135 regional headquarters. Using jeeps, motorcycles, horses or boats, these workers take the census, control communicable diseases such as malaria and intestinal parasites, vaccinate against tuberculosis, measles, tetanus, whooping cough, diptheria, poliomyelitis and smallpox, carry out maternal and child health programs involving family planning, maternal care and infant nutrition, treat or refer selected diseases, work to improve environmental hygiene in regard to water supply, latrines, waste disposal and education, and engage in community organization. Although this program has not as yet been evaluated, mortality trends related to certain communicable diseases indicate that the rural area is being well-covered. In Table 23.7, for example, we find a marked decrease in deaths preventable by vaccination which closely correlates with the establishment of the Rural Health Program in 1971.

TABLE 23.7

DEATHS DUE TO DISEASES PREVENTABLE BY VACCINATION
1965–1974

Year	Polio-myelitis	Diphtheria	Whooping Cough	Tetanus	Measles	Total
1965	8	26	131	239	186	590
1967	13	19	86	202	260	580
1969	22	19	36	164	322	563
1971	2	19	48	137	84	290
1973	1	5	50	103	61	220
1974	0	0	39	93	12	144

Community organization has also brought encouraging results. Some communities have established aggressive committees which, under the spur of "better health and welfare," have branched out into agriculture, road and bridge construction, and similar projects requiring greater capital and effort. In this way, "health for the people, by the people" (Newell 1975) may become "development for the people, by the people." This program has demonstrated that any intervention should incorporate subprofessionals and involve substantial community participation. It also offers an alternative to the increasing number of physicians and engineers needed to satisfy the demands of an industrial society. While such elements should be granted rational attention, what is needed is a holistic approach in the movement toward improved development, health and welfare.

While it is true that relative improvements have been made in the small nation of Costa Rica without following orthodox models, it is also true that we are experiencing certain deleterious cultural and economic transformations while still at some distance from our optimal goals. What seems to be of paramount importance at present is a review of the entire concept of national and international development in order to define exactly what we want in terms of human health and welfare without resorting to large-scale industrialization or a "growth race."

It seems quite evident that the present models of advanced nations are not appropriate for the underdeveloped nations. In this light, some of the problems discussed at this symposium by nutritional planners and other intellectuals may turn out to be mere academic exercises. The answer to the question "Can man's biological adaptation cope with cultural change, especially as regards nutrition" can be "Yes," *if* nations begin to work now, in full cooperation, to find alternatives to the orthodox models of development; *if* the developing nations effectively implement systems of social justice; *if* the wealthier nations can make significant contributions to the poor nations; and *if* most nations decide to control consumerism, unlimited growth and distortions of human nature. Since these conditions are quite utopian, a negative answer to the question may be unavoidable after all, at least for many countries in the not too distant future.

REFERENCES

COE, M. D. 1966. The Maya. Praeger Publishers, New York.

DE CERVANTES-SAAVEDRA,. M. 1605. The Clever Nobleman Don Quixote de la Mancha. J. García Soriano and J. García Morales (Editors). Aguilar. Madrid. (Spanish)

DÍAZ, C., and VARGAS, W. 1975. Nutrition Survey. Ministry of Health, Costa Rica.

DUBOS, R. 1959. Mirage of Health. Doubleday and Co., New York.

ILLICH, I. 1975. Medical Nemesis: The Expropriation of Health. Barral Editores S. A., Barcelona. (Spanish.)

INCAP. 1966. Nutritional Evaluation of the Population of Central America and Panama: Costa Rica. INCAP. Guatemala City. Guatemala. (Spanish)

JIMÉNEZ, E., and JIMÉNEZ, G. 1901. Hygiene of Homes and Water in Costa Rica. Typografía Nacional. Costa Rica. (Spanish)

KASS, E. 1971. Infectious disease and social change. J. Infect. Dis. *123*, 110–114.

MATA, L. J. 1975. Malnutrition-infection interactions in the tropics. Am. J. Trop. Med. and Hyg. *24*, 564–574.

MATA, L. J. 1976. The Children of Santa María Cauqué: A Prospective Study of Health and Growth. MIT-Cornell Press, Cambridge, Mass.

MATA, L.J., MOHS, E., ALBERTAZZI, C., and GUTIÉRREZ, R. 1976. Considerations on malnutrition in Central America, with special reference to Costa Rica. Rev. Biol. Trop. *24* (Supp. 1), 25–39. (Spanish)

MC LUHAN, T. C. 1971. Touch the Earth: A Self-Portrait of Indian Existence. Promontory Press, New York.

MEADOWS, D. H., MEADOWS, D. L., RANDERS, J., and BEHRENS W. W., III. 1972. The Limits to Growth. Potomac Associates, New York.

MESAROVIC, M., and PESTEL, E. 1974. Mankind at the Turning Point. E. P. Dutton and Co., New York.

MORRIS, D. 1967. The Naked Ape. McGraw-Hill, Inc., New York.

MOYA, L. 1975. Morbidity and Mortality Statistics. Ministry of Health, Costa Rica.

NEWELL, K. W. 1975. Health for the People. WHO, Geneva. (Spanish.)

PUFFER, R. R., and SERRANO, C. V. 1973. Characteristics of Infant Mortality. PAHO Sci. Pub. *262*, Washington, D. C.

RECINOS, A. 1950. Popol Vuh: The Sacred Book of the Ancient Quiché Maya. Univ. Okla. Press, Norman, Okla.

SIDEL, V. W. 1975. Medical care in the People's Republic of China. Arch. Int. Med. *135*, 916–926.

SMITH, G. H. 1973. Income and Nutrition in the Guatemalan Highlands. Ph. D. Dissertation, Univ. Oregon 1972. Univ. Microfilms, Ann Arbor, Mich.

STRUEVER, S. 1971. Prehistoric Agriculture. American Museum of Natural History, New York.

TURNBULL, C. M. 1972. The Mountain People. Simon and Schuster, New York.

VAN LAWICK-GOODALL, J. 1971. In the Shadow of Man. Dell Publishing Co., New York.

VILLEGAS, H., and VARGAS, W. 1975. Program of Rural Health. Ministry of Health, Costa Rica.

VON HAGEN, V. W. 1960. World of the Maya. Mentor, New York.

WADE, N. 1975. Third World: Science and technology contribute feebly to development. Science *189*, 770–776.

WAGNER, P. L. 1958. Nicoya, a Cultural Geography. Univ. Calif. Press, Berkeley, Calif.

CHAPTER 24

Hernán Delgado
Timothy Farrell
Robert E. Klein

A Design for Socioeconomic Intervention Programs in Rural Communities

We wish to present data which focus on the organization of a program of socioeconomic intervention in rural Guatemala. Our experience is based on a longitudinal study of the effects of an experimental, low-cost health and nutritional intervention program in four rural villages in eastern Guatemala. Also, we have evaluated the socioeconomic consequences of an independent community development program in the highlands of Guatemala. From these experiences, we have derived a generalized model for intervention programs that utilizes a system of curative and simple preventive medicine as a vector for operationalizing an integrated plan of community development.

HEALTH CARE AS A COMMUNITY ENTRY

There are several reasons why low-cost medical care programs are advantageous as points of initial entry in community intervention programs. In our experience, without exception, one of the most vividly perceived needs in rural communities is adequate medical care facilities. Mortality statistics for Guatemala are consistent with village perceptions in that they list the five principal causes of death as (1) acute respiratory diseases, (2) diarrhea, (3) malnutrition, (4) perinatal mortality, and (5) parasitic diseases (Ministry of Public Health and Welfare 1973).

A second advantage to beginning development activities around health and nutrition interventions results from the organizational structure and initial village responsibility for these activities. A health committee formed by village members serves as the basic organizational unit. The health care personnel associated with the program work directly for the village, and specifically for the committee. In this fashion, the village is involved in the initial planning and the continuing operation of their health program.

A third reason for focusing on health and nutritional intervention is that these areas best demonstrate the efficacy of modern medical care, and are also highly visible. As an example, a program in four villages in eastern Guatemala has reduced the infant mortality rate from 155 per 1000 to 85 per 1000 (Klein et al. 1973; Habicht et al. 1974). Figure 24.1 shows that a relatively modest caloric supplementation to pregnant women cuts the incidence of low birthweight approximately in half. Increases in birthweight are closely associated with reductions in infant mortality (Lechtig et al. 1975).

265

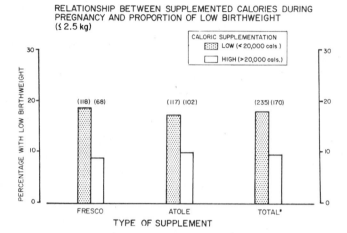

FIG. 24.1.   RELATIONSHIP BETWEEN SUPPLEMENTED CALORIES DURING PREG-
NANCY AND PROPORTION OF LOW BIRTHWEIGHT (≤2.5kg)

Finally, development programs organized around health and nutritional interventions have a better chance of being integrated into national health systems, which are usually well-organized and have clearly defined goals. Thus, there are important advantages, both at the community and at the national level, for beginning interventions of the type to be described here. In our experience, such programs are both feasible and desirable since they provide an entry for community-governed development programs, and consciously strive for articulation with national systems which have developmental goals.

ISSUES IN DEVELOPMENT INTERVENTION

An important component of health and nutritional interventions is that they have readily measurable objectives for evaluation. Assessment of development programs is necessary not only in terms of impact, but also because it provides for internal operational checks on the management of the program. Part of the experience upon which our preliminary model is based involves the evaluation of an independent program of community development in highland Guatemala.

This program has been in operation for over ten years, and has initiated numerous interventions aimed at socioeconomic development. While one of its components includes a medical clinic, the intervention agents have not used health care as an entry vehicle for other programs. The cost of the program in 1974 was about $150,000 in direct and indirect expenditures. Despite this financial input to a town of 6,000, our evaluation discovered some serious problems concerning its operation and impact. Specifically, we found that it lacks an integrated self-assessment component, and believe that various minor problems became serious because they were not detected early in the operation.

Our experience parallels that of developers internationally; that is, we recognize that evaluation—both operational and effectual—is essential to organizing and implementing a coherent system of designed intervention. We employ the concept of management-by-objectives as one structure around which we have designed our model. We understand, however, that structure is a static concept. Around the structural framework are vital operational issues which seem to govern the integration of development plans and operations. Substantive case studies of intervention programs reveal four issues thought to be salient to the success or failure of planned socioeconomic development projects:

(1) Conflicts between agents' goals and community-perceived or "felt" needs;

(2) Appropriate use and appreciation of traditional systems of social organization and leadership;

(3) Design and maintenance of appropriate systems and modes of communication; and

(4) Circumvention of the reality of economic constraints against the adoption of innovations (Arensberg and Niehoff 1971: Foster 1962; Goodenough 1963; Niehoff 1966; Spicer 1952).

We want to discuss these issues briefly and indicate some ways in which they have affected an intervention program in the Guatemalan highlands. We believe that close attention to these issues, the details of which can be identified through ethnographic research, permits the design of intervention programs which have a greater than usual probability of success.

By and large, problems in development are more complicated than those in primary medical delivery systems. The variation within and between communities with respect to modes of production, social structure and organization, as well as the traditions and beliefs interwoven with economic life, is often poorly understood. As is apparent from international development experience, technological assistance alone is insufficient to bring about desired results. Economic and ethnographic research provides programs of intervention with the information needed to integrate technological skills with social and cultural issues.

The operational issues can be conceptually organized into compartmental domains, but their reality is not amenable to such structure. There is considerable overlap among them, and their interaction is highly complex. We will discuss these issues separately, but wish to emphasize that their operation is simultaneous, their priority equivalent, and their integration essential.

Community Needs

The issue of community-perceived needs versus interventive goals is often a source of ongoing miscommunication, and can threaten the success of a program (Niehoff 1966; Spicer 1952). On one hand, the intervention agents may have an a priori agenda which conflicts with the perceived needs of the community. On the other, both the agent and the community may share a similar sense of what is needed, but the community may be unable to articulate a detailed solution. This is often because the solution itself involves latent—but real—needs, the technology and understanding of which may be unknown to rural villagers.

For example, a common response to a probe for felt needs is "more to eat" or a "source of money." The agent's technical response may be the introduction of an agricultural cooperative, an innovation which is often perceived as acceptable by a community. However, it also generates certain other needs, such as education in cooperative organization, literate officers, and a communal organization. These necessary component needs may not be perceived or understood by the community, and therefore stand the risk of being rejected.

Such a case occurred in the Guatemalan highlands after a cooperative organization was formed. Ninety small coffee growers initially subscribed and demonstrated their enthusiasm by paying an initiation fee of $30. Unfortunately, the intervention agents were unable to respond to the generated needs, and did not stress the importance of organizational behavior or provide appropriate training. The organization appeared to function smoothly for one year, but afterwards two serious problems occurred. One involved several members who sold their crops privately in advance of harvest, thus diminishing the unified power of the organization. The second was more severe and involved the theft of a substantial amount of cash (Farrell 1975).

The essence of the example is that, while working with felt needs is an imperative issue, agent goals and needs generated by the community are equally important. They cannot be dismissed or given low priority simply because they are not immediately perceived by the community. A major task, then, is to provide for the satisfaction of generated needs while simultaneously concentrating on perceived needs.

Social Organization and Community Leadership

As with the issue of needs, the literature on rural community development stresses the importance of working through traditional leadership and the formal or informal organizations it represents (Foster 1962; Goodenough 1963; Niehoff 1966; Spicer 1952). While we find this to be true generally, our data from the highlands suggest that these organizations may not be the most efficient vehicles for development interventions.

For at least three decades, there has been debate regarding the type of individual most likely to adopt innovations (Barnett 1953; Foster 1962; Linton 1936; Murdock 1956; Rogers and Shoemaker 1971). One theme of this debate has been that the most likely candidates are those of high social status. The other argues the reverse—that the discontented, disaffected and poor residents of a village are most likely to adopt innovations.

In rural communities, high traditional social status and village leadership correlate typically with age. Similarly, a positive relationship is usually found between high status individuals and adoption of an innovation. However, age itself shows no consistent relationship with behavioral innovation (Rogers and Shoemaker 1971). Our data suggest that one explanation for such apparent ambiguity is that the dimension of traditional status, respect and leadership is nearly orthogonal with more modern leadership roles and achieved status pathways.

In the Guatemalan highland intervention community, a few traditional leaders of high social status subscribed to various innovative programs. Their participation, however, can be generally classified as passive and individualized. In a program striving for self-sufficiency, these leaders were not providing dynamic or innovative direction. The intervention agents, however, recognized their value as a vehicle for gaining and maintaining a broad base of community support. Consequently, when programs involving paid on-the-job training in construction, experimental agriculture and animal husbandry were undertaken, a new group of individuals was named to managerial positions. In general, these men were younger, owned less agricultural land, and had less status in the traditional sense. However, they were selected in consultation with the traditional leaders.

Over time, these newly incorporated individuals have risen to positions of leadership, the domains of which are distinct from those of traditional high status leaders. Social network data collected on high status-respected individuals and modern opinion leaders support the argument that at least two dimensions of leadership exist in the community. These data appear in Table 24.1. We believe that the modern dimension is a product of agent intervention, and is noncompetitive with traditional domains of authority and respect.

Because of this, we believe that traditional leadership and organization play a significant role in the initial stages of an intervention. However, new leadership niches become available over time, and we contend that these are best filled by younger, more dynamic individuals who have the capacity and desire to maintain the impetus of intervention projects.

Intracommunity Interventions

The issue of communication is central to development (Batten 1965; Erasmus 1961; Goodenough 1963; Niehoff 1966; Rao 1966; Rogers and

TABLE 24.1

CHARACTERISTICS OF LEADERS

Factor	Traditional Leaders (Most Respected)	Modern Opinion Leaders
Age	Over 50	Under 50
Land	100% owned more than 10 acres	15% owned more than 10 acres
Traditional religious status	100% highest rank	100% low rank or no rank ever
Wealth	All identified as richest in community	Never identified as richest in community

Source: INCAP (75–1291)

Shoemaker 1971). Without adequate communication of its purposes, plans and operations, no program can hope for successful results. There are numerous channels of communication in a community, and these can work at cross-purposes to an intervention program. While we recognize that communication between agent and client is essential, we are also concerned with communication among clients themselves. In the highland case, a major communication problem has arisen. Daily briefings are held between agents and project managers. Information from these meetings is to be disseminated first to other program employees, and then informally throughout the community. However, small social groups composed almost exclusively of development program participants have been formed. As a result, much of the information designed to flow throughout the community is impeded. Table 24.2 shows that members of such groups tend to associate largely with each other and not with the general community. As a consequence, substantial information becomes the relatively exclusive property of a self-selected group.

Relatively little can be done by intervention agents to discourage the formation of such groups, and it is not at all clear that this would be

TABLE 24.2

SOCIAL INTERACTION PATTERNS AMONG COMMUNITY MEMBERS[1]

	Degree of Program Participation			
	High (19)	Low (19)	t	Sig.
% High participating friends	62.8	10.8	4.46	.001
% High participating drinking companions	57.3	8.5	4.47	.001

Source: INCAP (75–1292)
[1]N = 38

desirable even if possible. Our goal is to establish systems of formal and informal communication which provide for the ongoing interchange of information between agents and the community, and among the clients themselves. The logical vehicles for this are community health promoters, who have intensive personal contact with many community members each day.

Economic Constraints

The foregoing issues—assessment of and responses to needs, community organization and communication—broadly define the focus of a development intervention, outline a leadership structure, and anticipate potential impediments to the circulation of program information. The issue of economic constraints is more directly concerned with community and individual idiosyncrasies which (usually) mitigate against participation in the intervention (Dalton 1971). Evaluation of the Guatemalan highland program has isolated three principal economic factors which have prevented many individuals from taking advantage of projects they otherwise desire to enter: (1) time, (2) land-space, and (3) cash or readily available liquid assets.

Some general statements have been made to the effect that poor rural people have relatively large amounts of free time available for participation in projects (Niehoff 1966). Our findings indicate that this is not always the case, and time-available is a highly variable factor. In the highland community, an analysis of activities-by-time-spent revealed that the average total number of hours per day invested in economic activities was 10.83 (SD = 4.6, N = 85). Of this, about 2.5 hours are spent in walking to and from work, maintaining tools, and making household repairs.

The importance of time availability is clear. Individuals who spend large amounts of time in economic pursuits are poor candidates for programs in adult education, and probably for programs involving the donation of labor on a regular basis. Such individuals can best be served through on-the-job-training, individualized consultation during their work routine, or at home in the evening. This latter method has been used extensively in religious proselytization by both Protestant and Catholic groups; in fact, adult literacy training in many Guatemalan highland communities is often achieved through such Bible tutorials. We think that similar techniques can be used to disseminate technical information pertinent to intervention projects.

Additional constraints refer to land-space, and variation by community and individual is often dramatic. In some villages, most individuals own their house sites; in others, few have direct ownership. Even where house sites are owned, their size and secondary usage can be a limiting factor.

Development programs often aim to increase food availability by means of home garden plots or animal husbandry projects. If the site is not owned, such activity may be prohibited by the landlord. When the site is owned, but is small or involved in cash-crop production, the owner may be reluctant to engage in certain intervention activities. In the highland community, only 21% of the sample had project animals or gardens, but 80% of the remainder expressed a verbal desire to participate in such projects. Most said they were unable to do so because they lacked adequate space.

Absence of working capital also limits many areas of intervention. In the highland community, the overall average daily cash wage in 1973 was about 70 cents. This yields about 10 cents per day per person for food. Where family incomes are higher in this community, one finds greater allocations toward food and medical resources, and to maintaining children in school. Table 24.3 illustrates this pattern of wages and expenditures. Higher daily wages apparently are accompanied by greater expenditures toward family well-being, but little actual cash remains for capital investment after family needs are satisfied.

TABLE 24.3

INCOME AND EXPENDITURES AMONG HIGH AND LOW PROGRAM PARTICIPANTS[1]

| | Degree of Program Participation | | | |
	High	Low	t	p /
Average daily wage	0.80	0.60	1.95	.025
Average $ spent on food per week	4.25	3.11	3.41	.001
Average number of clinic visits per family per year	7.3	2.6	3.03	.004
Average percentage of school-age children in school	59.0	16.0	4.51	.001

Source: INCAP (75–1293)
[1]N = 85

One general solution proposed for the constraints of land-space and capital are agricultural cooperatives, through which a sizeable plot of land can be purchased for members' use as home gardens or animal pens. While this is satisfactory in some degree, the relatively high entrance fees may exclude the economically more marginal families. One solution involves credit cooperatives, which have relatively smaller initiation dues and can provide unsecured, short-term, low-interest loans. A program of this type was instituted in the highland community in 1969 with a capitalization of $600. In 1974, its working capital amounted to about $2000, most of which was employed in one-year loans to members.

The Guatemalan highland development program has served to help us focus on some relevant issues in operationalizing a model for socioeconomic intervention. We believe that some of the problems in that program could have been avoided by instituting a systematic evaluation component. Consistent assessment of both operations and objectives permits the controlled implementation of plans, and provides an ongoing quality control mechanism.

MEDICAL DELIVERY SYSTEM

As we noted earlier, a low-cost medical delivery system appears to be an ideal entry vehicle for programs of socioeconomic intervention. It meets real and perceived needs, and can serve as a preliminary channel of agent and community communication.

Several aspects of such a system warrant discussion. The first deals with the personnel involved, their level of training, and the techniques of supervision and quality control employed. These are cardinal considerations, and serious difficulties may occur if they are ignored.

Personnel

The personnel engaged in health promotion work are paraprofessionals. The requirements for such positions are literacy, motivation, and willingness to work in isolated rural areas. Formal training in treatment and health promotion takes about one month, and can be done in the context of regular clinic activities under the supervision of a nurse or auxiliary nurse trained in this system. We have found on-the-job-training to work extremely well and to be relatively efficient. With this simple preparation, the health promoter becomes an extension of the community health service system beyond the outpatient clinic. His role is to make periodic visits to the dwellings of the people in the region to be served, to maintain contact within the community, and to stimulate use of the outpatient clinic. A wide variety of other activities in health, nutrition and general development can be assigned to the health promoter, depending on the design of the intervention program and its stage of evolution.

The supervisory backbone of the health intervention aspect of the program is an auxiliary nurse. Auxiliary nurses are widely used in Latin America, and typically have some minimal level of formal hospital training. In the program described here, the auxiliary nurse received an additional six months of training in the diagnosis and treatment of common illnesses. We have employed auxiliary nurses extensively during the past six years, and have found that they perform extremely well with the training and close supervision described here.

In the present program, the auxiliary nurse is located at the village health center and her function is to treat patients, refer serious cases to a physician or hospital, and supervise the work of the health promoters in their efforts to extend health services beyond the clinic.

The person principally responsible for the overall direction, supervision and functioning of the health intervention is a registered nurse or physician. Such a person can supervise up to ten health centers, and is principally responsible for maintaining the quality of medical care.

This model, extending from the promoter up through the supervisory nurse or physician, has three distinct advantages over traditional systems:

(1) It extends health services beyond the health clinic and thus results in high coverage rates among the target population;

(2) It allows for the systematic collection of health data by the health promoters, both for epidemiological surveillance and the development of simple indicators to identify those individuals at highest risk of morbidity and mortality; and

(3) Through coordination with national health systems, the data collected by the health promoters and the auxiliary nurses can be channelled into the national epidemiological surveillance network, and thus contribute directly to national health planning and resource allocation.

Portions of this model have been tested extensively during the last eight years by members of a research team at INCAP. Specifically, we find that well-trained and supervised auxiliary nurses, using the physician's criteria, can adequately treat over 90% of the patients they see (INCAP-DDH 1973). Moreover, they can accurately refer those cases they are unable to treat. Table 24.4 shows the number of patients referred by auxiliary nurses to the supervising physician and to the hospital in six programs currently functioning in Guatemala. Data on adequacy of medical history, diagnosis, treatment and follow-up are regularly collected and provide the basis for continual quality control of the program.

We find high levels of acceptance and enthusiasm on the part of rural villagers for this type of treatment. In addition to expressed patient satisfaction, the number of visits per patient per year is over four, a number beyond that normally encountered in programs based entirely on patient decision (INCAP-DDH 1973).

TABLE 24.4

PATIENT VISITS AND REFERRALS PER YEAR

Program	Visits[1] per Inhabitant	Referred to M.D.	% Referred to Hospital
PROSA	0.5	All	Unknown
Micro.	1.7	All	0.9%
PPSR	1.8	Unknown	Unknown
DHD	4.2	1.0%	0.4%
Mkll	1.2	1.1%	0.5%
Behr	0.1	8.7%	2.1%

From Habicht et al. (1973).
[1]Only diagnostic visits.

Costs

In addition to such fundamental program characteristics as personnel, training, quality control and patient satisfaction, the issue of cost is crucial. Several investigators in our group have worked extensively on the problem of medical care costs in the context of simplified programs. We estimate that the cost per visit for planned intervention programs will be approximately 50 cents. This compares with a range of 64 cents to $2.03 across six other simplified medical care programs operating in Guatemala in 1972 (INCAP-DDH 1973). The low cost is principally due to savings from bulk purchase of inexpensive medicines, and relatively low expenditures on salaries for health and supervisory personnel.

The medical care and nutrition intervention model described here is admittedly a palliative activity. It will provide few (if any) long-term benefits for the village in terms of general development. Rather, it is a program specifically designed to provide information on initial organizational experience for the community, and a structure through which integrated development programs can proceed. Unless the larger issue of development is kept clearly in mind and the goals clearly articulated, it is highly possible that health intervention might become an end in itself, and in turn retard the general process of community development.

In service of the larger development program (and crucial to its success) is the careful and detailed collection of data directed toward two basic aims:

(1) Baseline date which allows for the ongoing evaluation of the effectiveness of the health and nutrition program, and for adjustments which are inevitably necessary; and

(2) The design of the larger development program and its detailed evaluation.

GENERAL MODEL FOR SOCIOECONOMIC INTERVENTION

The general model we propose to implement is presented in schematic form in Fig. 24.2. The abscissa represents time in undefined and arbitrary units, and the ordinate describes various stages of the program. It will be noted that evaluation has a primary role and is a continuing component of the model. Beginning at the bottom of the ordinate, Stage 1 comprises the formation of a village health committee. The village collaborates through the committee during Stage 1, which includes an initial diagnosis of the public health situation in the community. Data from this survey provides baseline information for initial planning of the health intervention, as well as for subsequent evaluation of the program and its impact. Personnel training (including health promoters and auxiliary health personnel) is also accomplished during this time, with specific reference to information provided by the initial baseline health survey. On the basis of the work by the

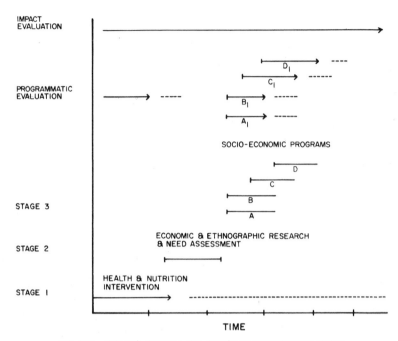

FIG. 24.2.   GENERAL SCHEMA FOR PROGRAM INTERVENTION MODEL

community committee and the intervention team, the program is to be implemented with objectives determined during the initial health survey.

Following the successful design and implementation of the health intervention, the proposed model provides for an intensive period of economic and ethnographic study and data collection. Specifically, such areas as religious and political structure, patterns of subsistence, beliefs, attitudes and behavior of the target population and cultural norms will be analyzed. The principal purpose for this is to assess real and perceived community needs, and to define a detailed program design.

Succeeding stages are defined in terms of the implementation of various aspects of the development program directed toward satisfying socio-economic, health and nutritional village needs. The specific programs and priorities are to be determined by the villagers themselves in coordination with the intervention agent. Careful and detailed work with respect to economic, ethnographic and needs assessment activities during Stage 2 provides the specific direction and timing for subsequent projects and their implementation.

Finally, each of the individual interventions (as well as the overall program) has its evaluation components, as indicated in the schematic. The operational evaluation of the internal organizational structure and administration is carefully implemented and closely tied to each discrete development intervention. The overall evaluation component is a continuing activity which seeks to measure changes and understand the success and failures of the programs. (It is represented by the continuous line in the upper portion of the schematic.)

It is our belief that an evaluation component of this general nature—tied both to operation and impact—is essential to achieve effective programs of socioeconomic, health and nutritional intervention. However, our goals extend beyond the boundaries of a specific intervention as we seek to understand the processes which govern contemporary sociocultural change. We believe that systematic evaluation of well-designed interventions provides the optimal strategy for achieving this end.

ACKNOWLEDGEMENTS

This research was supported by Contract NO1-HD-5-0640 from the National Institute of Child Health and Human Development, National Institutes of Health, Bethesda, Maryland.

REFERENCES

ARENSBERG, C., and NIEHOFF, A. 1971. Introducing Social Change. Aldine Publishing, Chicago.

BARNETT H. G. 1953. Innovation: The Basis of Culture Change. McGraw-Hill. New York.

BATTEN, R. T. 1965. The Human Factor in Development Work. Oxford Univ. Press, London.

DALTON, G. 1971. Economic Development and Social Change. Natural History Press, New York.

ERASMUS, C. J. 1961. Man Takes Control. Bobbs-Merrill Co., New York.

FARRELL, W. T. 1975. Economic Factors in the Process of Modernization in a Highland Guatemalan Town. Ph. D. Dissertation. Univ. Calif., Los Angeles, Calif.

FOSTER, G. M. 1962. Traditional Cultures and the Impact of Technological Change. Harper and Row, New York.

GOODENOUGH, W. H. 1963. Cooperation in Change. Russell Sage Foundation, New York.

HABICHT, J-P., GUZMAN, G., LECHTIG, A., and LOU, O. 1974. Community control and quality control of medical primary care personnel. Paper presented at the XIV Congress of Pediatrics, Buenos Aires, October 3-9.

INCAP-DDH. 1973. Delivery of primary care by medical auxiliaries: Techniques of use and analysis of benefits achieved in some rural villages in Guatemala. In Medical Care Auxiliaries, PAHO/WHO Sci. Pub. 278, 24–37. 278, 24–37.

KLEIN, R. E., HABICHT, J-P., and YARBROUGH, C. 1973. Some methodological problems in field studies of nutrition and intelligence. In Nutrition, Development and Social Behavior, Proceedings of the Conference on the Assessment of Tests of Behavior from Studies of Nutrition in the Western Hemisphere. D. J. Kallen (Editor). HEW Publication (NIH) 73-242, 61–75.

LECHTIG, A. et al. 1975. Maternal nutrition and fetal growth in developing countries. Am. J. Dis. Child. 129, 553-556.

LINTON, R. 1936. The Study of Man. Appleton-Century-Crofts, New York.

MINISTRY OF PUBLIC HEALTH AND SOCIAL WELFARE. 1973. Assessment of the health situation. Guatemala. (Spanish)

MURDOCK, G. P. 1956. How Culture Changes. In Man, Culture and Society. L. Shapiro (Editor). Oxford Univ. Press, New York.

NIEHOFF, A. 1966. A Casebook of Social Change. Aldine Publishing, Chicago.
RAO, Y. V. 1966. Communication and Development. Univ. Minn. Press, Minneapolis, Minn.
ROGERS, E. M., and SHOEMAKER, F. 1971. Communication of Innovations. Free Press, New York.
RYAN, B. 1969. Social Change. Ronald Press, New York.
SPICER. E. H. 1952. Human Problems in Technological Change. John Wiley and Sons. New York.

CHAPTER 25

Margaret Mackenzie

Discussion

The topic addressed in this section is "Man's Complex Culture Today and Tomorrow—Can Man's Biological Adaptation Cope with Cultural Change, Especially as Regards Nutrition?" Dr. Leonard Joy approached the problem from the perspective of international organizations, Mr. Sol Chafkin from the perspective of the developed countries, Dr. Leonardo Mata from the perspective of the underdeveloped countries, and Dr. Robert Klein from the perspective of those involved in nutritional intervention programs.

Let me begin with Dr. Joy. In speaking about Costa Rica, Dr. Mata thought the answer to the question we have been considering was "Yes—if nations begin working now . . . to find the alternatives to orthodox models of development." I regret, then, that Dr. Joy presented us with the orthodox model of homeostasis, equilibrating mechanisms and regulations which he feels were set up to enhance man's chances of survival. He said that he was making links with anthropology, and he was—particularly with the Radcliffe-Brown structuralist-functionalist models.

The problem is that we end up imputing functions without having any good criteria to assess the validity of the functions we've attributed to what we are analyzing. The homeostatic model, after all, is only a model. We can't be sure that man always actually works for survival. And so, with Dr. Mata, I worry about the fruitfulness of using such a model. Of course I find it attractive to adopt an argument like that of Dr. Jelliffe, who suggested that selective malnutrition may bring about good results; that by giving the best protein to the elderly, for example, we preserve them as data banks of knowledge. I'm sympathetic to the idea. But I worry about just where we are getting *analytically* when we do this sort of thing. How can we judge its accuracy?

Having discussed these homeostatic societies, Dr. Joy then said that such societies tend to break down under the stress of cultural change. The problem, it seems to me, is that he left "stress" as an unanalyzed black box, except for one health and two economic variables. The limited approach here worries me. And while he mentioned values a few times in passing, he never discussed them in depth. I would suggest here that American anthropology has something very important to offer us of British and British colonial extraction (to include myself), because I think we must face what the Americans *have* faced—that is, the role of symbols and meanings.

Anthropologists in the United States must be respected for having faced up to the importance of definitions, classifications and connotations; that is, to the meanings we give to our experiences and environments. I shall return to this point later on.

The stresses specified by Dr. Joy were (1) development of the market, (2) the external introduction of new technology, and (3) efforts in public health. When the breakdown resulting from these stresses occurred, he said that new regulators would come into play—specifically, the market and the government. And the result, he said, was goal-seeking societies. Now I suspect that I have been listening to an argument based on Economic Man, on man as a maximizer. This is an old fight between economists and economic anthropologists. Of course man maximizes, and the traditional analyses held that man was maximizing economic variables. But British anthropologists have argued that man maximizes other things as well, and that he may be maximizing values which really have nothing at all to do with categories which we would define as economic.

I feel somewhat hesitant about criticizing a senior professor, and I am wondering if perhaps I didn't hear what he meant to say, or if perhaps he didn't say exactly what he meant. But I think that we get into enormous trouble if we say that traditional societies are not goal-seeking. People *do* have purposes for their behavior, even though we may not always agree that they're doing things for the reasons they *say* they are. In almost any society, you will find goals and aims and hierarchies of values.

Dr. Joy also said that these stress-induced breakdowns have vast nutritional consequences as a result of changes in food production, food processing and dietary patterns. At this point, the problem of neglecting classifications and meanings seems to me very serious, because what we must recognize is that when we introduce new foods into a colonial society, we also bring about changes in the values of the traditional economic foods. The evidence (beginning with Dr. Heizer) is that prior to outside contact, societies from prehistory to the present have been nutritionally well adapted. What happens in the colonial setting, however, is that the local population notices, for example, the healthy children of the colonial expatriates in the administration, and notices as well that these administrators feed their children on different foods. As a result, the local people lose respect for their traditional foods.

Moreover, people in colonial societies discover that working for cash brings status, and therefore want to work for the administration. This, of course, leaves little or no time for cultivating their subsistence foods. In addition, they are paid very little for their labor; an American Samoan, for example, is paid about one quarter the wages paid to an American expatriate for the same work. As a result, the local worker cannot afford to buy all the foods that the expatriate can afford to buy, and usually spends his money on imported items such as white bread and spaghetti. Taking the case of Samoa again, we find a situation where Samoan mothers notice that American children are healthier than their own, and that American mothers feed their children milk powder. The Samoans want to emulate this pattern, but they haven't enough money to be able to feed their children the same concentration of milk powder as do the Americans. I think this example points up the role of status and value, and the fact that we must take a close look at the symbols and meanings which we export along with our administrations.

Dr. Joy also pointed out that the pressures of cultural change make it easier for people to "contract out," but he never defined what he meant by that term. I suspect he was saying that labor goes on the market and is employed with money, but I am not really sure what the difference is.

One argument on which Dr. Joy seemed to place a great deal of importance was the notion that feasts are equilibrating mechanisms, that they are levellers, that they prevent the accumulation of wealth, that they limit individual power, and that they insure cohesion and stability. Again I hesitate to criticize, but I am afraid that most anthropologists would say that the notion is mistaken. There is a great deal of anthropological evidence, particularly from Melanesia, to suggest that people clearly see feasts as a means of maximizing individual power. It is the big men who put on the feasts, the specific reason being to accumulate capital through the exchange system.[1] Even if that capital were to circulate, whether immediately or at a later time, the present aim of the exchange is to accumulate personal political power. Whether this system leads to stability or not is an open question. I do think, however, that we must be careful about saying how and where and when social stability occurs.

From here, Dr., Joy went on to attack the World Food Conference for its notion that increasing population was the most critical factor in the world food crisis. I am delighted to stop criticizing and agree completely. One of the problems with this theory is that we often tend to underestimate the achievements of the developing nations in regard to family planning. For example, *Agenda for Action*, a book produced in April 1975 by the Overseas Development Council, points out that 16 developing countries have reduced their birthrate by as much as 10 per 1000 since 1960. Also, *Agenda for Action* argues that the policy of denying aid to countries which have not reduced their populations is self-defeating.

At this point, I have a very serious argument with Dr. Joy. I realize that he did not specifically endorse triage or "lifeboat ethics," but he seemed dangerously close to that when he argued that, since we cannot provide aid to everyone, we will have to develop criteria for selecting those whom we

---

[1]Since many of the values are perishable, presentations can be interpreted as ways of storing accumulated capital because the recipients are obliged to reciprocate with other valuables at some later date.

do help. He suggested that we choose on the basis of self-help, but then admitted that we have no criteria for determining who is and who is not helping himself. If, as he said earlier, the heart of the problem is not involved with increasing population, and if population can be controlled successfully only when the living conditions improve, and if the American Congress is denying aid to those countries which have not decreased their populations, then we have to face that fact that we lack any real solution to the problem. I don't have an answer either, but I am much more sympathetic to Mr. Chafkin's idea that the problem is actually pan-human, and that "we/they" divisions only get us into trouble.

Dr. Joy went on to say that our greatest problem is not, as the World Food Conference seemed to think, an insufficient supply of food, but that large numbers of people in the Third and Fourth Worlds simply cannot afford to buy the food which is available. He saw the solution, therefore, as one of increasing the food supply in Third and Fourth World countries, and not one of providing "soup kitchens." I sympathize very much with this view, but I think we have to add another dimension to the problem. Let me quote from Lester Brown's *In the Human Interest* (1974): "Hunger does not owe its existence to man's inability to produce enough food even in the poor countries themselves, and we must face the economic and political limits of food production and of fuel and fertilizer."

I am not saying that I disagree with the idea that the problem lies with internal food supplies, but that I think we're putting blinders on if we put all the weight on the Third and Fourth World countries. I would like to explore the notion that the world food crisis is perhaps partly the fault of the affluent countries. Look, for example, at the selling policies of the United States: Kissinger was willing to sell 1.2 million bushels of wheat to the Russians, while limiting India (which wanted to buy an equal amount) to only 500,000 bushels. Consider also California farmers drowning chickens and farmers in the Midwest shooting 100,000 calves. Per capita grain consumption in the United States is 1900 lb per annum, most of it in the form of beef; India, on the other hand, consumes only 400 lb per capita.

At present, we are sending only one-sixth the amount of food abroad as we did ten years ago. Of the one billion dollars spent on food aid in the United States, over 70% went to our allies and satellites (such as Korea, Indonesia, Syria and Vietnam). Over half of our agricultural lands are being used to produce stock feed. Cattle in the United States are fed twice as much grain per annum as all of India consumes. We use three million tons of fertilizer a year for lawns and golf courses, which is more than India uses to grow crops. We spend four times as much money to pay U. S. farmers to keep 20% of the agricultural land out of production as we do in food aid for the rest of the world. Clearly, then, supply is not the sum total of the food problem—there is also a problem of distribution throughout the world.

I think the United States is using food as a weapon, and it seems to be no accident that the ultimate control of food has now been transferred to the National Security Council. I think we could also look at protein imperialism. In the United States, for example, we import large quantities of fish meal from Peru which we then feed to livestock. The blame, of course, does not lie entirely with the United States; the Netherlands imports most of the peanuts from Africa to feed its livestock.

Dr. Joy stated that international aid might be valuable, but that it could just as easily not be helpful if its focus were merely on increasing the GNP. You can increase a country's GNP by developing large agricultural estates and completely ignoring the individual small farmer. Here again, I think we have to face the entire colonial and neocolonial situation. Prior to European contact (and I'm using my own value judgments here), the Third and Fourth Worlds showed a magnificent diversity in their food supplies and in the methods used to obtain them. Colonialism brought about the destruction of much of that diversity in return for a dependence on monolithic crops and technologies. People began to spend most of their energy in the cultivation of single cash crops (among which we might include tourism) which were then exported. They received cash in return for their labor, but only enough to buy low quality imported foods.

To put all of our attention on increasing the food supply in the Third and Fourth Worlds is, in a sense, to ignore the consequences of colonial and neocolonial history. There are sobering facts to recall, such as the fact that food aid increases to those countries in 1975 were completely wiped out by increases in the price of oil. And too, the symbols we export, such as hamburgers and Coca-Cola. Nutritionists overseas are inclined to advise the consumption of animal protein in societies where the traditional foods were largely vegetarian. We export values such as competitiveness, and single technological solutions.

In the last analysis, Dr. Joy felt it must be national governments which take the action. But he didn't tell us why that was so, nor did he say what those national governments could do. He talked about the problems of the large estates, about the displacement of labor and how that displacement will exceed absorption capacities, about a world in which so many people are born without an opportunity to be productive at any time, about how these people are actually rejected by governments which see themselves as no longer responsible for them, and he asked how we could make these people productive and self-reliant. He had no answer, and I have no answer.

He told us again that governments must make the reduction of malnutrition a goal, and that they must mobilize political support for such a cause. But he didn't tell us how. And finally, he addressed the question of United Nations capabilities. He talked about setting up data banks, ordering priorities, and the identification, design and implementation of projects.

His conclusion was pessimistic. We need knowledge, he said, and we don't have it. Nor, he believed, did it exist anywhere in the world; thus, it can't be mobilized. He said it had to be developed, but that he didn't think there was sufficient understanding or willingness to even begin such a project.

The solution, as Dr. Joy saw it, was to reach a point where it became clear that malnutrition was both undesirable and unnecessary, and that the remedies were costless. We would all be better off, he said, if we believed this. I agree. But no one seems to have a model which would allow us to achieve this at an international level. And certainly that model is not one based on equilibrium vs goal-seeking.

I would like to turn now to Mr. Chafkin, who began his presentation with the phrase "Nutrition is good but money is better." By that he meant that those countries with serious nutritional problems also had severe internal and external financial problems, and that they were forced to protect themselves financially at the cost of social solutions.

He then made the point that, as governments become increasingly sophisticated, they tend to bring about the atrophy of those traditional organizations which looked after local problems. Yet, he said, effective nutritional intervention requires vigorous community organizations, which provide a basis for continuing commitment and may even take responsibility for handling the money involved. The problem was exacerbated, he said, by the export of planning skills (for better planning allowed governments to further their outreach at the local level), leading to greater atrophy in the community itself. As a result, he was highly skeptical of the benefits of centralized planning.

As did Dr. Joy, Mr. Chafkin argued that the soup kitchen was no solution. Instead, he focused on the problem of consumer education; that is, how can we educate the consumer so that he can make the best nutritional use of his added income? He talked about ways to decrease the displacement which Dr. Joy had mentioned, and to stabilize food prices for the city dweller while increasing the income of the small farmer. He then discussed several models, such as the People's Republic of China, for reorganizing economic and political power (but added that outsiders usually do not succeed in telling governments what to do). And he laid out for us Iron Laws in regard to financial survival and bureaucratic functioning, and said that he thought these laws were perhaps more universal than basal metabolism.

The nutritional consequence of this, I think, is that we have discovered that the local inhabitants of various countries differ in their nutritional requirements and in their biological ability to adapt to their food supplies. I refer here to the imputed ability of the New Guineans to derive more protein from sweet potatoes than a European could. So it may well be that the "universal" requirements which so many of us depend on may not in fact be an answer.

Mr. Chafkin then focused on the $7 billion aid program being conducted in the United States, pointing out that it is probably the largest food aid program in the world and one in which no attempt has been made to evaluate the results. This, he said, was an example of the arrogance so prevalent in the developed world: We insist that other nations evaluate their food programs, but see no need to examine our own. In regard to our food stamp program, I remember seeing a slogan which read "The United States is not fighting a war against hunger—it's fighting a war against hungry Americans." The United States too often ignores the Fourth World in its own backyard. (Britain, too, has a Fourth World composed of Indian and Pakistani immigrants.)

These points led Mr. Chafkin to suggest the fruitlessness of seeking "we/they" solutions, as opposed to seeing the problems of nutrition as a "pan-human" phenomenon. He concluded by citing three universal principles which seem to be part of every country's priorities: (1) meeting balance of trade requirements; (2) keeping prices as low as possible; and (3) providing farmers with enough incentives to maximize food production.

Having heard so many pessimistic approaches to the problems of nutrition, it was delightful to hear Dr. Mata point out that there are in fact countries which have taken great strides in health care and which are relatively free of nutritional problems. Dr. Mata supported his argument with data concerned with decreased mortality, increased life expectancy, improved health and nutritional status, emphasizing that all of these had been accomplished without large scale studies or nutritional intervention. But while I think we should applaud the note of hope which comes to us from Costa Rica, I think we must also remember that the outlook in many other countries is nowhere as promising.

What I am talking about here is the Fourth World, a term which I think was first used in 1967, and which applies to those countries with a low literacy rate, poor transportation systems, rapid urbanization, poor material resources (some or most of which they must export), a life expectancy of less than 50 years, a 10% infant mortality rate and negligible government expenditures for health, education or welfare. In 1974, the United Nations defined 33 countries as being members of the Fourth World: 21 in Africa, six in Southeast Asia, four in Latin America and two islands (Western Samoa and Haiti). All of these countries are former colonies, and the Overseas Development Council estimates that their individual growth will certainly be less than 1% over the next decade, and may actually decline into negative figures. These countries have few channels for investment, and even with all the sources of aid available to them will not be able to solve their problems.

Dr. Mata also emphasized that malnutrition is a man-made problem, and that its causes are primarily social. At this point, I would like to record my respect for the overall theme of these discussions because I think its effect has been to force us to view malnutrition as something other than a biochemical phenomenon; we have seen the problem from the perspective of history, culture and biology. The value of this wide perspective was highlighted, I believe, by Dr. Mata's emphasis on the fact that the improvements in Costa Rica were not the result of solely nutritional programs.

In concluding his presentation Dr. Mata challenged the notions of unlimited growth which were accepted until just a few years ago. He did not see an indisputable value in technology, chemicals and machinery. Citing DuBos, he expressed his doubts about the value of increased industrialization, pointing out such undesirable side effects as an increase in the number of battered children, increased drug and alcohol dependency, increased dependency on imported foods and exported cash crops, decreased physical activity and increased anxiety. He also pointed out the challenges to liberty which such systems introduce, and the effects upon human attitudes. Hope, he said, depended on finding alternatives to orthodox models, on diverting resources from the rich countries to the poor, on a concern with social justice, and on a decision to put the brakes on economic growth. He admitted that his views were utopic, but he was hopeful nonetheless.

Finally, we come to Dr. Klein's paper on problems in Guatemala. It seems significant to me that the most optimistic papers have come from those countries which we think of as having the greatest problems. Dr. Klein was both helpful and encouraging in outlining the organization, implementation and evaluation of nutritional intervention programs which use low-cost medical care and community health involvement as the means of bringing about change. His example involved four subsistence agricultural communities in Guatemala, where two received protein/calorie supplementation and two received calorie supplementation. All four received high-level medical care.

Most encouraging was his documentation for the notion that, if you increase the level of nutrition during pregnancy and lactation, there is a statistically significant improvement in the rate of infant mortality until one year of age. He also pointed out that you can identify those women who run a high risk in terms of infant mortality, and can plan a supplementation program which counteracts that risk. Other improvements brought about by such intervention were documented by data drawn from psychological testing.

He then talked about programs with specific and feasible aims built on community participation. Improved medical care, he argued, was a good way to begin such programs, since most communities have very good health infrastructures, and the results are both rapid and visible. He said that mere technical assistance was not enough because attention must be paid to the felt needs of the community (taking into account the fact that their goals and those of the intervener may be different). Communication has to be built into the system, perhaps even to the point where the program might be able to articulate those needs which the community could not articulate for itself. Techniques are needed to circumvent the major economic constraints. He stressed the use of local personnel, selected in consultation with community leaders so as not to clash with traditional status systems while providing new leadership opportunities.

He mentioned the economic restraints that could be identified in Guatemala (time, land space and cash) and the ways in which they could be changed. I suspect that this identification of specific constraints and the means of handling them offer us great hope. The modesty and feasibility of the program he described is something I think we should all focus on when we talk about applied programs. He concluded by discussing the problems that even such a hopeful program as that in Guatemala has created—specifically, the risk of creating a dependency. Certainly the program was dependent on introduced funds, but its ultimate aim was to promote independence in such a way that the improvements in nutrition could be sustained without further external intervention.

REFERENCES

BROWN, L. 1974. In the Human Interest: A Strategy to Stabilize World Population. W. W. Norton, New York.
OVERSEAS DEVELOPMENT COUNCIL. 1975. Agenda for Action. Overseas Dev. Coun., Washington, D. C.

RESPONSE BY DR. LEONARD JOY:

It is flattering to have so much critical attention directed toward one's words, but I found it very disturbing to discover how serious a communication problem I was facing. I hope that a review of the transcript will sort out some of these points.

First of all, in regard to homeostasis, I certainly did not mean to imply that "traditional" societies were stable or stagnant, that there was no change and no conscious goal-seeking, or that their state was either desirable or undersirable. I did not wish to impute particular values, nor to impute either purpose or desirability to mechanisms or their outcomes. I explicitly denied teleology in my argument. I was concerned with the significance of the behavior of these societies in terms of results, and I believe that my very crude summary of partial aspects of what I referred to as the *jajmani* system, and my example of the *rwot kweri* system in Northern Uganda were valid in the terms that I suggested. I was interested to hear that further study has suggested situations in which feasts are in fact used to increase disparity in communities, but I am not sure whether that makes them more or less stable. My references drew upon Dalton and Adelman.

I found it difficult to absorb Dr. Mackenzie's point about symbolism. No doubt it is important to understand the role of symbolism in order to understand the dynamics of social change. Understanding symbolism is also important for our sensitivity to objectives and values. I hope that in failing to discuss symbolism, among other things, I was not committing the fallacy, highlighted by Dr. Churchman, of assuming that I knew what the problem was.

I am sorry that I was interpreted as someone who sees man as *homo economicus*—the economic maximizer. If you look at my writings, you will see that I have very explicitly criticized the limitations of this view. I have also denied the usefulness or the validity of the characterization of governments as maximizing social objective functions. My arguments were simply that there are social mechanisms—expressed in behavior, responses and interaction—which have nutritional consequences that are not in any sense necessarily optimal from the points of view and the values now implicit in our discussion. I argued further that these patterns of interaction and these mechanisms change, that they break down under such stresses as I outlined, the most significant in terms of nutrition being the process I summarized as "displacement and absorption." Of course, values change too, and any models we build to predict changes in malnutrition must incorporate value changes as endogenous variables so as to model their interaction with economic and other changes. The process I am discussing is very clearly modeled in my mind and in my writing.

I think that my characterization of the development of modern nation states in terms of the development of commercial economies and national governments, and my emphasis, therefore, on the roles of government and the market in the aggravation of malnutrition, is important and essential. I did not try to contrast nation states as goal-seeking and traditional societies as non-goal-seeking. But I do argue that economic, social and political power in new nation states is generally in the hands of the well-nourished, and that this tends to result in deprivation for some people, including nutritional deprivation. Explicit goal-seeking behavior on the part of governments is necessary to counter these inherent outcomes.

Dr. Mackenzie asked a number of specific questions about things she did not understand. One of these was "contracting out." What I meant, within that context, was the denial of traditional rights and obligations; that is, the denial by some people of their interdependence within the community. I think that I illustrated the concept by citing the refusal to participate in reciprocal digging parties, and the refusal to recognize obligations to retainers.

I would certainly not wish to be identified with the triage lobby, even by accident. I want to explicitly disassociate myself from it. The key element in the triage argument, as I see it, is that there is only limited room in the lifeboat, and if we try to rescue anyone else, we shall sink ourselves as well. I do not accept this way of looking at the world's malnourished. But I do think that we have an unavoidable responsibility to be discriminating in our choice of where and how to direct our life-saving efforts. We should not support "solutions" which actually aggravate the problem. We must clarify our values and our views concerning the nature of the solution. I agree with Dr. Churchman that we have to be humble when asserting values and not presume that our values are the proper ones. But to deny the assertion of *any* values or priorities must certainly be wrong.

I did not understand Dr. Mackenzie's point about the transfer of food from rich to poor countries, and I am not sure that she understood mine. However, the point at issue seems to be the question of to what degree the solution of the problem rests with the developed countries. She seems to question the idea that the fundamental action must rest with the poor countries. But I think the fact that the problem must ultimately be tackled by the poorer nations is made quite clear by what I was saying. If we agree that it is the improper distribution of social, economic and political power within these countries that produces the problem as we define it, then it follows that these nation states must act to change this situation, or at least to minimize its effects on the nutritional status of the people. External aid might be used to aid in this endeavor, but it might just as easily be used to resist such changes. Those influences brought to bear from the outside will either ease or aggravate the problem, depending on what the nation states do in response. That was my point.

Dr. Mackenzie said that I did not provide any answers as to how to make people productive and self-reliant. I am sure that she does not want a prescription. Indeed, there isn't one. If she was looking for a discussion of how one makes planning more human and more a part of the political process, I might reasonably plead that this is not what I was asked to do (although it is a subject on which I have a well-defined position).

I was a little shocked to hear Dr. Mackenzie reflect my pessimism concerning the UN and its ability to effect an immediate and effective response to the challenge it has set for itself. I think my assessment of the probabilities is a reasonable one, and I will stick to it. I am not sure whether she was telling me that my assessment was *un*reasonable, or merely that I should not make such gloomy predictions. Certainly what I said was not delivered in a spirit of pessimism, but from a sense of realism.

As regards the question of the "costlessness" of "solutions," I think the point is that solutions are not likely to be costless to some people as they perceive their own interests. The key question, however, is who perceives it as a cost, and who judges which is a greater cost? We have to explore the alternatives and we have to explore our own values as well.

CHAPTER 26

C. West Churchman | Five Planning Fallacies

I would like to address myself to the fallacies and pitfalls of planning, with a special emphasis on nutritional planning. It seems to me that there are five essential fallacies:

(1) Segregationist planning, or the attempt to isolate the problem;

(2) Planning in one's own image;

(3) Planning without any consideration of how such plans might be implemented;

(4) Planning which tries to evade the question of values; and

(5) Planning from a superior position.

Each of these will be considered both in general terms, based on my own experience in planning, and in its specific relationship to the problems which have been discussed at this symposium.

SEGREGATIONIST PLANNING

When I first became interested in nutrition, it seemed to me that nutritionists were very definitely trying to isolate the food problem by addressing it in strictly nutritional (or malnutritional) terms. The consensus of this symposium, however, seems to be that such an approach is erroneous. Dr. Leonard Joy, for example, pointed out that it is a mistake to view the problem of malnutrition in terms of a gap between population and available food, urging instead that the problem be seen in cultural and economic perspective. I applaud his wisdom, and hope to expand on his point of view.

As a result of my contacts with various Federal government projects, I have begun to believe that the attempt to isolate problems is one of the most serious flaws in our national planning. Take, for example, the case of a Federal irrigation project on a Navajo Indian reservation. The plan was put into effect, essentially, because one person knew where there was a lot of water and another knew where there was a wide expanse of desert land, and they decided that the two elements ought to be joined in some way. As a result, the Bureau of Reclamations dug an 80-mile ditch from Navaho Lake into the reservation. At no time, however, did anyone consider what the project might mean to the Navahos themselves. For example, no one considered the long-range implications of forcing the Navahos, who traditionally live at some distance from one another, to spend their lives in close proximity with their fellows.

Like that irrigation system, the problem of nutrition is deeply linked to every aspect of a social system, whether cultural, educational or political. And there is one other aspect which ought to be but has not been considered: The psychological symbolism of what we eat and drink. I don't think that the intense psychological implications of food can be confined under the rubric of "culture."

So I would have to ask, "Is the problem really one of malnutrition?" Obviously there is a problem which must be handled, but is a heavy emphasis on malnutrition really suitable from a planning point of view? Why concentrate on this one view of a world problem? Isn't the problem, after all, more economic than nutritional? In many ways, it seems as though it would be necessary to solve the world's economic problems before attempting to isolate the issue of malnutrition.

I am not saying that planners should not set boundaries for themselves. They must; otherwise the problem blows up into all mankind for all time. But planners ought to realize just how they set those boundaries so that they can change them when it is necessary. (In fact, one of the reasons that boundaries are set in certain ways is precisely to allow for alterations.) This shift in boundaries is an on-going process, and there is no "common sense" to set the rules. They are set by judgement, and altered when experience proves that judgment wrong.

PLANNING IN ONE'S OWN IMAGE

In a sense, this is a problem of disciplines, since each discipline tends to view the world the same way it views its own problems and investigations. An economist sees everything from an economic point of view. All human activity (including literature and the arts) becomes a vast economic model. Biologists see everything as a function of biology or biochemistry. As for anthropologists, they have gone out into the world, investigated it and discovered that it is essentially anthropological in nature. And of course there are the nutritionists, who fully realize that food is what troubles the world. Everyone, in short, has his own idea of how the world is run. In fact, Jay Forester at MIT has constructed a world model called "Dynamo," and it depicts the world in terms of electrical engineering. Need I tell you what his background is?

As planners, therefore, we all run the risk of simply projecting our own world view onto the situation. How does one avoid this particular mental set? I would suggest that philosophy holds the key, since that happens to be *my* field. As everyone knows, philosophers can get themselves out of any mental set because they happen to be so skilled at dialectics. However, I won't push that particular point here.

The real answer, I think, is that you *can't* get out of your own frame of reference, but you can try to maintain an awareness of the fact that there are other ways of looking at reality, and a number of other planning images. This attitude will not only help in framing one's own plans, but will help one to be more receptive to what others might have to say. Thus, I would again ask, "Are you sure the problem is one of malnutrition?"

IMPLEMENTATION-FREE PLANNING

The fallacious strategy here goes something like this: You try to solve a problem the best way you can, using your own intellect, background and experience, and then deliver the plan to decision-makers in as clear and concise a manner as possible. That, says this fallacy, is the end of your responsibility; the actual decision-making can be left to someone else. It's an attractive strategy for dealing with social issues, because it allows you to steer clear of all the major roadblocks (such as politics) and permits you to interact with your colleagues at a lofty intellectual level.

In terms of practical planning, however, we have come to learn that, while such a position may be very comfortable, it doesn't accomplish anything. In fact, it's the worst possible strategy to follow if you are really interested in seeing your intellectual efforts translated into reality. In my own field of operations research, we estimate that between 95 and 99.9% of the projects concocted by operations researchers are never implemented in any real sense, in large part as a result of this fallacy. Such implementation-free planning has been at the root of many of the planning disasters which have occurred in communities, corporation, nations and the U.N.

But in order to discuss this fallacy further, I think I should first define what planning is. In the most general terms, planning is the attempt to use one's intellectual capacities in order to secure improvements in the human condition. In this sense, planning is not confined to professionals; we all do it. No one could conduct his daily life sensibly without doing a bit of planning first. Implementation is connected to the phrase "in order to *secure*"; that is to say, planning is not simply a process of thinking or data-gathering, but an attempt to put intellectual activity into action.

Over the past two decades, a number of people (myself included) have worked intensively on this problem of implementation. We have even conducted experiments using human subjects in our attempt to discover the sociological, psychological and political determinates of implementation failure. And if I were to summarize all of the efforts up to the present time, I would have to say that we really don't know how to implement the best laid plans of mice and men, nor do we understand the process by which intellectual effort is transformed into action and change.

Not surprisingly, however, we *do* know that politics play an essential role in regard to implementation, despite the fact that politics are probably the antithesis of rational planning. In some ways, of course, the two may be complementary, but there is a very deep sense in which they are enemies. This means that we must understand how politics work in a community, or a state or a nation or, indeed, throughout the world, and how various political powers relate one to the other in the obstruction or perversion of rational planning.

Let me ask yet again, "Is the problem really one of malnutrition?" Or is it perhaps a problem of understanding how world and national politics work *before* we can try to bring that political system into accord with the dictates of rational planning? I am aware that such a statement makes it appear as though I think planners should control politics; actually, I think the evidence indicates that the planner ought to be the tool of the politician. He is, for example, one of the tools a politician uses to help insure that his own proposals are approved and funded. In Washington, D. C., a "cost-benefit analysis" is definitely a plan for securing certain political programs.

The problem, then, is not how to alter politics, but how to bring planning activities into some harmony with the political process. Until this happens, I fear that the serious problem of malnutrition will remain with us.

VALUELESS PLANNING

By using this tactic, the planner hopes to escape the extremely difficult problem of making value judgments. For once he or she has made those values explicit, the planner may be accused of trying to assert a certain (and uncomfortable) role in the process, especially since basic human values are not well-established. As a result, the question of values is generally evaded, usually by posing the problem in crisis terms. If, for example, I can convince you that 20% of the world's population is going to starve to death in the next 50 years, I may be able to talk you into believing that prevention of that event is the only value of any concern. Any other value considerations become irrelevant.

To be strictly philosophical for a moment, the fact is that there is really no such thing as a crisis. Human beings make judgments, and a crisis may emerge as a consequence. But if we are to consider the question of death from starvation, we are forced to ask if mankind, as presently constituted, ought to survive, and if so, in what way? That is a sensible philosophical issue, and the "crisis" merges into a basic problem of philosophical values. What is man as a species? What is natural about the species, and how can we behave in a natural way toward other species?

Of course we don't have the answers to such questions, but I think we all have to face such basic questions of value if we are to plan in a rational way. The topic under consideration here happens to be malnutrition, but it could as easily have been transportation, education or the arts. In each case, we would expect those involved to act as though that one issue were central to human survival; they might even suggest that money be diverted from nutritional research in order to further their own programs, which they assume to have greater value.

I think all planners are (or ought to be) applied ethicists; that is, their job is to apply ethical principles (as they understand them) to life. If a planner insists that he is trying to solve a crisis, he has made an ethical commitment which he may not be able to defend. So again I ask, "Is the problem really one of malnutrition?" Isn't it a problem of what the human species is and how it behaves? Doesn't the problem involve the destiny and purpose of humanity?

I thought that Dr. Leonard Joy might suggest that, were we to use the homeostatic model, we could expect a certain portion of our "tribe" to perish along the way in order to maintain stability. Certainly that is one answer: The destiny of man is to maintain a "steady-state." It is not a particularly grand or joyful perspective, but it represents one way to handle the problem. We have been presented with grand perspectives throughout human history—the Chinese *I Ching*, for example, or Plato's *Republic* and Aristotle's *Ethics*. In the 18th century, we find people like Rousseau and Kant who attempted to understand the human condition in order to make suggestions concerning what mankind should do. In neither case were those suggestions concerned with happiness. Instead, they felt that the basic purpose of human life was to obey a moral law derived from ourselves in a free and open "kingdom of ends" where everyone is king; thus, rules and regulations wither away and equity prevails. Clearly, the question of what we ought to do as a species is not an easy one; it requires a tremendous— but necessary—commitment of the part of the planner.

PLANNING FROM SUPERIORITY

This is perhaps the toughest pitfall to avoid, but a planner should never adopt a position clearly superior to those he is planning for. At one point in my life, I served on a National Academy commission of science and rural poverty. The commission spent two years "studying" rural poverty and talking endlessly about the rural poor. After a while, it dawned on me that all of us who were trying to help these poor people were speaking of them as though they were machines or cattle. They were always the people "out there" for whom something had to be done; or, as Mr. Sol Chafkin put it, there was always a clear division between "we" and "they." It is amazing how often the word "we" crops up in planning literature.

The Federal government has been trying to convince the Navahos to let it build coal gasification plants, so "we" sit "them" down and explain that if "we" construct the coal gasification plant, "they" will have wood floors in their hogans (instead of dirt) and running water and refrigerators and television sets. "We" try to convince them that "they" really want all these things. What happened was that the Navahos simply stared at "us." And when "we" asked how many of "them" wanted all of those items, not a single hand was raised. Naturally, "we" assumed that "they" didn't understand, so "we" went through it all again, and still no hands were raised. Finally it dawned on "us" that perhaps some of "them" actually didn't want this new technology. And when "we" asked who *didn't* want the coal gasification plant, everyone raised his hand.

I might also cite a conference which "we" held in Paris. Being modest, this group of planners titled its conference "Toward a Plan of Action for Humanity." In the middle of one of the plenary sessions, a gentleman from Africa got up and said, "I have spent three days listening to you talk about the developed and the underdeveloped nations, but you miss the point: *We* are developed and *you* are overdeveloped." In this man's sense, those planners concerned with "developing" other nations are themselves under-developed.

As another example, during one of our meetings on rural poverty, a rather famous engineer said, "I have been listening to a lot of loose conversation here. As an engineer, I like to define things precisely. Now, it seems to me that there are two kinds of people out there in the country—the old and the young. Why don't we simply paint the houses and fix the toilets so that the old people can live out their lives in comfort. Then we move all the young people into the cities and find them jobs in a factory. That way the problem is removed." And someone else said, "I'm getting on in age myself, and I don't think I'd like it if something like that was done to me." The engineer was baffled by the notion that someone might actually object to such a scheme.

Even worse is the rather well-known "Nobel" scientist who suggested, at a conference devoted to the scientific solution of world problems, that instead of sending criminals to prison for, say, fifteen years, we radiate them to the point where they are fifteen years older, thus saving us the costs of incarceration and them the dreariness of life in prison.

Since this is a conference on nutrition, I might say that these gentlemen are badly in need of spiritual nourishment, and what they ought to be developing is a set of human feelings. I think it is extremely important that planners learn to appreciate what other people are saying and the reasons they have for saying it the way they do, even if it strikes him as irrational. We must avoid the sort of attitude displayed by the scientist who suggested radiation as a means of eliminating prison costs. When he was asked by another participant, "Don't you think a love of humanity ought to play some role in this?", he answered quite simply: "Love is merely an instinc-tual relationship between the male and female of a species." That handled another problem!

What I am talking about, essentially, is humility. The problem with rational planning is that it seems to force us to embrace wide per-spectives—in this case, world malnutrition. And we begin to think that we can grasp this perspective better than anyone else. Obviously, then, we are in a superior position. Perhaps what is needed is a period during the day in which "we" become "they" and "we" admit that we really don't know anything, that we are really quite inferior to the world's poor, that we have a lot to learn from them, and that it is really we who need *their* help. So what I would ask in conclusion is this: "Is our problem really one of malnutrition, or is it one of learning how to make planners more human?"

CHAPTER 27

Asok Mitra

Revolution by Redefinition of Parameters

Governments have developed their own ways of solving gnawing problems. Trying to keep up with the revolution brought about by rising expectations, they proclaim blueprints for radical solutions designed to transform gross inequalities and bring about ideal distributions in record time. As time passes and the relationships based on current power structures set more solidly, they water down the original solutions, yet take pains to make it appear that they have been carried out in full. Land reform is an apt example of this point.

Minifundia and latifundia are at the root of most social, economic and cultural ills in many countries, yet in very few cases (even in those nations avowedly committed to rapid economic and social progress) have even their gross manifestations been eliminated. Instead, the original intention degenerates into mere tokenism through a continuing series of edicts. The government, of course, tries to convince the people that land reform has indeed been enforced. This is what I would call "revolution by redefinition of parameters," for what the government does is to redefine the original plan by successive stages until its original outlines have been lost.

This may well be the fate of the young nutritional movement being launched by multilateral and bilateral agencies. Originally conceived as a small, manageable program confined to infants, young children, pregnant women and lactating mothers (i.e., a relatively small portion of the total population), it has instead opened up a Pandora's box which cannot be closed with the limited amount of resources, administration and management originally envisaged. The implications of malnutrition now embrace virtually every aspect of social and economic life, from birth, death and family planning to efficient schooling and social welfare investments to problems of increasing productivity and technological change. The enthusiasts of yesterday are sober men today. Daunted by the unfolding enormity of the problem, they have sought alternative paths to contain it, and many programs have already fallen prey to tokenism. Some of the uncomfortable problems are explained away in terms of immutable cultural variations or differences in activity norms and demands.

What the countries of Asia, Africa and Latin America need today, if they are to catch up with social and economic progress, is to accelerate, not merely perpetuate, the level of activity which obtains among the young in

297

their traditional or prevailing environment. With the existing level of activity and technology, they will decline in economic and social well-being, not improve. Anyone who cites adaptive capacities to argue that current levels of protein and calorie intake among lower activity and income deciles in the lesser developed countries (LDCs) is sufficient in terms of their prevailing low levels of activity and employment must be found guilty of trying to solve the nutrition problem by merely redefining its parameters.

The report of the April 1975 Informal Meeting of the FAO/WHO Gathering of Experts is an honest enough statement of how inadequate and patchy our knowledge of human nutrition is, not only in respect to LDCs but in respect to developed countries as well. The report also offers guidelines for the interpretation of adaptability to nutrition availability, as well as pointing out just what constitutes a misinterpretation of this term. When a human body receives more protein and energy than the standard norm demands, it adapts itself to the excess by eliminating it. A good example of how excess food is disposed of by the adaptive human body is the marvelous range of exercises and games which have evolved for the purpose of burning away excess fats and the cholesterol ingested with rich foods.

But since the gap between normality and the sort of extreme malnutrition exhibited in kwashiorkor is so great, the dividing line between adaptation and response to stress, or between normality and disease, is by no means clear. Under certain cultural conditions, it is difficult to determine significant statistical differences between 100% of normal and 80% of normal, even though it might be possible to attribute any voluntary or involuntary reduction of activity within those limits to human adaptation. But while immunocompetence (in terms of cell-modulated immunity and intestinal absorption) can be measured, learning ability is difficult to gauge within the 60–80% of normal range (a state of mild or moderate deprivation).

The first sign of impeded adaptation is growth retardation, which may be exhibited in the unique form of "nutritional dwarfs." In such cases, weight for height appears to be normal and nothing (including learning ability) seems impaired, but the bodies remain short and slight. Such persons may display great energy, activity, intelligence and learning ability at certain times, but there is little or no reserve strength; that is, while they may be able to build themselves up for a certain task, having conserved all their energy by a long process of adaptation, their ability to stretch themselves beyond that task is limited.

Differences in nutritional status and the true meaning of adaptation can be revealed when a person is given the option at the end of a day's work to choose (whether voluntarily or involuntarily) between physical rest in front of the TV set or a vigorous game of tennis. True indifference would qualify for the term "adaptation," while a statistically marked preference (again, whether voluntary or involuntary) for sedentary activity would mark the choice as a response to stress.

In order to implement their social, economic and technological goals, the LDCs do not need children who are merely larger or fatter. To make up lost ground and find themselves equal to the task of national regeneration, these children must be more energetic and active. In this context, the fact that Ugandan children require less energy intake to develop bodies comparable to those of English or Scottish children is a trifle beside the point. More pertinent is the question of whether that English or Scottish child, given the same intake of energy and protein as the Ugandan child, would exhibit his customary energy in work or play, or lapse into the involuntary sedentism of the Ugandan child. For a nation engaged in the task of reconstruction, energy, activity and learning ability are more important than an apparently healthy physique achieved by such involuntary sedentism.

Viewed in this light, the findings of the April 1975 Joint FAO/WHO Experts Committee seem more relevant to LDCs than the findings in the opening article of the Proceedings of the Symposium sponsored by the Malnutrition Panel of the U. S.-Japan Cooperative Medical Sciences Program (October 1974), published in the volume titled *Influence of Environmental and Host Factors on Nutritional Requirements*. The human body adapts to energy deficits by cutting down on work, as happens involuntarily to the Ugandan child. But this reduction of physical activity serves neither the individual nor the national interests of the LDCs, which, by any measure, must put in more physical labor each year just to maintain the status quo.

The case with protein is even worse, for one cannot adapt to protein deficiencies by simply not working. The consequent rise in protein-calorie ratio and in protein requirements during situations of restricted energy intake has been discussed at length by the Joint FAO/WHO Committee in its report of April 1975. And here's the rub, so far as the LDCs are concerned: In a situation of low physical activity, the protein requirement increases along with the rising protein-energy ratio. At the same time, all forms of protein, whether animal or vegetable, are far more expensive (both individually and nationally) than the energy available in the form of grain. Should the proportional (if not absolute) protein intake rise as a consequence of reduced energy intake, the cost to the nation is much greater— and there is no equivalent return in the form of increased activity. An emphasis on desired height and weight alone is not enough. Given the more expensive diet, the nation sees its costs go up and its returns decrease.

Moreover, when there isn't even enough grain to go around (grain being cheaper to produce then animal or vegetable protein), it seems highly unrealistic to talk about producing and distributing more protein. It is like asking people to eat cake when they cannot even afford bread. Even a low protein diet will cost more than a high calorie diet. Therefore, it is not in the best interest of the poor nations to achieve a high protein-energy ratio in return for moderate or low activity. Low energy diets, involuntary sedentism, underemployment and unemployment are all components of a vicious circle. Since the poor nations need higher levels of activity and enterprise, their efforts must be directed toward raising caloric intakes to the same level as that of available protein.

It is much more important for the LDCs to plan in terms of caloric needs in order to get the most from their populations in terms of nation-building; they cannot let their young people remain idle or sedentary while building tolerably good human frames. Of course, this does not mean that protein needs will automatically take care of themselves once energy demands are met. But as the demand for calories begins to be satisfied, protein require-ments will insist on a similar satisfaction. (At least, this has been borne out by successive National Sample Surveys of family consumption.)

It does little good to explain away the low energy intake among LDCs in terms of social and cultural variables, for most of the patterns reflected in reduced physical and intellectual activity are not wholly desirable. Nor can they be seen as conscious choice. Who would choose to keep 15–20% of the population unemployed, and an equal or greater number underemployed? Who would choose to keep 30% of the young people in what amounts to a state of suspended animation? The leadership of the LDCs knows very well that active, restless and exercised children are good for the future of the nation. Activity breeds curiosity, the desire for change, the will to experi-ment, the wish to choose, to take risks, to create new technologies and new demands, to unsettle or overturn the present scheme of things. Increased energy among the older people calls for new social and cultural relation-ships and values, for new modes of ownership and production, new systems of distribution, for the acquisition of knowledge and the transformation of traditional systems.

On the other hand, a voluntary or involuntary reduction in the level of activity among the young produces excessive docility, respect for age and tradition, and unwillingness to question the established order of things—a condition which is often characterized, whether with respect or contempt, as resignation, a Buddha-like calm, and uncritical acceptance. In point of fact, however, even the most restless, turbulent and innovative nations of the Western world would develop the same Buddha-like calm if they were forced to make do with a Ugandan or Ecuadorean diet. Conversely, it is quite possible that if the calorie-protein intake were increased among the LDCs (and this has happened among the Punjab and Haryana of India), the people would become as restless, innovative, migratory and colonistic as any northern European nation.

The most urgent need of the LDCs is to improve the learning abilities of their children so that they can become vehicles for change in educational and behavioral norms, in the acquisition of knowledge and technology, in productive relationships, and in the industrial, social and cultural structures of the society. At the root of this is an increase of physical activity among the young, which leads to a more intimate acquaintance with the physical world and its productive forces. Thus, improvements in learning may be brought about by a better energy balance—which also happens to be the least expensive path for the LDCs to follow.

How this desirable economic choice at the macro level is instinctively made at the micro level is illustrated in Tables 27.1–27.3, based on the National Sample Survey of India for 1960–61. Looking at them, we can see how the income elasticities in the demand for foodgrains vary (1) in quantity in respect to foodgrains alone, and (2) in relation to other food items like vegetables, oil, fats, milk and animal protein. The tables also illustrate how the demand for protein builds up only after an income level has been reached at which energy satisfaction is attained. Below that level, to think about supplying protein in preference to grain through nutritional intervention programs in the hope that such a population will create a self-perpetuating level of protein intake is to give in to illusion.

In an exploratory discussion at the National Commission of India on

TABLE 27.1

PER CAPITA DAILY CONSUMPTION OF FOODGRAINS AND SUBSTITUTES
AT CONSUMPTION LEVELS BELOW THE AVERAGE (1960-61)

Monthly Per Capita Expenditure (Rs)	Per Capita Daily Consumption of Foodgrains and Substitutes (g)		Price of Foodgrains and Substitutes (price per kg)		Urban Price as % of Rural Price
	Rural[1]	Urban[2]	Rural[3]	Urban[4]	
0–8	356	332	39.3	40.8	103.8
8–11	480	377	42.3	45.3	107.1
11–13	560	388	43.4	49.4	113.8
13–15	616	412	44.2	51.6	116.7
15–18	625	418	47.8	55.0	115.1
18–21	675	445	48.4	54.0	111.6
21–24	705	485	49.0	55.9	114.1
24–28	690	506	51.7	55.9	108.1

From Poverty in India (Dandeker and Rath 1971)
[1]Data from Table 1.9.0, National Sample Survey No. 138, Sixteenth Round, July 1960-August 1961, Tables with Notes on Consumer Expenditure.
[2]Data from Table 2.9.0, NSS Survey No. 138.
[3]Data obtained by dividing the monetary expenditure on foodgrains in Table 1.8.0 by the corresponding quantity of foodgrains in Table 1.9.0, NSS Survey No. 138.
[4]Data obtained by dividing the monetary expenditure on foodgrains in Table 2.8.0 by the corresponding quantity of foodgrains in Table 2.9.0, NSS Survey No. 138.

TABLE 27.2

DISTRIBUTION OF RURAL CONSUMER EXPENDITURE BY MAJOR ITEMS AT
CONSUMPTION LEVELS BELOW THE AVERAGE (1960-61)

Monthly Per Capita Expenditure (Rs)	Population[1] (%)	Annual Per Capita Expenditure[2] (Rs)	Percentage Distribution of Total Expenditure[3]				
			Foodgrains and Substitutes	Other Food Items	Fuel and Light	Clothing	Other
0–8	6.38	79.3	64.42	18.25	8.74	1.23	7.36
8–11	11.95	116.6	63.57	17.43	8.56	2.51	7.93
11–13	9.88	147.2	60.25	19.09	7.36	5.70	7.60
13–15	9.82	170.8	58.12	20.44	7.48	4.63	9.33
15–18	13.79	200.0	54.50	23.66	6.93	5.23	9.67
18–21	11.44	237.3	50.31	24.10	6.67	6.97	11.95

From Poverty in India (Dandeker and Rath 1971).
[1]Data from Table 1.6.0, NSS Survey No. 138.
[2]Data from Table 1.4.0, NSS Survey No. 138.
[3]Data from Table 1.7.0, NSS Survey No. 138.

Agricultural and Nutritional Policy, it was asked why the national average for calorie and protein requirements should be uniformly set at 2400 g and 56 g respectively, instead of taking observed regional variations into account. It was argued that if such regional variations were respected, the targets for grain production by 2000 A.D. could be reduced, thereby saving money which could be diverted into the production of capital goods

TABLE 27.3

DISTRIBUTION OF URBAN CONSUMER EXPENDITURE BY MAJOR ITEMS AT
CONSUMPTION LEVELS BELOW THE AVERAGE (1960-61)

Monthly Per Capita Expenditure (Rs)	Population[1] (%)	Annual Per Capita Expenditure[2] (Rs)	Percentage Distribution of Total Expenditure[3]				
			Foodgrains and Substitutes	Other Food Items	Fuel and Light	Clothing	Other
0–8	2.15	77.6	63.79	17.87	8.93	0.63	8.78
8–11	5.49	118.3	52.67	26.65	8.23	1.13	11.32
11–13	7.19	145.0	48.32	27.35	8.64	2.27	13.42
13–15	6.86	169.7	45.73	29.11	8.03	2.87	14.26
15–18	10.71	201.2	41.72	31.37	7.38	3.57	15.96
18–21	11.40	235.7	37.17	33.40	7.49	3.41	18.53
21–24	9.68	271.7	36.45	33.81	7.12	3.94	18.68
24–28	11.03	315.4	32.72	34.56	6.91	5.29	20.52

From Poverty in India (Dandeker and Rath 1971)
[1]Data from Table 2.6.0, NSS Survey No. 138.
[2]Data from Table 2.4.0, NSS Survey No. 138.
[3]Data from Table 2.7.0, NSS Survey No. 138.

and other enterprises. These regional variations were something like 1832 g for 10 eastern and southeastern states (including Tamil Nadu), 2468 g for 4 northern states, and 2187 g for 6 central and western states. At the national level, this amounts to a difference of approximately 35 million tons of grain by the year 2000.

However, it is difficult to accept such an argument because it not only perpetuates (or even strengthens) fictions concerning ethnic or cultural stock, but also widens regional disparities in consumption and income. It would also consolidate regional differences in industrial and cultural enterprise that could not be concealed under the mystique of sociocultural uniqueness in terms of environment and cultural milieu.

II

The compartmentalization of disciplines in modern times has led to various attitudes which impair progress. For example, despite the fact that public health scientists have demonstrated the enormous costs borne by a nation as the result of holes in the human nutritional bucket caused by chronic and acute infections which impair intestinal absorption and lead to national waste (Scrimshaw *et al.* 1975), nutritional scientists would still have us believe that it is cheaper to plug these holes with protein and energy delivery, failing to appreciate the fact that this process merely delays the long-term effort needed to eliminate such holes.

The perpetuation of chronic and acute infections brings with it such undesirable cultural features as apathy, listlessness, fatalism, resignation and voluntary or involuntary decreases in the level of physical activity. It also has deleterious effects on infants, child and maternal mortality, and family planning. These effects involve not only intestinal absorption, but immunocompetence and learning capacity. They reduce man's ability to *adapt* to lower protein and energy levels. (In such cultural or economic environments, the phrase "adaptation to lower intakes" degenerates in response to stress.)

This impaired learning ability reduces the response to the needs of technological change and the challenges of production, thereby perpetuating traditional, low-level technologies. Thus, the nation's path toward modernization of attitudes and socioeconomic change can be seriously blocked. The distinction between the continuance of chronic and acute infections and their elimination accounts for a great deal of the social and cultural differences between the developed and underdeveloped worlds, and explains the differences in the utilization of capital of all kinds between those two worlds. The costs to the LDCs of neglect in this area, both overt and covert, are immense.

For some years (and particularly since Mr. Robert McNamara's address to the World Bank in 1971), there has been some concern over the amount of return to be expected from the direct delivery of nutrition to target groups, particularly in the underdeveloped countries. In the past two or three years, comparatively large sums of money have been earmarked for positive nutrition programs, along with relatively small amounts for the public health aspects of the main delivery system. It seems that such programs are essentially designed to treat symptoms, ignoring the actual cause of the disease. This course of international activity closely resembles the family planning programs of the late 1950s and 1960s, in which the emphasis was placed on the distribution of contraceptive materials, with little regard to what might actually induce people to *practice* birth control. The underlying philosophy was that the success of family planning was the direct function of an available contraceptive technology. Such, however, was not the case.

Such programs require trained manpower, organizational skills and administrative machinery far in excess of the results achieved. Moreover, underdeveloped nations lack precisely these sorts of manpower resources. But since these programs tend to be prestige areas for international funding, underdeveloped nations often find it hard to resist even those aspects of an outside intervention which do not fit into their own scheme of social and economic priorities. This, too, creates problems.

There is yet another area which needs attention. It is generally assumed that nutrition will automatically improve if food production accelerates at a comfortable pace. Even in ordinary years, all underdeveloped countries probably produce more food than is needed for nutrition, if the amount of foodgrains produced is divided on a per capita basis. In fact, many underdeveloped nations produce enough food to allow for seed, feed and unavoidable wastage incurred through storage and transportation. The real problem is distribution, which is further complicated by income disparities. In the past 20 years, many countries have found that, while food production has increased enough to keep ahead of population growth, the level of nutrition remains as low as ever (or perhaps even lower). Thus, the level of nutrition depends less upon the amount of food production than upon the extent of inequality (aggravated by a lack of education and community organization) prevailing in the area.

There seems to be enough historical evidence to show that six processes have been more responsible for improving nutrition and reducing mortality than any public health services or nutritional intervention programs. These are:

(1) Literacy and formal education;

(2) The eradication of communicable and helminthic diseases, and the elimination of intestinal parasites;

(3) Immunization;

(4) Protected drinking water supplies;

(5) Environment sanitation; and

(6) The employment of women in work, preferably outside the home.

I would not for a moment argue that there is no need for positive nutrition programs or for the distribution of contraceptive materials. On the contrary, I believe that such programs are valid in any situation, even when the conditions are premature. But unless they are accompanied by measures designed to eradicate the disease itself, these programs do little but scratch at surface symptoms. Nutrition works best when it is part and parcel of the process of modernization.

ACKNOWLEDGEMENTS

The author acknowledges his debt to Dr. C. Gopalan for his valuable discussion and for his comments on the draft of this paper. However, Dr. Gopalan is not responsible for any of the arguments contained in it.

REFERENCES

SCRIMSHAW, N. S., GARZA, C., and YOUNG, V. R. 1975. Human protein requirements: Effects of infections and calorie deficiencies. *In* Influence of Environmental and Host Factors on Nutritional Requirements. U.S.-Japan Cooperative Medical Sciences Program. Univ. of Calif., Berkeley, Calif.

CHAPTER 28

John Platt | Summary

For several years, I have been a member of the Club of Rome, an international group of scientists, businessmen and civil servants who are concerned with the global *problematique*, that is, with the problem of problems. It is clear to us, as it is to you, that global problems cannot be limited to finite sets. Human society, after all, is at least as complicated as an automobile, and a car has some 15,000 parts, each of them designed and redesigned by research and development teams. The same is going to be true of our social R&D teams, although we might hope that the rate of failure will not be quite so high.

Moreover, no part has priority over another in the design of a car. You cannot say that the steering wheel is more important than the brakes. In the same way, we cannot assign priorities to human problems. As we move from villages and nation states toward what must be a more integrated global system, we must either design or drift by accident into a society in which all the parts fit and work together smoothly.

The Club of Rome has listed five major areas in its *problematique*: (1) peace-keeping, (2) the gap between the rich and the poor, (3) resource development (which includes both food and energy), (4) pollution and ecological maintenance, and (5) population control. The purpose of the Club of Rome is to raise the consciousness of governments and the general population in regard to these problems and their possible solutions.

There has been a flood of new developments in the past ten years which speaks well for the future. A good deal of new literature has been generated in such fields as agriculture, medicine, nutrition and education. In particular, I might mention the fascinating reports from the International Development Research Center in Canada, which may be the largest publicly funded center for research and analysis of global problems. Rather than try to tell other governments what to do or what to work on, the IDRC responds directly to requests from the field, working to set up conferences and technical assistance studies.

We have seen the rise of a new awareness of global problems, and new attention paid to such things as ecology, women's rights and contraception. And we discover, for example, that the birth rate in the United States has declined steadily. This was accomplished not by putting contraceptives in the water supply, or taxing children, or sterilizing people who had more than two children, or by any of the other fascistic methods our liberal friends seem eager to adopt when they lose their understanding of the democratic process, but by the voluntary actions of millions of married couples.

I might also cite *The Limits to Growth*, a study sponsored by the Club of Rome and published by MIT in 1972. Despite the fact that it is fairly technical, this book has been translated into 30 languages and has sold 3 or 4 million copies. We have seen more and more communities decide to limit their growth, for good reasons and bad. They have limited the heights of buildings, the use of cars in the city, the construction of suburbs and so on. In a way, they have begun to think in global terms, to realize the need for a transition to a sustainable society for the entire world.

I think it is important to realize that we are in fact in the midst of an enormous social revolution. In scale, it is perhaps like tying the Industrial Revolution to the Protestant Reformation and letting it all take place within a single generation. Obviously it is a very dangerous period. It is a moment of metamorphosis during which the caterpillar we have been for so long suddenly becomes a butterfly. We find ourselves beset with internal stresses as old structures cease to be appropriate, while those which might replace them are as yet undeveloped.

While I don't always agree with McGeorge Bundy, I found his article in the August 1974 issue of *The Saturday Review* quite fascinating. Looking back at us from a point 50 years in the future, he depicts us as facing enormous crises over the next 10 years, some of them verging on catastrophe. An incident of nuclear terrorism, perhaps, which will force us to change our attitudes toward nuclear energy and the control of plutonium. Or perhaps a famine which brings about the death of 50,000,000 people. In his view, these crises—if they are not so overwhelming as to write an epitaph for the planet—will produce in their wake a series of "global covenants." In other words, these catalytic crises will mobilize human energy and money into the creation of global management structures to control such problems as nuclear power, food and population.

Bundy predicts that by 1989 the nations of the world will be united under a "Great Covenant," by means of which we shall create (if we are to survive at all) the global structures needed to handle the problems which are too great for any single nation to deal with. While 1989, being the bicentennial of world democracy, is rather a magic date, I think Bundy's figure is accurate within a few years either way. And I think that this conference has moved us one step closer to that date with its emphasis on the scientific research, study and analysis that will be needed to create these structures.

A lot has been said about values in discussing this topic, and I would like to say something about a book called *A Theory of Justice* written by John Rawls of Harvard University. It is a difficult book, but well worth the effort. While I am not sure that I agree with all of his conclusions, I feel that Rawls has produced the sort of modern examination of justice we need in this high-information, high-education society. The old ideal of communitarianism or socialist equality in which everyone gets an equal amount of everything doesn't seem to be a practical model for any real society; there are still enormous inequalities in Russia and in Red China. Nor, it seems to me, can we rely on utilitarianism, which aims for the greatest good to the greatest number. In a sense, this means that it is all right for the rich man to gain ten if the poor man only loses nine, because the average for the population has been raised. Clearly this is an intolerable view, and any nation which tried to adopt it would be destroyed by terrorism, assassination or revolution.

What Rawls has done is to ask, "What would our principles of justice be if we came together as equals before the game had started. Knowing that some of us would get a good role of the dice and some bad, what would we agree upon in terms of justice?" And his answer is that we would want some such rule as this: That each of us would want to be protected against the worst possible catastrophes, and that inequality could be justified only if it benefited the worst off among us. In other words, the lucky ones agree to minimize the misfortunes of the unlucky. This principle can be seen at work in Red China, where if you are lucky enough and intelligent enough to become a doctor, you are obligated to serve the people who need your services the most. This is also the principle behind our own affirmative action programs, which represent a Federal determination to upgrade the lot of those who have been left out for decades.

We also see this principle at work in the demands of Third and Fourth World countries for "affirmative action" to correct the colonial injustices under which they have suffered for so long. I think that the Rawlsian banner is going to be flying over the barricades on both sides during the great debates of the next 20 years. The rich will claim that their inequality is justified because it is used to benefit the poor, and the poor will demand those measures of inequality needed to benefit themselves.

What I think this means is that we are going to have to behave, on a global scale, as though we were a family. Within a family, it is the child with special needs who gets most of its mother's attention. It is true, of course, that this principle has its limits when one reaches the point of absolute survival, and it is here that the triage principle takes its place. But we are a long way from the point where someone is going to have to be thrown overboard so that the others can survive. We are not in a lifeboat, but in the captain's cabin on a large ocean vessel, and there are people down below who are starving. We must treat them, as we must treat the rest of the world, as though they were members of the family in an affluent society.

Index

Other AVI Books

AGRICULTURAL AND FOOD CHEMISTRY: PAST, PRESENT, FUTURE
  Teranishi
CARBOHYDRATES AND HEALTH
  Hood, Wardrip and Bollenback
DIETARY NUTRIENT GUIDE
  Pennington
DRUG-INDUCED NUTRITIONAL DEFICIENCIES
  Roe
ELEMENTS OF FOOD TECHNOLOGY
  Desrosier
ENCYCLOPEDIA OF FOOD SCIENCE
  Peterson and Johnson
ENCYCLOPEDIA OF FOOD TECHNOLOGY
  Johnson and Peterson
EVALUATION OF PROTEINS FOR HUMANS
  Bodwell
FOOD FOR THOUGHT
  2nd Edition   *Labuza and Sloan*
FOOD MICROBIOLOGY: PUBLIC HEALTH AND SPOILAGE ASPECTS
  deFigueiredo and Splittstoesser
FUNDAMENTALS OF DAIRY CHEMISTRY
  2nd Edition   *Webb, Johnson and Alford*
FUNDAMENTALS OF FOOD FREEZING
  Desrosier and Tressler
NUTRITIONAL EVALUATION OF FOOD PROCESSING
  2nd Edition   *Harris and Karmas*
PROGRESS IN HUMAN NUTRITION
  Vol. 1   *Margen*
PROTEIN RESOURCES AND TECHNOLOGY
  Milner, Scrimshaw and Wang
PROTEIN AS HUMAN FOODS
  American Edition   *Lawrie*
SOYBEANS: CHEMISTRY AND TECHNOLOGY
  Vol. 1 Proteins   *Smith and Circle*
TECHNOLOGY OF FOOD PRESERVATION
  4th Edition   *Desrosier and Desrosier*
THE STORY OF FOOD
  Garard
WORLD FISH FARMING: CULTIVATION AND ECONOMICS
  Brown